NOTES FOR THE MRC

Dr. Hel
Portobello
14 Codrington Me
Tel: 020-7727-5800/2
Practice Code: E87005

Notes for the MRCGP

K.T. PALMER
MA BM BCh MRCGP DRCOG AFOM

SECOND EDITION

OXFORD

Blackwell Scientific Publications

LONDON EDINBURGH BOSTON
MELBOURNE PARIS BERLIN VIENNA

© 1988, 1992 by
Blackwell Scientific Publications
Editorial Offices:
Osney Mead, Oxford OX2 0EL
25 John Street, London WC1N 2BL
23 Ainslie Place, Edinburgh EH3 6AJ
3 Cambridge Center, Cambridge
    Massachusetts 02142, USA
54 University Street, Carlton
    Victoria 3053, Australia

Other Editorial Offices:
Librairie Arnette SA
2, rue Casimir-Delavigne
75006 Paris
France

Blackwell Wissenschafts-Verlag
Meinekestrasse 4
D-1000 Berlin 15
Germany

Blackwell MZV
Feldgasse 13
A-1238 Wien
Austria

First published 1988
Reprinted 1989 (twice), 1990
Second edition 1992

Set by Excel Typesetters Company,
Hong Kong
Printed and bound in Great Britain
by Hartnolls Ltd, Bodmin, Cornwall

DISTRIBUTORS

Marston Book Services Ltd
PO Box 87
Oxford OX2 0DT
(*Orders*: Tel: 0865 791155
          Fax: 0865 791927
          Telex: 837515)

USA
Blackwell Scientific Publications,
    Inc.
3 Cambridge Center
Cambridge, MA 02142
(*Orders*: Tel: 800 759-6102
          617 225-0401)

Canada
Times Mirror Professional
    Publishing, Ltd
5240 Finch Avenue East
Scarborough, Ontario M1S 5A2
(*Orders*: Tel: 416 298-1588
          800 268-4178)

Australia
Blackwell Scientific Publications
    (Australia) Pty Ltd
54 University Street
Carlton, Victoria 3053
(*Orders*: Tel: 03 347-0300)

A catalogue record for this book is
available from the British Library

ISBN 0-632-02909-9

Contents

Preface to the Second Edition

I suspect there is a tradition that compels authors to preface revisions of their book by commenting on how much things have changed since last they wrote. I would not wish to break with tradition — and in all honesty I have no need to do so. It is fair to say, after *Working for Patients*, the new contract and a major revision of the Red Book, that general practice has received its biggest shake-up for two decades. The MRCGP examination has altered in tandem: two new sections have been added, one removed, and others updated to reflect the new emphasis.

The impact on this new edition can be judged by the fact that there are 15 new sections, 29 new tables and figures, more than 90 new references and one entirely new chapter. At least a quarter of the text has been rewritten in an attempt to reflect fully what has been radical enforced change.

I hope the result will continue to meet the needs of MRCGP candidates wherever they may be.

Preface to the First Edition

The MRCGP examination is one of the fairest of postgraduate examinations, and given reasonable preparation candidates stand a good chance of success in it. The chief challenge arises from the breadth of the syllabus, which draws on many areas of medical practice — clinical, psychological, social, administrative, interpersonal, legal and ethical. In preparing for my own examination I became aware that while there were several excellent books on each aspect and several study books that worked their way through sample examination papers, there was no concise revision text that tried to encompass the whole broad canvas of the syllabus. This is not really surprising when you consider the limitless scope the examiners have and the wide range of reading material available. Nevertheless, examination candidates in the latter stages of their preparations often express a need to have a fact-packed concise revision source around which to formalize their thoughts. I hope this book will meet their needs.

Adopting the 'short notes' format leaves an author open to the accusation that his coverage is superficial, arbitrary or dogmatic. Brevity naturally promotes a didactic style and I hope I will be excused this failing in the cause of a greater good. Certainly the 'facts' and opinions in this book are not written on tablets of stone and candidates should be sensitive to the eternal cycle of debate and change which characterizes general practice.

In selecting my material I have deliberately concentrated on those aspects of practice which are non-clinical — the running of a business, communication and counselling, the social and legal aspects, the 'wider issues' — almost to the exclusion of 'pure' clinical medicine. There are two major reasons for this: first, most candidates by this stage already have a strong foundation in clinical matters from their hospital training, and to duplicate this material would make the book unnecessarily cumbersome; second, experience suggests that the non-clinical areas pose a greater obstacle to candidates, a fact examiners recognize in setting their questions. The book concludes with some useful statistics, further reading, and the examination itself: the syllabus, the format and my personal ideas and suggestions on examination technique. I hope this approach will help the candidate to steer a steady course to examination success. Happy navigating!

Acknowledgements

In the preparation of this book I found the following to be valuable sources of information: *Running a Practice*, R.V.H.Jones, K.J.Bolden, D.J.Pereira Gray & M.S.Hall, Croom Helm; *Practising Prevention*, BMA publication; *Preventive Medicine in General Practice*, eds M.Gray & G.H.Fowler, Oxford Medical Publications; *Sociology as Applied to Medicine*, eds D.Patrick & G.Scambler, Baillière Concise Medical Textbooks; *Common Dilemmas in Family Medicine*, ed. J.Fry, MTP; *Common Diseases*, J.Fry, MTP; various editorials and articles from the *Journal of the Royal College of General Practitioners*, notably those by A.McPherson (May 1985), C.Freer (June 1985), J.Cohen (Sept. 1985) and D.Tant (Nov. 1985); and the *Update Clinical Debate* series (1985). The series *Trainee's Guide to Practice Management* by Dr M.Mead proved especially helpful in the writing of Section 1.3 and I am indebted to him: his discussion of practice record-keeping is so expert and comprehensive that little extra of value has been or need be added.

The new chapter on epidemiology and statistics would not have proved possible but for the lucid teachings of Dr R.McNamee on behalf of Manchester University's Distance Learning Course for occupational physicians. Thanks are due in special measure to her for all that is good in this chapter. The failings, if failings there be, are mine alone.

I would also like to thank my former tutors for their advice in the book's first edition, and in particular Dr R.Coles for his helpful suggestions. Thanks are also due in large measure to my father-in-law for his knowledge and to my wife for her fortitude and forbearance.

1 Practice Matters

1.1 THE BUILDING

Types of ownership
Premises are in two major categories:
1 Owner-occupied (i.e. owned by one or more partner or a close relative).
2 Rented.

Each category can be subdivided according to the premises' origins: (a) purpose-built (i.e. newly built as a surgery or a substantially altered existing property not previously used for medical practice); (b) adapted (i.e. not originally intended for medical purposes but now approved for them by the Family Health Service Authorities (FHSA)).

The capital costs of practice premises
In the case of *rented* premises the capital cost is borne by the owner and not the GP. Purpose-built rented premises are usually Health Centres — since 1982 the responsibility of District Health Authorities (DHAs) and built by NHS capital specifically to rent to GPs; alternatively private developers or the General Practice Finance Corporation (GPFC) may do the same with FHSA agreement.

In *owner-occupied* premises the capital is raised by the partner(s), either from private funds or a loan from the GPFC, high street banks or building societies. The interest on the loan for purpose-built premises is usually covered by the cost-rent scheme (see below).

The running costs of practice premises
In rented premises
The 1966 GP Charter undertook to provide rent and rate reimbursements to GPs. In Health Centres this is essentially a formality: a rental is charged and reimbursed 100%, making it a book transaction only.

In other rented premises a 100% reimbursement is also available, provided that the rent charge is 'reasonable'. What is 'reasonable' is determined by an employee of the Inland Revenue called the *District Valuer* (who inspects and compares it with the current market rent charged on comparable properties in the same area).

In owner-occupied premises
If these are purpose-built under an approved cost-rent scheme, the rent and rates are again entirely reimbursed.

1

If the premises are adapted, the owner-doctor is compensated for the capital he or she has tied up in bricks and mortar by the payment of a *notional rent*, i.e. although he pays no actual rent, he receives an annual payment comparable to the current market rent of similar local property (the sort of rent he could have received himself if the premises were used otherwise). The value of the notional rent is set by the District Valuer and reassessed every 3 years or when any change occurs. (GPs who dispute the District Valuer's assessment can employ an independent valuer to argue their case, and can ultimately appeal to the Secretary of State.)

Note that the GP's Terms of Service (see Section 7.12) impose the responsibility of providing 'adequate' surgery premises and FHSAs can withhold reimbursements if premises are substandard.

Running costs other than rent and rates are *not* reimbursable although they are tax-deductible — GPs in Health Centres pay a quarterly consolidated service charge (covering use of heat, light, cleaning services, etc., in proportion to their overall use of the building), and other GPs pay their own service expenses as they arise.

The cost-rent scheme

This scheme is controlled by the FHSA and covers the cost of three categories of purpose-built premises:

- the building of completely new premises;
- substantial modification of existing practice premises;
- the acquisition of premises 'for substantial modification'.

The *principle* is that the partners raise the capital and the FHSA meets the interest payments on the loan. Several *practical* points apply:

1 In all cases prior FHSA approval and consultation are needed as well as planning permission (future funds for this purpose are cash-limited and allocated on the basis of priority);

2 Strict Red Book schedules exist regarding allowable expenditure, e.g. acceptable building costs per square metre, architects' fees, planning consent costs, etc.;

3 The final rent reimbursed is called the *cost-rent* and is calculated from the capital costs of the project and the interest rate charged (This interest rate is linked to the GPFC's rate and the loan may be at a fixed or variable interest rate.);

4 As the cost-rent is a scheduled percentage of the building cost, there comes a time when the revalued notional rent exceeds it. At the next triennial review the practice can then opt to switch from cost-rent to notional rent.

This is a simplified account of a very complex area of practice finances. In April 1990 cash limits were imposed on the scheme. In 1991 a civil service report labelled the scheme 'archaic and complex'. Fewer new projects have been approved lately and the scheme appears to be heading for an overhaul.

Improvement grants
These are available from the Department of Health (DOH)
provided that:

- there is prior FHSA approval;
- work is on facilities for staff and patients (and *not* primarily on
doctors' accommodation);
- the grant is to improve 'what already exists' and not to provide
new premises.

Projects should normally comply with the standards of accommodation in Para. 56/Schedule 1 — Red Book. Payments may be
up to two-thirds of the total cost, but there is:

- a minimum project cost;
- an overall cost limit and maximum grant per doctor;
- a condition that tax relief claims are forfeit on capital costs met
by grant (Para. 56/Schedule 1 — Red Book).

A cost-rent is also available (assuming the usual conditions of the
cost-rent scheme are satisfied).

   Part of the grant is repayable if premises stop being used as an
NHS surgery within 3 or (depending on grant level) 4 years.

Pros and cons of Health Centre and owner-occupied premises
See Table 1.1.

Branch surgeries
Many practices, especially those in rural areas, have branch surgeries; these often arise from the historical amalgamation of separate practices.

Advantages
1   The major advantage is to patients in rural areas who have
shorter distances to travel, and do not have to depend on infrequent rural bus services to see doctors.
2   Home visiting to this group of patients is reduced by encouraging them to attend a surgery.
3   GPs in rural areas are able to sustain a higher list size, with
consequent increase of profits.

Disadvantages
1   Facilities are often primitive compared with the main surgery.
2   There is a duplication of administrative and running expenses
which drains practice profits (unless GPs dispense from branch
surgeries the net result is usually a financial loss).
3   Various practical problems are posed, e.g.:

- the security of largely unattended premises with drug
stocks and confidential records;
- how to run an appointment system and staff the premises;
- where to house clinical records (which cannot exist in both
premises at once!).

Table 1.1 Pros and cons of Health Centre and owner-occupied premises.

		Health Centre	Owner-occupied
1	Initial financing	By the DHA; the GP only invests minimally in practice equipment	By the partners; this means capital is needed early in a GP's career, and may cause him problems in expensive areas with high housing prices
2	Capital growth	None for the doctors	Appreciable long-term investment (especially since the cost-rent scheme effectively grants an interest-free loan)
3	Control of premises	Limited: (a) consultation on the initial design may be limited, (b) substantial alterations may prove difficult to obtain (funds come from the DHA's community budget and compete directly with other community projects and services: delays in decision-making and the 'drying up' of funds are common problems); (c) maintenance and redecoration are the DHA's responsibility; unless covered by prior agreement the timing can be a source of dispute between GPs and the DHA	(a) Design is in the hands of the GP and his architect; (b) Alterations are easier to make (and can be covered by improvement grants and the cost-rent scheme); (c) Maintenance decisions are in the hands of the Principals
4	Staff employment	Staff may be shared with the DHA by joint appointment or entirely employed by the practice. If they are on the DHA payroll, the administrative burden of calculating and paying salaries is borne by the FHSA, but the GP sacrifices control over their activities and may find himself in dispute with the DHA over shared staff	The GP hires and fires his own staff and has control over their wage levels and work activities
5	Running costs	A service charge is set by the FHSA; this varies considerably and GPs may find themselves in dispute over the level set	These are more directly under the control of the GPs and dependent on their management policies. They are usually higher than those of average Health Centres
6	Allowed use of premises	At present virtually unrestricted, except that if private work comprises more than 10% of total income, reimbursements are reduced in proportion and stopped if 50% is private. However, since the property is not owned by the partners it is conceivable that further conditions could be placed upon its use	As for Health Centres (although security of future use is possibly greater)

4 They cannot be closed save by permission of the FHSA. Since branch surgeries are jealously defended by consumers and local communities, it often proves difficult for doctors to terminate this responsibility once they have undertaken to provide it.

1.2 THE PEOPLE

Recruiting staff

When a vacancy occurs, the following steps need to be taken:

1 A *review* — does the post need to be filled?
2 The preparation of:
 (a) a *job description* (main function, task and scope of job);
 (b) a *profile* of the person required (e.g. qualifications and experience, potential, personal qualities, commitment).
3 A search for applicants — this can be:
 (a) by word of mouth (this is cheap and simple, and draws in candidates with local ties and loyalties, but may pose problems if dismissal or confidentiality become issues);
 (b) by advertisement (e.g. local newspaper);
 (c) by checking with local colleges and career services.
(Application forms add to administrative costs and lengthen the selection procedure but do allow *direct* comparison of applications.)
4 *Short-listing* — should someone carry out a preliminary sift?
5 The *interview* — establish beforehand:
 (a) who is on the interview panel?
 (b) what points do they want to clarify/cover?
 (c) who will ask the questions?
 Avoid interruptions, insufficient time and repetition of questions. The London Business School recommends a formal approach:
 • draw up a checklist of desirable qualities;
 • allocate particular questions pertaining to this list to particular interviewers in advance;
 • ask candidates similar questions, at least some of the time, so that the answers can be directly compared;
 • score the candidates' answers as they are given: this allows some objective comparison to be made.
6 *After the interview* — if in doubt, defer the appointment. Otherwise:
 (a) confirm the job offer by letter (stipulating the starting date and the main headings of the contract to follow);
 (b) plan an induction period and an induction plan for the new employee;
 (c) produce a contract (as outlined below).

Employees' rights

Contracts

1 More than 50% of GPs fail to issue their employees with a contract, presumably because they forget, or it takes too much time, or they feel it is formal and intrusive.

2 Legally, as employers, they should provide for any employee working more than 16h per week a written statement of the main employment terms within 13 weeks of commencement. Employees working 8 or more hours a week for 5 years also have this right.

3 The contract must include certain items, including:
    (a) the names of the parties;
    (b) the job title;
    (c) the date of commencement and continuity of contract;
    (d) a statement of hours, pay and holiday;
    (e) a statement of sick pay and pension;
    (f) a statement of notice, grievance and disciplinary procedures.

4 Even where there is no legal obligation to provide a contract, it is still advisable, in anticipation of possible future labour– management disagreements.

5 Where no *written* contract exists, the law may still deem a *verbal* contract to exist and interprets its conditions on the basis of pre-cedence and practice.

Employment law
This is a very complex field, with frequently changing legislation. The *principles*, however, change more slowly, and are described in Table 1.2.

Staff finances

Reimbursements
The Red Book makes provision for the reimbursement of the major part of the expense of employing staff. Prior to April 1990 the following costs were reimbursed for qualifying staff (an approved quota performing approved duties):

1 70% of salary paid (less any Statutory Sick Pay paid).

2 100% of the employer's National Insurance (NI) contributions.

3 Contributions paid by the employer to the NHS or certain private superannuation schemes.

4 70% of the costs incurred in approved extra-practice training of staff.

However, following the introduction of a new Red Book and Terms of Service, these reimbursement arrangements exist only on a transitional basis for staff in post on 1 April 1990. For replace-ments and new appointees fresh conditions apply. Essentially reimbursements are still available in respect of **1** to **4**, as well as

Table 1.2 The main principles of employment law.

	Rights	Conditions
1 Notice	To receive a minimum period of notice	After 4 weeks' employment; also an employee's obligation after 4 weeks to *serve* a minimum notice
2 Contract	To receive a contract	After 13 weeks (if employed for 16 h/week) or after 5 years (if employed for ≥8 h/week)
3 Pay statement	To receive an itemized pay statement, including all deductions	
4 Time off	To have reasonable time off for: (a) approved trade union duties; (b) certain public duties; (c) to look for a new job if redundancy is impending; (d) antenatal care	Unpaid Unpaid After a minimum period of employment Employers can demand certification of pregnancy (form FW8), and proof of antenatal appointments
5 Discrimination	The right *not* to be: (a) discriminated against on grounds of sex or race; (b) unfairly dismissed; (c) discriminated against because of union activities (or to be forced to join a trade union)	 After 26 weeks' employment
6 Redundancy	To receive redundancy pay	After a minimum period of continuous employment (104 weeks). Pay is based on a statutory formula. (The employer can claim a rebate of half this from the State Redundancy Payment Fund and the balance from the FHSA)
7 Maternity	The right to: (a) keep one's job;	No dismissal on grounds of pregnancy alone, as long as the employee has been employed for a certain minimum period and can still do the work
	(b) receive maternity leave and pay;	These rights depend on the duration of employment in relation to the expected week of confinement and the number of hours worked per week. Claimants must also furnish written notice of maternity leave and a certificate of expected confinement (form Mat BI)
	(c) return to work after maternity leave	The same conditions as for (b) above. In addition: • 3 weeks' written notice of intention to return; • a time limit of 29 weeks (postnatal)

Table 1.2 *Contd*

	Rights	Conditions
8 Safety	Health and safety at work rights place on the employer several obligations: (a) to display a statement of safety policy; (b) 'as far as reasonably practicable' to ensure a safely maintained workplace; (c) to notify certain categories of accident to the Health and Safety Executive; (d) to keep an accident book; (e) to take out insurance against accidents to staff, and to display the insurance certificate. (The Health and Safety Executive inspectorate also have the power, 'at a reasonable time', to enter and inspect premises to ensure they comply with the Health and Safety at Work Act)	If five or more ancillary staff are employed e.g. Those involving death within a year, hospital admission for more than 24 h and major fractures
9 Statutory Sick Pay (SSP)	Employers are responsible for paying SSP to employees who have made qualifying class 1 National Insurance contributions	For first 28 weeks
10 Pensions	From April 1978 it became obligatory to offer full-time employees either the State Pension Scheme or an approved private one	

for redundancy payments and absences for 'reasonable' holiday, sickness, maternity leave and training.

But:

1 The extent of approval and degree of reimbursement are at the discretion of the FHSA, and is said to depend on the FHSA's:

(a) perception of need;

(b) own development strategies, budget and priorities;

(c) evaluation of the proposed job description (role, objectives, contractual and training needs) and job candidates (minimum qualifications and experience).

2 Decisions on these discretionary reimbursements can be reviewed at intervals of no less than 3 years.

All GP principals are now eligible (whether part-time or full-time). No quota system operates, nor is there a stipulation regarding the type of staff or their activities, other than that there should be local approval.

Prior to these changes, the subsidy was underused (in 1984 each GP in the UK employed the equivalent of only 1.062 full-time ancillaries against a quota maximum of 2 per head). The removal of qualifying restrictions has been trumpeted as a move to encourage more staff and a wider range of duties while at the same time targeting more precisely according to need and in the light of local job markets. Early indications are that the converse has applied: reimbursements have fallen because of downward pressure on FHSA expenditure and competing claims for its limited funds.

Salaries
1 A good guide to the minimum acceptable pay levels is provided by the appropriate Whitley Council rates paid to Health Authority employees doing the same jobs. (Arguably the rate should be higher, since Health Authority employees receive an index-linked pension, and a good sick pay scheme, whereas relatively few GPs make these provisions for their staff.)
2 As an employer, the GP is obliged to deduct income tax and class 1 NI contributions before giving employees the balance of their pay. The deduction is calculated using NI contribution and tax tables; then, on or before the 14th day following the end of the month, a cheque is submitted to the tax collector including total tax and staff and employer's NI contributions. The reimbursement of salary and employer's NI contributions is claimed quarterly from the FHSA.

The health visitor
Qualifications and training
1 Always SRN.
2 Often state-certified midwife as well.
3 Must possess:
    (a) an approved obstetric certificate;
    (b) a health visitor's certificate (obligatory).
4 Must undertake a year's full-time study in preventive and social medicine and human development to obtain the health visitor's certificate.

Employers
Employed by the DHA and accountable to the nursing managers.
    Attached to 88% of practices (Cartwright & Anderson 1981).

Possible roles
The health visitor has a very broad potential brief, which includes some *statutory* duties.
1 Postnatal home visiting: this is a statutory duty from the day the midwife stops attending (usually the 10th day), and follow-up

usually continues until the child attends school; the function is to educate and support the mother in basic baby care, common postnatal problems and minor childhood illness and developmental milestones. Similar advice is offered at child health clinics.

2   Child developmental and screening work, undertaken in the home or at the child health clinic, and including simple tests of sight, hearing and development.

3   Case work — the specific surveillance and support of at-risk groups, e.g.:

(a) single-parent families;
(b) cases of potential non-accidental injury;
(c) the handling of children with emotional and behavioural problems, or physical and mental handicap;
(d) marital counselling.

4   Preventive work and health education:

(a) immunizations;
(b) health education (including antenatal/parentcraft and relaxation classes, weight-watching groups, etc.);
(c) visiting/screening the elderly;
(d) family planning advice.

5   Advisory and liaison work:

(a) advice on local resources, e.g. mother and toddler groups, day nurseries, self-help groups;
(b) advice on home safety, home helps, welfare benefits; liaison with GP and social worker.

Workload
In practice the work is mainly with the *young* and much less with the old; for example in one study:

- 65% of the clientele were under 5 years old;
- 13% were over 65 years old;
- although these two groups commanded nearly 80% of the health visiting caseload, they represented only 20% of the practice population.

There is, however, a new and growing breed of health visitor with a special interest and expertise in the elderly, the geriatric health visitor, whose role may have to expand to meet the needs of the increasing elderly population.

The district nurse
Qualifications and training
1   Usually SRN but may be SEN.
2   SRN needs:
(a) 2 years post-registration experience;
(b) a 9 month training course in community nursing (DN).
3   SEN needs the National Certificate in District Nursing (DEN).

Employed by the DHA and accountable to the nursing managers.

Attached to approximately 70% of practices (Cartwright & Anderson 1981).

Possible roles

There is a broad potential overlap with other members of the primary health care team but the natural training and experience of the district nurse favour clinical nursing in the community above other roles.

1   General nursing care including:
    (a) prevention of pressure sores;
    (b) bowel care and catheter care;
    (c) treatments, e.g. injections and dressings;
    (d) venepuncture;
    (e) rehabilitation, etc.
2   A special role in the care of the elderly, disabled and terminally ill. In addition to general nursing care (above) this includes:
    (a) psychological support to patients and family;
    (b) mobilization of resources, e.g. incontinence aids, commodes, ripple beds, night nursing and bath nurses, etc.
3   Assessment, referral and liaison work:
    (a) with GP, health visitor and social worker;
    (b) advice to patients on local resources and voluntary associations.
4   Preventive work, for example:
    (a) monitoring at-risk groups by home visiting;
    (b) health advice;
    (c) influenza vaccinations.
5   Assistance in the surgery's treatment room (with any of the tasks listed below under **The practice nurse**).

Workload

In practice 95% of the district nurse's time is spent in practical nursing and only 5% in educational work. Much of the caseload comprises the elderly, chronically sick and severely disabled.

The practice nurse

Qualifications and training

There is no fixed or standard requirement. The practice, as the employing body, can choose according to its own needs and from the local material available. Most practice nurses are experienced SRNs who value part-time work, fixed hours and general practice-based responsibilities. Many now have family planning training.

Employers

When Cartwright and Anderson surveyed general practice in 1977, 35% of practices employed their own nurse. However, over the past few years the number of practice nurses has doubled, making this the fastest-growing group of health personnel in the UK.

Possible roles

The role of the practice nurse depends in part on personal interests, confidence and experience, and also on the degree of responsibility and freedom encouraged by the GP employers. At one extreme is the nurse-practitioner, who sees and vets minor illness, provides an alternative appointment system for the patient and refers to the GP at her discretion. Whatever the degree of freedom allowed, the GP remains ultimately responsible for the practice nurse's decisions and must take steps to ensure that:

- the nurse is adequately trained for the job;
- the boundaries of responsibility are defined and understood.

The most commonly performed tasks are:

1 Basic nursing procedures: e.g. dressings, venepuncture, injections, immunizations, basic observations (weight, blood pressure, urine testing), suture removal, ear syringing, taking swabs, etc.

2 The management of minor accidents.

3 Special clinics (e.g. wart clinics, diabetic clinics, hypertensive and well-woman clinics).

4 Pill checks and taking cervical smears (family planning trained nurses).

5 Assistance with various procedures (e.g. intrauterine device fitting, minor surgery, insurance medicals, ECG recordings).

6 Regulation of treatment room stock and other paperwork (e.g. filling in item-of-service claims).

7 Health education and advice.

Advantages

The advantages of employing a practice nurse are:

1 The service is relatively inexpensive. Part of the salary may be reimbursable and the remainder allowable against tax. Increased income from item-of-service work undertaken in the treatment room and health promtion clinics may help to pay the difference.

2 It saves the GP time, thus leaving him free to do other work.

3 Patients express a high level of satisfaction with the facility and appreciate it.

Disadvantages

1 Practice nurses need adequate training which the GP may have to provide, especially when the nurses are asked to take on new responsibilities.

2 There is a problem in defining the boundaries of responsibility — a GP who delegates must live with the possibility that he may, at some time, be answerable for someone else's error. It is difficult

to provide a fail-safe referral policy that covers all possible circumstances. The GP must also satisfy himself that the correct decisions are being made without appearing to question his colleague's professional competence — this is a difficult balance to achieve and the relationship hinges on it.

3   The facility often generates *more* work when its convenience is appreciated. In particular, patients may use the practice nurse to bypass the appointment system, then causing the GP's surgery to be interrupted because a doctor's opinion was really required.

4   If a practice nurse is employed, this generally means (because of the limited quota of reimbursable salaries) that one fewer receptionist is employed.

Trends
There has been an expansion in the number of practice-employed nurses in recent times because they have two clear advantages over community nurses using the treatment room:

1   The GP has tighter control over their activities when he is the employer than when they are answerable to the DHA.

2   It circumvents the awkward problem of asking DHA-paid nurses to undertake item-of-service work, the profits of which go to the practice.

The Cumberlege Report makes it clear that the Royal College of Nursing (RCN) opposes the growing trend of practice-employed nurses. However the utility of the present scheme is such that it is likely to continue, possibly with even more work delegated. In the meantime the RCN, British Medical Association and Royal College of General Practitioners have expressed particular concern over the lack of formal training and the possible medicolegal ambiguities which this system encourages.

The practice manager
Qualifications and training
In the past qualifications and training for practice managers have been ill defined but there are now three bodies, the Association of Medical Secretaries, Practice Administrators and Receptionists (AMSPAR), the Association of Health Centre and Practice Administrators (AHCPA) and the Guild of Medical Secretaries, who provide recommendations on training. AMSPAR also organizes a diploma course in practice administration. In general, however, it is left to the partnership's discretion to select someone of managerial material. Broad requirements are:

●   personal qualities such as innovative thinking, tact and sensitivity, patience and persuasiveness;

●   administrative skills;

●   training and experience in managing personnel, books and record keeping, and the business side of general practice.

Pre-employment and in-service training are reimbursable (see Red Book Para. 52.8).

Responsibilities

Responsibilities can and often must be delegated, but the practice manager retains overall control of six broad categories of administration — staff, finances, administrative work, premises and supplies, future planning and liaison.

1 *Staff*:
   (a) hiring and firing;
   (b) induction and training;
   (c) rotas and holidays;
   (d) contracts;
   (e) grievances and problems.

2 *Finances*:
   (a) monitoring (and maximizing) all sources of income;
   (b) monitoring (and controlling) all outgoings;
   (c) paying staff salaries, pensions, NI, outside bills, petty cash;
   (d) record keeping, accounts preparation, cash-flow analysis, interpreting the Red Book, etc.

3 *Administration*:
   (a) ensuring all forms are completed and submitted to the FHSA as required;
   (b) organization of basic administrative tasks concerning records, filing, appointments, repeat prescribing, the age–sex register, reception and office procedures, FHSA returns, item-of-service claims, etc.

4 *Premises and supplies*:
   (a) stock control — stationery, forms, bottles, etc.;
   (b) purchase and maintenance of equipment;
   (c) maintenance of decorations, building, fixtures and fittings.

5 *Future planning*:
   (a) monitoring activity statistics and current practices — to anticipate change or improvement;
   (b) ensuring that the practice is developing towards its goals;
   (c) reviewing journals for new ideas;
   (d) investigating new equipment and approaches, e.g. computers;
   (e) helping to plan building changes.

6 *Liaison work*:
   (a) consultation with staff and doctors;
   (b) arranging meetings, minute-taking, circulating information, notifying others about policy changes;
   (c) liaison with accountants, workmen, drug company representatives, the FHSA and other agencies;
   (d) handling staff and public complaints (public relations work).

Computer literacy is now a prerequisite for many of these managerial tasks.

The reception staff

Qualifications and training
There are no statutory qualifications; again, personal qualities (e.g. manner, aptitude, motivation, flexibility) and experience/clerical ability are the only guidelines. Staff job descriptions are available from the Guild of Medical Secretaries and training courses through the Association of Medical Secretaries.

Responsibilities
Approximately 40% of the work involves direct patient contact. The main responsibilities are:
1 *Reception duties*:
    (a) making new and repeat appointments;
    (b) receiving and directing patients, and answering their enquiries;
    (c) taking visit requests.
2 *Telephone duties*:
    (a) answering the telephone and taking messages;
    (b) operating the switchboard.
3 *Filing and record duties*:
    (a) locating patient records for surgeries and re-filing them after use;
    (b) dealing with the post;
    (c) filling in claim forms and collecting fees for different certificates;
    (d) registering new patients, obtaining their records from the FHSA and returning obsolete records;
    (e) updating clinical records and the age–sex register;
    (f) administering the repeat prescribing system.
4 Numerous *general duties*, e.g.:
    (a) handling waiting room problems and tidying the waiting room;
    (b) maintaining and distributing stationery stocks;
    (c) opening and closing the premises;
    (d) delivering messages, etc.
5 *Specialist secretarial duties*, e.g.:
    (a) shorthand dictation and typing;
    (b) maintaining files and indexes;
    (c) taking agendas and minutes of meetings;
    (d) organizing clinics and patient recall;
    (e) liaison work — transport, social services, community nurse, private appointments, etc.

The social worker

Qualifications and training

Various training paths can be followed by those wishing to become social workers: courses are through colleges, polytechnics and universities, and are open to graduates, non-graduates and post-graduates; relevant degrees may shorten the training period; field experience is also required.

The Central Council for Education and Training in Social Work (CCETSW) currently recognises two qualifications: the Certificate of Qualification in Social Work (CQSW) and the Diploma in Social Medicine. (The examination leading to the CQSW is to be phased out by 1995).

Employers

Social workers are employed by Local Authority Social Services, i.e. they are independent professionals not answerable to health authorities or GPs. Their caseload therefore includes public self-referrals.

Workload

The four basic areas are:

1 *Individual casework,* e.g.:
   (a) counselling those individuals and families with financial and personal problems;
   (b) marital and bereavement counselling;
   (c) counselling disturbed children and their families;
   (d) follow-up and support for the mentally ill.
2 *Advice and allocation of resources:*
   (a) home helps and meals-on-wheels;
   (b) social service day centre places;
   (c) advice to the impoverished, disabled and homeless (to whom a wide range of support resources are available — home adaptations, telephone installation grants, welfare benefits, legal housing rights, voluntary and self-help groups, etc.).
3 *Statutory responsibilities (and work with legal implications):*
   (a) supervision of children in care;
   (b) supervision of adoption, fostering, childminding and day nurseries;
   (c) the management of child abuse cases;
   (d) the compulsory admission of mentally ill patients under the Mental Health Act (1983);
   (e) responsibilities for the handicapped under the Disabled Persons Act (1970).
4 *Liaison work,* e.g. between clients and primary care, social services, hospitals and occupational therapists.

Social work and general practice

1 There is a wide overlap in the caseloads of primary care and the Social Security Department (many patients have social and

emotional problems, while many of the DSS clientele have physical or psychological problems).

2   Despite this overlap, the relationship between social workers
and GPs is infamous for its hostility and antagonism.

3   This has been explained in terms of the obvious differences of
age, training and knowledge, ideology and priorities.

4   It is said that the typical GP has a stereotyped impression of
social workers as:

(a) young and unqualified;

(b) constrained by bureaucracy;

(c) lacking energy and effectiveness;

(d) lacking a general practice perspective and loyalty.

The typical social worker, by contrast, perceives the average GP to
be:

(a) resistive to change and blinkered in outlook;

(b) arrogant;

(c) overpaid and overrated;

(d) a prescriber when he really should be a counsellor;

(e) lacking a social worker's perspective.

5   Various attempts have been made to improve liaison with
primary care basically by adopting one of two possible straegies:

(a) *attachment schemes* — in which the social worker takes referrals from GPs using practice premises as base; his commitment
to practice policies outweighs his other Social Work Department commitments;

(b) *liaison schemes* — social workers visit practices at certain
times and collect referrals or discuss cases; their work for the
practice is second in priority to the Department's needs.

Surveys indicate that more than 50% of local authorities participate in these schemes. The liaison system is preferred by all
parties because it promotes more effective communication and
mutual trust and education.

6   The *disadvantages* of these schemes are:

(a) to the *social worker*: the risk of professional isolation, divided
loyalties and abuse by GPs who refer inappropriately or use
the social worker to offload their problems;

(b) to the *team*: time must be found for regular structured
meetings;

(c) to the *GP*: there is a problem with confidential information
— should social workers have access to clinical records?

Despite these disadvantages social workers have important skills
to contribute to the GP's daily practice, so it is to be hoped that
these liaison schemes will flourish.

1.3 THE RECORDS

The current state of records in general practice
Standards are generally *poor*, e.g.:

1 Tulloch (1976) reviewed 400 incoming records over a 6-year period:

(a) more than 50% were not in chronological order;

(b) there was no attempt to highlight important information in 85%;

(c) less than 5% had any form of indexing;

(d) only 33% of patients taking the Pill had this fact recorded and up to 25% of records missed essential information (including open heart surgery, deep venous thromboses, renal failure and hysterectomies!).

2 Moulds (1985) reviewed 1000 new patient records coming into the practice:

(a) only 92 had letters/reports in chronological order and only nine had *all* notes in order;

(b) only 15 had summary cards;

(c) only eight had drug cards in the notes.

3 Other criticisms of records include the following:

(a) vague and firm data are mixed and diagnoses recorded without evidence;

(b) objectives are seldom noted;

(c) there is a failure to assemble *all* relevant factors (especially family and social histories).

Requirements of a record system

The traditional *functions* of clinical notes are several:

1 *To improve patient care*, e.g. to:

(a) make diagnoses clearer;

(b) make management decisions clearer;

(c) make follow-up more systematic, especially in chronic illness;

(d) avoid simple errors (e.g. drug interactions and sensitivities, unnecessary repetition of investigations, prescribing that is inappropriate to the patient's past history).

2 *To aid communication*:

(a) between doctors (especially in large group practices and those without personal list systems);

(b) in the primary care team (e.g. by keeping immunization cards);

(c) with outside agencies (medical reports, referral letters, legal correspondence, etc.).

3 *As an aide-mémoire*:

(a) of main events in the patient's life (physical, psychological, social) and of his family;

(b) of what was said and done at the last consultation.

4 *As a tool* in:

(a) audit, research, epidemiology;

(b) teaching;

(c) planning of patient services.

5 *As a medicolegal record* (important in a climate of increasing litigation).

6 *As a means of maximizing income,* by recording when items of service are undertaken and when claims are due.

Some authorities have questioned GPs' reasons for note-taking — *not* for others to read if they are largely illegible and *not* to record the consultation accurately when they often write init-ial remarks rather than balanced conclusions. Are these notes idiosyncratic? Are they just a personal habit?

The requirements of a good record system are:

1 A complete database.

2 Information recorded at the level of certainty.

3 Important information indexed and highlighted.

4 Clear progress notes (in order!) recording objectives.

Improving clinical records

Many doctors now feel that the minimum requirements are:

1 Continuation cards in chronological order — treasury-tagged.

2 Hospital letters and reports arranged likewise.

3 Pruning of irrelevant, duplicated and illegible material.

4 A summary card.

5 A drug record card for patients on repeat prescriptions.

6 An immunization/vaccination card.

7 Tagging of the record envelopes with Royal College of General Practitioner colour-tags: blue — hypertension; brown — diabetes; yellow — epilepsy; red — drug sensitivity; green — tuberculosis; white — long-term maintenance; black — attempted suicide; chequered — measles.

Useful additions to the notes include:

1 A card to summarize the patient's personal, social and family history.

2 Flow sheets for specific conditions (e.g. graphical records of blood pressure or blood sugar control on hypertensive or diabetic record cards; cards covering the geriatric, new registration and periodic medicals).

3 Highlighting of diagnoses and investigations (e.g. by writing investigations in red and marking diagnoses with a box).

In future the computer will play an increasingly important part in record keeping, although manual and electronic systems are bound to coexist for some time to come.

The different record systems

Traditional — Lloyd George records (FP5/6)

Introduced in 1911. The commonest system. The records are the property of the Secretary of State.

1 *Advantages*:
   (a) pocket-sized:
   - easy to carry around on visits;
   - require less shelf storage space;
   - may encourage brevity;
   (b) it is the status quo — any change involves thousands of records and is a big administrative undertaking.
2 *Disadvantages*:
   (a) lack of space — leads to cramped illegible entries which may end up *too* brief;
   (b) hospital letters, now A4, must be folded. This leads to bulky records and a reluctance to unfold, read and refold them in consultations.

A4 records
In 1973 the DHSS agreed in principle to conversion of records to A4 but progress has been slow.
1 *Advantages*:
   (a) plenty of space to make entries;
   (b) better layout:
   - space for summary cards, flow sheets, etc.;
   - indexing is easy;
   - hospital letters can be filed unfolded and hence may be read more easily;
   - facilitates research and audit.
2 *Disadvantages*:
   (a) storage space:
   - A4 records occupy 1½ times more space;
   - almost half of GPs could not therefore accommodate them without building changes;
   (b) secretarial costs of transfer (approximately one full-time secretary per principal for 2 years);
   (c) the cost of stationery (£1500 for 3000 folders) has to be met by the GP (FP 5/6s are free);
   (d) in the transition period there would be difficulty in transferring records between practices using different systems;
   (e) A4 records, by definition, do not slip readily into the pocket!
   (f) more writing space may encourage verbosity!

Problem-orientated medical records (POMRs)
Proposed by Lawrence Weed (1969). There are three main ingredients:
1 Problem list (active and inactive, medical and social).
2 Background information package:
   (a) fixed information, e.g. sex, date of birth, personal and family history, immunizations, etc.;

(b) changing information, e.g. marital status, job, address, screening tests, etc.

3 Progress notes (mnemonic — SOAP):

(a) *s*ubjective — the patient's observations;

(b) *o*bjective — the doctor's observations and tests;

(c) *a*nalysis — the doctor's understanding of the problem;

(d) *p*lans — goals, further information needed, action, advice to patient.

• *Advantages*:

(a) encourages logical thought and approach; information is recorded at the level of understanding;

(b) makes records much clearer to other readers;

(c) records can easily be audited and are a better research and teaching tool;

(d) the database is more comprehensive;

(e) orderly notes allow planning of preventive care.

• *Disadvantages*:

(a) space and time (really needs A4 record space to avoid bulkiness);

(b) SOAP is long-winded and inappropriate for straightforward problems;

(c) it makes sensitive information clearer as well, raising worries about confidentiality.

The age–sex register

What is it?

The age–sex register consists of a series of cards (blue for males, pink for females) for every patient on the list. Each card records the patient's name, date of birth, address, date of entry into the register and anything else desired (e.g. last cervical smear date). The cards are filed, males and females separately, alphabetically under the year of birth.

How to set up a manual age–sex register

1 Cards and filing cabinets can be purchased from the Royal College of General Practitioners or commercially.

2 Required details are then transferred on to the cards for every list patient — either manually or by computer (some FHSAs will oblige).

3 Make a member of staff responsible for setting it up and maintaining it (adding and removing patients, changing addresses, etc.).

4 Record somewhere what you have done (e.g. tag the notes when the patient is entered; untagged notes can later be checked to make sure they have not been forgotten).

No direct FHSA reimbursement is available, but staff salaries can be recouped in the usual way (see Section 1.2, **Staff finances**). In addition and until 1993 there is a reimbursement scheme for new or updated computer systems (see below).

Uses of the age-sex register
There are four main categories of use:
1 *Screening and recall*, e.g. planning a child surveillance clinic, an over-40s blood pressure screening clinic, home visiting for the over 75s or whatever.
2 *Improving practice income* — by identifying patients who qualify for items of service separately payable. Examples might include over 25s' cervical cytology or immunizations at key ages (pre-school, school entry, school leaving, rubella vaccination of all 10-year-old girls). An age–sex register also allows you to check that FHSA capitation payments are in accordance with the age profile and list size of the practice.
3 *Research*, e.g.:
   • easy to generate age–sex-matched controls, and
   • to identify at-risk groups by age and sex.
4 *Planning*, e.g. identifying changes in the age–sex structure of the practice and hence its changing needs.

Morbidity registers
Constructed to identify groups with special needs for chronic care, e.g. all practice diabetics, all patients on maintenance thyroxine.
   Simple morbidity registers can be constructed:
• using tagged notes;
• from partners' memories;
• from repeat prescription cards;
• opportunistically (records passed on to the secretary for entry after the patient attends for something else);
• by manual search of all records (laborious, but obviously faster if there are summary cards);
• by computer search (the best method).
   More elaborate registers include the E book. This is a loose-leaf ledger, filled in after every consultation with a code number corresponding to the diagnosis. When analysed the ledger provides comprehensive local and national morbidity statistics that assist research and planning.

Advantages
1 They allow the audit of prescribing, compliance and other measures of standards in primary care.
2 They allow the planning and implementation of change in services (e.g. by identifying special-risk groups who could benefit from preventive activities).
3 They greatly simplify research.

Disadvantages
1   Time involved (for doctors and secretarial staff).
2   The need for a high level of motivation and cooperation — they need to be maintained and all new diagnoses (hospital or surgery) need to be entered or amended.
3   Unless run on a computer system there is often a limit to the number of conditions for which registers can be set up, stored and maintained.
4   Registers cannot be guaranteed to be accurate: diagnoses are often tentative or simply wrong.

Computerized records
Because of its unique ability to shuffle and re-sort information rapidly the computer's uses go much further than manual systems.

Uses
1   As a clinical *prompt*:
    (a) in opportunistic screening;
    (b) in long-term maintenance.
For example, appointment lists can be printed with reminders that cervical smears, blood pressure checks, tetanus vaccinations, digoxin levels, thyroxine levels or glycosylated Hbs are overdue; surveillance clinics can be organized and word-processed letters printed; geriatric home visiting lists can be drawn up, etc. Furthermore, computers can sort into 'degree of overdueness' so that with limited resources a start can be made according to priority.
2   As a source of *information*:
    (a) drug formulary information;
    (b) warning of drug interactions or contraindications;
    (c) a guide to the Red Book;
    (d) a word processor and printer of patient information pamphlets.
3   In *record keeping*, e.g.:
    (a) summary cards;
    (b) age–sex registers;
    (c) morbidity registers;
    (d) patient lists.
4   As an *administrative* tool, e.g.:
    (a) computer-run repeat prescribing systems;
    (b) accounts and workload analysis;
    (c) as a claim prompt;
    (d) as a check of FHSA returns.
5   In *audit, research* and *epidemiology*.

Disadvantages
1   Capital costs are presently high, although help is available from the Government until 1993 (see below).

2 Cost-effectiveness in strict financial terms has been questioned (although new stricter performance-related payments increase the computer's attractions).

3 The administrative work needed to transfer patient records on to a computer is considerable (especially since many records are not orderly to begin with).

4 Staff must be trained to use the new equipment.

5 Confidentiality of records is a source of concern.

6 Government legislation concerning computer-held data may eventually give patients right of access to computer records.

There are also worries that technological changes are rapid and today's equipment may be tomorrow's 'white elephant', or that power cuts in an influenza epidemic may paralyse a practice, or that operator error may erase vital records!

The practical considerations of choosing a computer system are considered in Section 1.4.

Access of patients to their records

Patient access to records became an important issue because of bodies like Campaign for Freedom of Information and a climate of increasing litigation and accountability. The Data Protection Act gave patients access to computerized health records, and the Access to Health Records Act 1990 accorded similar rights in the case of manual health records (see Section 7.8, p. 220).

Advantages

Advantages include:

1 Open, 'nothing to hide' approach may help patient's confidence.

2 May improve the doctor–patient relationship (patients are on a more equal footing).

3 It may provide reassurance.

4 It may act as a reinforcing cue to the doctor's advice. ('It must be important, since he's written it in the notes.')

5 Shared understanding and more patient involvement may improve compliance.

6 Casual, prejudicial remarks are less likely to appear in the notes.

7 Factual errors can be corrected by mutual cooperation.

8 The Act's proponents would argue in an open society that it should be a patient's *right*.

Disadvantages/possible consequences

1 More questions will be raised and a lot of time used in unnecessary explanation.

2 Patients may misinterpret notes.

3 The doctor–patient relationship may be harmed if the patient resents what is written.

4 Alternatively honest notes and honest impressions may not be written. Doctors may feel less secure under threat of public scrutiny (and possible litigation) but lack of frankness in the notes may be to the ultimate disservice of a patient if those notes are used by another doctor.

5 The notes may create unnecessary alarm, e.g. early speculations about multiple sclerosis.

6 Problems arise with sensitive information that doctors feel it is sometimes in their patients' best interests not to read, e.g. mention of cancer.

7 Sometimes loyalties are divided — is it right that patients should read medical insurance reports without the permission of the insurance company?

Case for patient-held records
Finally, patient-held records have their advocates because:
1 Up to 10% of doctor-held records get lost.
2 Doctors often fail to locate notes when they most need them (e.g. out-of-hours calls, temporary residents, new registrations, soon after hospital discharge).
3 50% of patients leaving hospital do not understand their discharge diagnosis and 30% cannot name their treatment!

Repeat prescribing
The scale of repeat prescribing
GPs issue 13 000 scripts each per year (a budget per doctor of £50 000 per year). 30–50% of these are repeats and a majority are for the elderly, psychotropics making up more than a third of these drugs.

Problems
Problems with repeat prescribing include:
1 Failure to review patients properly:
  (a) the drug may be inappropriate or the diagnosis questionable;
  (b) the patient's needs may have changed;
  (c) side-effects, interactions and problems of compliance cannot be assessed;
  (d) the *illness* for which the drug was given is not reviewed (e.g. diabetes).
2 The doctor–patient boundary may be widened.
3 Repeat prescribing is time-consuming.
4 Scripts written by ancillary staff contain errors.

Advantage
Advantage is convenience to patients and doctors, especially in chronic illness where repeated consultations may be unnecessary.

Requirements of repeat prescribing system
Important components in a good system are that:
1 Patients should receive scripts promptly, e.g. within 24 h.
2 Scripts should be accurate and error-free.
3 The system should be simple and cheap.
4 It should have a built-in recall system, clear to all.
5 It should be auditable.
6 A doctor using the records should know what the patient is taking and when last supplied.
7 A doctor should be able to gauge compliance and/or abuse.

Systems of repeat prescribing
The commonest system for repeat prescribing is the card which the patient keeps. Pitfalls are that:
● the cards often fail to make clear how many repeats are 'allowable';
● patients lose their cards or turn up without them;
● points 6 and 7 above are not covered unless a duplicate record is kept in the notes.

Many practices therefore include a separate drug card in the clinical records and mark both cards when each script is issued.

There are several alternatives to this commonly used system:
1 Repeat registers — a ledger kept at the front desk. This is easily adapted to audit and recall and is popular with staff (as it saves time extracting and refiling the notes) but the doctor still needs a duplicate record when he consults.
2 Computers. These will:
　(a) print scripts;
　(b) indicate recall frequency;
　(c) check compliance;
　(d) carry out automatic audit;
　(e) update the records;
　(f) minimize written errors and free staff time;
　(g) warn of drug interactions and contraindications.
(Disadvantages of the computer are covered under **Computerized records**, see above.)
3 Abolish repeat prescribing altogether and see all patients. Scott (1985) and others have tried this approach and commend it. There is an initial increase in number of consultations needed but this is partly offset by those cases in which unnecessary medication can be stopped, and by the freeing of staff time. In appropriate cases large prescriptions (e.g. a 6-month dose) are issued each time (which actually saves the NHS money on container and dispensing fees). It should be said that some doctors have reservations about prescribing such large stocks of drugs to patients, who could misuse them.

Audit

There is some confusion over the terminology employed when people discuss quality of care: various expressions such as 'audit', 'peer review' and 'assessment' are used, and a distinction is often drawn between audit and 'research'.

Mourin (1976) defined audit as an enumeration of past events or items. According to this definition audit is essentially a counting exercise (the *number* of patients screened for hypertension in the last 5 years; the *percentage* of the target population vaccinated, or whatever). In *Working for Patients* the Government defines audit as: 'the systematic critical analysis of the quality of medical care, including procedures used for diagnosis and treatment, the use of resources and the resulting outcome and quality of life for the patients'. This implies a process more active than mere counting — there should be self-improvement through standard-setting, measurement, change and remeasurement.

The scope of audit

Two major categories of activity are of consummate interest:
1   Audits of process (examining records, appointment books, immunization records, to see *how* patients are being treated).
2   Audits of outcome (mortality, morbidity, patient satisfaction — looking at the *results* of treatment).

The exercise can take one of several forms depending on the nature of the study:

(a) periodic random review of clinical records (with peer group discussion);

(b) the enumeration of process variables (workload, diagnosis, referral rates, waiting times, visiting rates, use of investigative facilities) and analysis of their trends;

(c) adverse outcome reviews (a post-mortem on cases with undesirable outcomes, to see if a better result could have been achieved);

(d) outcome surveys;

(e) patient satisfaction surveys;

(f) peer group structured practice inspections (of the sort undertaken for training approval).

The principal steps of the audit cycle

The essential steps in performing an audit are to:
1   Define objectives (what needs to be measured and why).
2   Agree ideal performance standards (these may come from the consensus statements and guidelines of expert bodies or, where available, the conclusions of formal clinical trials).
3   Define methods (how the data are to be collected and analysed).
4   Perform the audit.

5   Compare the outcome with performance criteria.
6   Agree and implement change — to bring expected and actual
performance closer together.
7   Repeat steps **4–6**, remeasuring and improving until the agreed
standards are achieved.

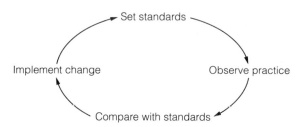

Fig. 1.1 The audit cycle.

This is the so-called virtuous cycle (Fig. 1.1). Steps **4–7** are essential to 'close the feedback loop' and to effect beneficial change. In philosophy this should be continuous and never-ending.

Audit comes of age
Doctors generally accept and the Government now requires that self-improvement through self-examination should be an everyday part of medical practice. More specifically:
● the NHS Bill requires GPs and hospital staff to engage in regular audit;
● the Royal Colleges and Faculties require evidence of audit when accrediting posts for specialist training;
● Medical Audit Advisory Groups (MAAGs) have been set up by FHSAs to assist the process (see Chapter 9).

Cost, benefits and problems of audit in general practice
There are some basic problems with general practice research:
● GPs deal in small patient numbers;
● studies tend to be descriptive rather than fundamental;
● scientific controls are often not possible;
● insufficient knowledge of natural history, placebo effects and clinician bias leads to shortcomings when audit is compared with more formal research.

Critics have complained that audit is limited, local and parochial. Patterson (1985) however points out in defence of the process that — provided honest, cautious and realistic conclusions are drawn — it shares in common with formal research important beneficial characteristics:
● the promotion of logical thought;

- the need for a rational and controlled approach;
- the quest for rational policies;
- establishing a starting point for wider thought.
  In practice several other benefits have been forthcoming, e.g.:
- improved standards of medicine;
- improved morale;
- improved income;
- improvements in practice management and planning of patient services.
  Several *costs* need to be counted as well. Audit demands:
- time and effort;
- commitment (which may not be shared equally in a partnership);
- a willingness to be inspected;
- a receptive attitude to constructive criticism and the flexibility to change.

Notwithstanding these limitations and costs, over the last 20 years research in primary care has gone a long way of filling in the gaps in our knowledge and has fostered in GPs a new willingness to improve by self-examination. The Royal College of General Practitioners has been an instrumental force in this spirit of change.

The problem of measuring quality of care is considered in Section 4.12 and the ethical aspects of medical research are covered in Section 7.11.

1.4 THE EQUIPMENT

In the Log Diary section of the MRCGP viva, reference is made to the equipment the candidate's practice possesses. Note that you are expected not only to be familiar with your own practice's selection and the use made of it, but the full range of possibilities and what others do in other practices. Also be critical of the value of equipment — does it really make a difference to your management? If your practice were to be given a lump sum by a local charity, which equipment purchase would receive priority?

An example — ECG machine
Many practices have an ECG machine, which may be used for:
- the diagnosis of acute chest pain;
- the assessment of an irregular pulse or palpitations;
- screening hypertensives for left heart strain;
- investigating confusional states, shock, collapse or breathlessness.
  Its *advantages* appear to be:
- high patient convenience (rapid access to a service in their own surgery);

- savings to the overworked local ECG department (and NHS budget);
- doctor satisfaction: more complete personal care and preservation of previously acquired skills through use.

However, there are *disadvantages* as well:

- high capital expense;
- machines that are either not robust enough or which are robust but bulky and non-portable;
- running costs (ECG paper, servicing);
- ECGs are time-consuming for doctors or practice nurses to take;
- expertise is needed to read ECGs — could a GP be liable if he missed something important? Does he do enough to maintain his skills?

Does an ECG alter management?

1 *In myocardial infarctions?* — In chest pain at home this is doubtful, since machines are not very portable, delays in transfer to hospital may be unacceptable and decisions can be made on clinical probability (10% of myocardial infarctions do not show typical ECG changes anyway) and the clinical state of the patient. It could confirm angina, or diagnose the persistent ST changes of post-myocardial infarction aneurysm, but cannot be said to make a big difference to management at the present time (if thrombolytic treatment becomes fashionable in primary care this view may need to be reconsidered).

2 *In hypertension* — certainly, evidence of end-organ damage would make treatment more important. Also ECGs are more sensitive than chest X-rays in detecting left ventricular hypertrophy (and this is much cheaper for the NHS if practices do them). However, the yield may be small and largely confined to difficult cases bound for the outpatient department anyway.

3 *In arrhythmias?* — Assuming a doctor has the expertise to read these difficult ECGs and then the expertise to treat them, a practice ECG machine *is* valuable. It may also be easier for patients with paroxysmal arrhythmias to get to a practice machine at the time than to a hospital one.

The pros and cons of possessing a practice ECG machine can be debated. Other equipment should also be considered critically, especially for the purposes of an exam viva.

Computers

The following points should be considered in selecting and installing a computer system:

1 *Requirements*. With more than 30 suppliers to choose from, the

General Medical Services Council (GMSC) has emphasized that doctors should think carefully before taking the plunge:

(a) is there the capacity to extend the system if requirements grow?

(b) is the supply company of adequate financial standing?

(c) does it provide a suitable after-sales service?

(d) will the system satisfy the demands of the new contract?

Broadly speaking it should be able to:

- check capitation lists;
- identify populations attracting target payments;
- monitor immunization, cytology and new-patient registration take-up;
- operate a repeat prescribing system (ideally monitoring pre-scribing patterns);
- log practice activities (referrals, investigations, admissions) to assist in audit and compilation of the practice report;
- generate word-processed correspondence.

2 *Selection.* In practical terms partners should:

(a) decide on what functions are required;

(b) short-list systems matching their criteria;

(c) obtain a demonstration (or visit other practices with computers already installed);

(d) establish what training, support and updating facilities are available;

(e) obtain quotes and investigate financial options (bank loans, leasing, rental, FHSA reimbursements etc.);

(f) select a system and agree an installation date.

3 *Installation:*

(a) identify sites which are clean and dry, ventilated, not subject to extremes of temperature and humidity, out of direct sunlight, yet accessible to a power source and convenient to staff;

(b) provide adequate desk space;

(c) remember that central processing unit-based tasks (disk housekeeping) need peace and quiet, whereas terminals need to be in the midst of the action;

(d) make provision for insurance and security;

(e) consult and train the staff at every stage (experts recommend appointing a computer key worker with special responsibilities);

(f) establish a working database:

- either manually from Lloyd George envelopes (very time consuming);
- or by down-loading computerized FHSA age–sex data on to the computer (quicker, but the FHSA register is believed to have an error rate of up to 25% and needs to be

checked against the practice age–sex register). This step is very labour-intensive.

4   *Reimbursements* — Part of the cost of installing new computer equipment may be reimbursed (see Section 1.6).

Other equipment

1   *Nebulizers* are unquestionably valuable but are they safe in all circumstances (see Section 4.6)? Their indications and disadvantages need to be defined.

2   *Glucometers* are quite expensive and their accuracy, when compared with a laboratory blood sugar, is very much dependent or reproducible technique: can a practice process enough samples on a regular basis to obtain meaningful results? (The same can be said of haemoglobinometers.)

3   *Audiology equipment* — many practices that possess audiometers *and* ECG machines find that they use the former more often.

4   *Peak flow meters* — simple, cheap and very useful, e.g.:
- to establish a *diagnosis* of reversible airways disease;
- to establish the *severity*;
- to establish the benefits of treatment;
- to monitor daily patterns (and hence assess night-time control and the occupational element);
- to alert patients at an early stage to the need to see a doctor.

But peak flow meters have some *limitations* as well, e.g.:
- they cannot be used by young children and often not in the elderly;
- even after careful instruction some patients cannot master the technique and give unreliable readings;
- the more mobile mini-meters are not quite as accurate and not so durable.

In conclusion, if your practice has equipment, ask how it is used, whether it helps and whether there are any shortcomings, pitfalls or problems with it. Did you use it on your Log Diary patients? (If not, why not?) Be aware of what others do as well.

1.5 THE MANAGEMENT

Management and teamwork
Principles of teamwork
According to Gilmore the characteristics of teamwork are:

1   The members *share a common purpose* which binds them together and guides their actions.

2   Each member understands his own function, the contribution of other professions and their common interests.

3   The team works by pooling knowledge, skills and resources, and shares the responsibility for outcome.

Other authors also emphasize the importance in effective teamwork of:

- Pooling;
- Delegation;
- Specialization of function;
- Multidisciplinary discussion and peer group support.

Advantages and disadvantages
In principle the patient should gain from the coordinated action of specialists with a common plan, and effective teamwork should bring harmony, order and a group of self-supporting workers. However, there are practical problems as well:

1 Teamwork needs time and frequent meetings. This may encroach on the time needed for face-to-face patient care.

2 It requires commitment and agreement.

3 There is a danger that no one person will accept overall responsibility (the so-called 'collusion of anonymity' described by Balint 1957); alternatively, if one member assumes overall charge (primacy) there is a danger that personal status and pecking order will diminish the team's harmony and effectiveness.

4 There is a problem of size: large teams contribute more skills and viewpoints, but dilute and delay decision-making and make communication harder.

5 Primary health care teams suffer the problems common to any group of workers — jealousies, prejudices, fears of exploitation or discrimination, peer group rivalry and competition. In particular, differences in training, status and remuneration have traditionally been a disruptive influence. Good will and a desire to get on are the most important elements of teamwork.

Management models
Management models vary between two possible extremes:

1 In the *egalitarian* model primacy and pecking order are minimized and equality of personal status is encouraged.

2 In the *hierarchical* model primacy is clearcut and the chain of authority is clearly and rigidly defined.

Both extremes (and various shades in between) exist in general practice, both have their advocates and may be appropriate in different contexts. A hierarchical management system is commonest in practice, because under his Terms of Service the GP assumes the ultimate responsibility for outcome.

Certain ground rules aid the task of management:

1 The decision-making process should be clearly defined and not haphazard.

2 Important rules (and the reasons for them) should be known to all.

3 The processes of information-sharing, feedback and griev-ance-airing should be encouraged.

Practice meetings

It is all too easy for busy doctors to concentrate on clinical prob-lems while neglecting longer-term plans. Practice meetings serve several purposes:

1 To ensure that necessary decisions are made.
2 To review policies and agree standards of care.
3 To improve communication and morale.
4 To review budgetary provisions.
5 To make contact with team members.
6 To educate and inform (e.g. by holding journal clubs).

The steps involved in organizing a practice meeting are:

1 To define its purpose.
2 And hence its agenda and participants.
3 Then to make decisions, draw conclusions and communicate them effectively.
4 To identify necessary action and those responsible for doing it. Then to give feedback to the next meeting on the outcome.

Experienced campaigners advocate a formal agenda, such as: apologies for absence; minutes of the previous meeting; matters arising; items for discussion; any other business. Someone should act as chairperson and someone should record the minutes.

There are potential benefits from this chore:

● groups in discussion often reach better decisions than an individual would acting alone;

● communication is more efficient and complete, avoiding the piecemeal approach.

Personal lists?

At present the majority (perhaps 75%) of GPs adopt a shared or combined list system. Under this system, while the patients' wishes are accommodated wherever possible and doctors try to follow up illness episodes themselves, patients have the freedom to choose a new doctor at every consultation and the practice has the freedom to direct patients and visits to doctors in a way that spreads the workload and speeds the throughput.

In personal list systems, by contrast, the aim is for patients to stay with the same doctor as closely as the system will allow and on a long-term basis.

The merits of the two systems have been much debated and the principal arguments are summarized below.

Advantages

1 To the patient:
   (a) he sees the same doctor each time — he can therefore get to

know him and to choose a doctor whose qualities suit and
inspire confidence in him;

(b) he also feels the doctor knows and understands his particular problems; unnecessary repetition is avoided; polypharmacy and outright errors are minimized;

(c) the patient is more likely to receive consistent information, and the doctor to implement a consistent plan; this may
facilitate compliance;

(d) patients who call late or have a difficult problem or personality are not passed around from partner to partner.

2 To the doctor:

(a) he gets to know the patient and his problems and this
eventually saves time; he is more likely to understand the *real*
reason for consultation and to judge the urgency/necessity of
visit requests;

(b) he does not inherit patients who are 'shopping around', or
patients who have been managed by a colleague in a way that
he finds he disagrees with;

(c) assuming similar list sizes, it encourages approximate
equality of workload;

(d) the doctor gets more feedback on his performance, which
may promote higher standards and professional satisfaction;

(e) personal care may promote a better doctor–patient relationship, more mutual tolerance (and hopefully less litigation!).

3 To ancillary staff: they know which doctor to speak to;
responsibility is clearly defined and there is no argument.

Disadvantages

1 To the patient:

(a) it makes it harder to 'sample' all the doctors and make an
informed choice;

(b) it removes his choice in individual appointments — in
practice patients may wish to take particular problems to a
member of their own sex; some prefer to take an embarrass-
ing problem to a strange doctor and others to a familiar one:
should they not have this choice?

(c) doctors may get stuck in a groove and a second opinion
occasionally helps; sometimes different doctors within a practice offer different skills and referral to a partner who, for
example, injects varicose veins, may save an outpatient visit;

(d) waiting times for appointments may be lengthened. This is
frustrating to a patient with a straightforward problem and no
particular doctor preference.

2 To the doctor:

(a) the vagaries of demand may mean an uneven workload,

day-to-day, with one doctor inundated with appointments and visits, and another empty-handed;

(b) to be effective:

- a doctor must make himself personally available as much as possible, e.g. he should field the late calls that could go to the duty doctor in a combined list system;
- he should minimize all outside commitments, e.g. assistantships, committee posts, etc.

This represents some sacrifice of personal freedom and ties doctors to a telephone.

(c) personal-list doctors are less aware of their colleagues' working patterns and will learn less from them; their experiences can only be shared in general terms; practice policies are harder to implement; professional isolation may be increased.

3   To the ancillary staff:

(a) personal lists sometimes mean uneven waiting times for puzzled and therefore irate patients — the brunt of this is borne by the receptionist;

(b) it is difficult for training practices to provide trainees with a personal list.

Deputizing services

Out-of-hours (evening, night and weekend) visits make up only 1–3% of GP consultations, but more than 40% of these are carried out by deputizing services.

Doctors have mixed views regarding these services:

1   Some studies indicate that 80% of users have found care 'satisfactory'.

2   However Cartwright and Anderson's survey (1981) found that 52% of doctors felt deputizing to be a *disadvantage* to patients.

The public image of deputizing services is poor:

1   Some deputizing services have clearly employed staff with inadequate experience.

2   Medical disasters involving deputizing services have been given prominent press coverage, causing the public to react with predictable concern.

3   A questionnaire by Sawyer and Arber (1982) tried to quantify feelings:

(a) 94% of patients were satisfied if seen by their own doctor;

(b) 91% were satisfied if seen by a doctor who knew the practice;

(c) 58% were satisfied when deputizing was used.

Recurring worries were:

- lack of relationship, trust and familiarity;
- concern that their past medical history was not known;
- greater difficulty in contacting deputies;
- deputies with a poor command of English.

4 Other surveys also indicate a preference for non-deputizing arrangements.

Advantages
1 The personal freedom of doctors to enjoy a social life out of hours and escape the pressures of work at antisocial times. This creates less personal and family strain in a profession already showing signs of it (higher than average rates of alcoholism, drug abuse and suicide).
2 (Arguably) a better standard of care in the 97–99% of day-time consultations since doctors are fresh, alert, motivated and refreshed by a break.
3 Deputies who start the night-shift fresh may make better decisions than tired doctors who have already worked a full day.
4 The personal availability of deputizing doctors is high: surveys suggest they are likely to respond to a call by visiting, while the GP is more likely to give telephone advice.
5 Deputies can provide cover under difficult practice circumstances (e.g. for the single-hander in need of an annual holiday; prolonged sickness in a small practice).

Disadvantages
1 Patients mistrust and are dissatisfied with deputizing (which may also affect their compliance).
2 There is a risk of inadequately qualified deputies (note that, except when the deputy is already a principal on an FHSA's list, the responsibility for omissions and errors by a deputy rests with the employing GP under his Terms of Service).
3 There is no continuity of care — patients are all unfamiliar and there is limited or no access to their notes. It has therefore been suggested that deputies:
    (a) make more errors;
    (b) refer and treat inappropriately;
    (c) have a tendency to visit, prescribe and refer more when patients are unknown; this involves unnecessary repetition and may also encourage patients to be less independent in the longer term; it also overuses hospital resources;
    (d) because they lack personal knowledge of the patient often fail to appreciate the hidden agenda — the real reason for the call — so the problem is deferred but not resolved.
4 Deputizing incurs some sacrifice of earnings.
5 Many bodies oppose deputizing on principle. Changes in the system of remuneration now penalize users of the service and a future ban is possible. Even if this does not happen, the standing of general practice and its fight to achieve recognition as a specialty in its own right may be damaged if others believe, rightly or wrongly, that standards are being compromised.

The facts on deputizing

Relatively few studies have been done:

1   They confirm deputies visit more often.

2   Deputies do not always treat inappropriately, e.g. Stevenson (1982) revisited 57 of his patients after a deputy and judged their care was satisfactory.

3   Studies suggest that most deputizing services reply fairly promptly.

4   Studies from Portsmouth Hospital, where a whole-town extended rota operates, found referrals to be no more frequent and no more inappropriate from the deputizing service than from practices outside the scheme (Bain 1984).

The alternatives

1   Doctors can accept that they should be on call more.

2   They can share on-call in a larger rota (in some large towns a large cooperative exists pooled from the local practitioners; in some of these use of the service is conditional on contributing to it, and standards are maintained by using only practising GPs; and night visits still attract the higher-rate payment if there are not more than 10 participants in the rota).

3   They can employ only deputies personally known to members of the practice (e.g. ex-partners, local part-timers).

Appointment systems

In a 1951 survey 2% of practices used an appointment system. In Cartwright and Anderson's survey of 1981 the figure had changed to 88%.

Advantages

The principal advantage is efficient use of time, space and resources but there are others:

1   Patients know when they will be seen and (hopefully) do not suffer an unpredictably long wait. (This may, in turn, encourage them to come to the surgery rather than request a home visit.)

2   Doctors know their timetable: they do not experience unpredictable surges of demand and troughs of idleness. Their workload is spread, regulated and adjusted to fit their personal timetable; follow-ups can be planned around their duty and leave rota.

3   In practices that favour common (shared) lists, the appointment system allows the workload to be spread.

4   An efficient use of limited consulting-room space may be planned.

5   Less waiting-room space is needed (only about five seats per GP consulting).

6   Where appropriate, consultations can be planned so that

relevant team members (e.g. practice nurse or health visitor) can attend.

7 Consultation lengths can be planned in some instances according to their needs (e.g. cervical smear or coil-fitting appointments; double appointment space for counselling).

None of this advanced planning is possible if demand is not spread and GPs do not know with any certainty when their surgeries will begin and end.

Disadvantages

1 The administrative workload increases: staff are needed to run the system and they, in turn, need training and salaries.
2 In some branch surgeries consultations may be too few to justify the system.
3 Appointments are *not* convenient for some customers, e.g.:
- the elderly, who have to make separate trips to a phone and to the surgery;
- rural patients who rely on infrequent bus services.

Inevitably there are other patients who abuse the system and do not 'play ball'.

4 Most important of all is the worry that appointment systems are perceived as an extra barrier between patient and doctor. Rigid and inflexible systems could deny access in cases of true urgency, while inefficient systems could result in long delays before an appointment is secured.

Running an appointment system

When patients are balloted by their doctors on proposed changes to the system they tend to prefer the status quo (appointments if they already have them, open access if they do not).

Practices running appointment systems need to review them periodically:
- how long do patients have to wait for non-urgent consultations?
- how often are patients denied the right to see a doctor the same day when they request it?
- do appointments run to time?
- are enough consultations on offer, or do surgeries always run over because of 'extras'?
- what provision is made to allow urgent cases to be seen promptly?

Length of appointment

What effect does the length of the appointment have on its outcome? And to what extent is this determined in turn by list size? A study where booked time was used as an experimental variable has helped to clarify the benefits of longer consultations (Morrell *et al.* 1986; Roland *et al.* 1986). This study compared patients

allocated at random to surgeries booked at 5, 7.5 and 10-min intervals respectively, using taped consultations. In 5-min appointments patients were no less likely to be examined, and no more
likely to receive a prescription, be referred to hospital or asked to
return again, but in longer consultations the doctor did:

- identify more problems;
- carry out more preventive procedures;
- spend more time listening and explaining.

Patients were more satisfied.

In other studies longer consultations resulted in more attention
to lifestyle and screening (Wilson 1989), and extra time to consider
psychosocial issues (Howie *et al.* 1989). In the latter case address-
ing these problems led to a fall in antibiotic prescribing. The
authors ascribe the difference in outcome to time management
decisions rather than inherent differences in clinical behaviour.

Several sources indicate that when doctors have smaller lists
their patients consult more often and spend more booked time
with their doctor.

Some doctors have experimented with allowing patients to
choose their own length of appointment. This has the advantage
that patients share with their doctor from the outset an idea of
the amount of time available, and have had a say in setting it.
Published studies suggest that patients are generally good at esti-
mating their requirements and do not request overlong appointment times (Lowenthal & Bingham 1987).

Telephone advice

Some authors have considered the role of the telephone in out-of-
hours care. While 95% of patients who seek help want a doctor to
visit (Dixon & Williams 1988), some doctors think that more than
half of cases may be managed without detriment by giving advice
over the telephone (Marsh *et al.* 1987). If so, differences between
public and medical perceptions need to be reconciled.

Home visiting

Current figures

The average number of home visits per patient per year is in the
range of 0.3–0.5. According to Cartwright and Anderson (1981),
81% of patients require none and 10% require one. More than
75% of the visits are to patients aged over 75 or under 1 year.

Variation between doctors

The variation between doctors is striking and not entirely
explained:

- Fry (1973) found a 32-fold variation in a study of 14 doctors;
- a Birmingham GP research group (1978) found a 26-fold variation between 22 doctors.

There has been a dramatic decline in home visiting rates; for example, Fry found from his personal records comparing 1949 and 1971 that there were 60% fewer visits per person per year. The decline in home visiting has been viewed with dismay by some doctors and with approval by others.

This trend has been explained in a variety of ways:

1 Improved community health (e.g. fewer serious childhood illnesses through effective immunization and sanitation policies).

2 Changes in the attitudes of doctors *and* patients:

(a) general practice is perceived more as a business, with the emphasis on efficiency: patients are under pressure to justify their request;

(b) patients have telephones and cars, and (either through goodwill or coercion) tend to use them;

(c) patients and doctors expect higher standards of diagnosis and treatment in the surgery;

(d) changes in working arrangements (appointment systems with less waiting time; more hospitable premises; doctors' attempts to be flexible) have encouraged patients to come to the surgery;

(e) possibly patients are more knowledgeable and more self-reliant;

(f) possibly the primary health care model has resulted in more *delegated* visiting (by nurses or health visitors for example).

Advantages

1 *Public relations*. Home visiting is a good public relations exercise and helps to cement rapport in the doctor–patient relationship. These benefits are intangible but real.

2 *Humanitarian and screening benefits*. It is kinder to the elderly and infirmed, and allows surveillance of 'at-risk' patients who might not otherwise attend and 'waste the doctor's time'.

3 *Fuller assessment*. It allows whole-patient assessment — the chance to see the family together in the home environment may provide important social information that could not be gathered in the surgery. It also allows compliance to be gauged (drawers full of untouched pills tell a useful tale!).

4 *It is the safest option*:

(a) serious conditions cannot easily be excluded by telephone;

(b) patients are poor judges of serious and trivial illness;

(c) 'failure to visit' is one of the more successful complaints that patients bring against doctors in Service Committee hearings.

Disadvantages

1 *Time*. The average surgery consultation lasts 5–6 min, but a home visit needs at least 15 min from the surgery and perhaps

30 min from home. Time spent in a car travelling is at the expense of other patients — through their taxes, through the loss of surgery services they *could* have had (e.g. extra clinics) and through fewer of the 'efficient' surgery appointments on offer per day.

2 *Standards.* Poor lighting, low beds, lack of diagnostic facilities and equipment potentially lower the standard of care.

3 *Costs.* These are not readily calculated. At the simplest level there are travelling expenses, but more home visiting may actually mean that the exchequer employs more GPs, which is clearly expensive to the NHS (who wish to pay doctors to consult, not travel!).

4 *Inconvenience.* Many patients who request home visits do so *either* on social grounds (lack of transport, difficulty getting an appointment, lack of babysitter, bad weather), *or* through erroneous medical beliefs (e.g. fear that a febrile child will catch a chill en route). A smaller proportion are genuinely not fit to visit the surgery or are elderly and infirm. If the visit is in the former category, who should bear the inconvenience — the patient, who sees a doctor on average three to five times a year, or the doctor, who runs a business, has 2500 other clients and conducts between 22 and 76 other consultations each day?

5 *The fostering of incorrect attitudes.* More motivation and self-reliance might follow if doctors rationed their visits to genuine emergencies.

Medical assessments
General Practitioners are required to perform three new kinds of medical assessment as a part of their Terms of Service:

1 *The new registration medical:*

(a) *Offered to* all newly registered patients over the age of five;

(b) *format of the offer:* in writing, or if verbal, confirmed in writing (the date of invitation should be recorded in the notes);

(c) *timetable of the offer:* the appointment must be offered within 28 days of registration. Patients can refuse the invitation. In order to attract payment it must be performed within 3 months of registration, except:

• where a large number of patients are inherited at once, giving grounds for deferment;

• when all reasonable efforts were made and the medical was performed as soon as possible.

(No registration fee can be paid unless the patient actually undergoes the consultation).

In fulfilling this obligation, the GMSC recommends that practices should:

• develop a standard invitation for each registration;

• include a simple questionnaire with the written invitation, to be completed prior to consultation;

- delegate wherever possible or incorporate appointments into a well-person clinic.

2 *Patients not seen within the last 3 years*:

(a) *offered to* all patients aged 16–74 not seen by any doctor in the previous 3 years;

(b) *the format of the offer* is the same as that for new registrations.

3 *Patients aged over 75*:

(a) *offered* annually to all patients over 75;

(b) *the format of the offer* is similar to that for new registrations, except that a domiciliary visit must be offered.

The content of these medicals is described in Table 8.2, p. 235; their clinical merit is examined in Section 3.3. (It is widely rumoured that the 3-yearly medical will in future be dropped from the Terms of Service.)

Leaflets, reports and directories

A further innovation of the general practice Terms of Service requires practices to produce leaflets and annual reports, and FHSAs to maintain accurate local directories on their principals.

Practice reports

Required annually by FHSAs. The minimum content is dictated in GPs' Terms of Service (Table 1.3).

Many doctors regard this scheme with suspicion, fearing that information on referrals and prescribing will be used to contain NHS costs rather than to improve quality of care. However, annual reports in some form have been advocated and produced by enthusiasts for a number of years prior to this contractual obligation. Keeble *et al.* (1989) have emphasized its potential as the

Table 1.3 Ingredients of the annual practice report.

Employed staff
Number, individual principal duties, hours worked, qualifications and relevant recent training

Surgery
Changes (introduced or imminent) in floor space, design and quality

Referral data
A breakdown of total numbers referred, as inpatients and outpatients, with reference to specialty and to hospital; also self-referrals the doctors learns about

Outside work
Posts held and work undertaken as a medical practitioner (annual hourly commitment)

Patient feedback
The nature of arrangement set up to receive patients' comments

Prescribing
Doctors' repeat prescribing (and where applicable, dispensing) arrangements

hub of objective setting and performance review, and the dissemination of information throughout the practice. Others accept that vital statistics must be collected before health services can be planned, justified or improved, and can be a useful educative exercise.

Discretionary information that some practices produce for internal use includes:

1 Demographic data:
   (a) number of list patients;
   (b) age–sex structure;
   (c) morbidity profiles.
2 Workload figures:
   (a) numbers of consultations;
   (b) numbers of visits (and night visits);
   (c) numbers of telephone calls;
   (d) numbers of temporary residents seen.
3 Performance data:
   (a) numbers failing to attend;
   (b) screening uptake;
   (c) prescribing figures;
   (d) clinical outcomes.
4 Statements of practice policy and practice objectives.
5 The results of specific audit projects.

Table 1.4 Ingredients of the practice leaflet.

Doctor details
Name, sex, registered medical qualifications, date and place of first registration

Working arrangements
Consulting hours and appointment arrangements
How to obtain non-urgent and urgent appointments
How to obtain non-urgent and urgent domiciliary visits
Out-of-hours arrangements
Repeat prescribing and dispensing arrangements
Practice area (as defined in an FHSA-approved map)
Arrangements for receiving patients' comments

Services and facilities offered
Maternity services
Contraception
Child health surveillance
Minor surgery
Special clinics (purpose and time of operation)
Access for the disabled

Practice structure
Employed staff (numbers and roles)
Whether a partnership is in operation
Whether trainees, medical students and assistants are likely to be in attendance

---

From January 1990 FHSAs became obliged to compile and publish
a local directory of family doctors. The intention is to provide
patients with the information needed to make an informed choice
of doctor. The directory is revised annually and sent free to community health councils, libraries and citizens' advice bureaux.

Principals are listed alphabetically with details of:

- their sex;
- registrable qualifications;
- age (or date of first full registration);
- normal surgery hours and special clinics;
- other relevant aspects of their practice (e.g. staff job descriptions; employment of assistants, trainees or deputies).

Supplementary information can be provided on a voluntary
basis, for example, other languages spoken and doctors' special
clinical interests.

Practice leaflets
The minimum content of the practice leaflet is now prescribed by
GPs' Terms of Service (Table 1.4). All principals must make this
information available to the FHSA and to their list patients, and
update it annually as appropriate. Some doctors have taken the
opportunity to include general health information and advice
on self-management of minor ailments; others have sought and
obtained commercial sponsorship, including advertisements, in
their leaflet.

Practice budgets
The NHS and Community Care Act 1990 made it possible from
April 1991 for general practitioners to hold and control a budget to
fund primary care services.

Principles
The scheme involves:
1 Negotiating a budget with the Regional Health Authority to
cover a range of:
    (a) hospital care;
    (b) NHS medicines;
    (c) practice staff costs.
2 Negotiating 'best buys' for hospital care with chosen hospitals.
3 Administering the system by:
    (a) checking hospital bills;
    (b) monitoring prescribing costs;
    (c) switching funds between the three general areas of drugs,
    staff and hospital services, as appropriate to need;
    (d) maintaining a separate budget account with monthly re-
    ports and an annual statement to the FHSA;

(e) allowing accounts to be audited (every 3 years) by the Audit Commission.

The following services are specifically excluded from the scheme:

- emergency treatments;
- maternity services;
- certain screening and direct-access services;
- patient care exceeding £5000.

Eligibility

This depends on:

1 *List size* — ideally at least 11 000 patients, although practices with 9000–10 000 patients will be considered individually and smaller practices may now group together to meet the size requirement. From April 1993 those with more than 7000 patients can join the scheme.

2 *Ability* — practices have first to be assessed by the FHSA and Regional Health Authority who will consider their current performance standards, computer support provisions and general competence.

(It is rumoured that health officials and the GMSC are examining plans to extend fundholding powers to *all* GPs.)

Potential benefits

1 *Financial* — Inducements include:

(a) a start-up fee (currently up to £16 000 over the first year);

(b) a managerial allowance (£32 000 per annum);

(c) more assistance with computer costs than for non-budget-holding practices (50% more for maintenance, purchase, leasing or upgrading);

(d) the opportunity to use budgetary savings for approved uses (additional staff or hospital services; improved premises; new equipment; better patient facilities — but not personal income).

2 *Administrative and professional* — Budget-holders may be able to exercise more control over their own affairs and those of their patients. For example; they may:

(a) offer their patients more choice or negotiate shorter waiting times for them;

(b) exert more influence over the availability and standard of local services;

(c) take on staff with new skills.

In short, they may be able to cut their cloth according to their own needs.

Potential problems

1 *Financial* — Balancing a large budget is a complex operation. Overspending will be investigated by the FHSA and may result in

sanctions, including the removal of budget-holding status. However:

(a) initial estimates of budgetary need by the Department of Health were embarrassingly inadequate;

(b) Enthoven (1989) suggests that a list size of 11 000 will be too small to cope with random fluctuations in demand on an annual basis and yet keep within the 5% of budget suggested in the Government's prospectus (the author suggests at least 50 000–60 000 patients are needed to iron out this random factor);

(c) pilot studies are in the pipline, but no data is presently available.

To some extent this is uncharted territory and many fear that current information systems are not up to the task.

2 *Administrative and professional* — The volume of work necessary is considerable, involving frequent practice meetings, extensive doctor and accountancy time, reporting, phoning and negotiating, collecting and endorsing receipts, and so on.

3 *Legal and ethical*:

(a) *from the doctor–patient viewpoint*: a patient's trust and confidence could be undermined if a doctor was thought to have a pecuniary interest in the outcome of the consultation; the doctor might be perceived as a gatekeeper saddled with a conflict of interests.

(b) *from the partnership's viewpoint*: the GMSC's lawyers suggest that budget-holding is a fundamental change in practice arrangements and that unanimity between partners would be required contractually to change status. This would in any case be prudent in the interests of practice harmony.

Fears have been expressed that GPs will be caught between their contractual obligation on the one hand to 'render all necessary and appropriate personal services' to their patients and cash-limited funds to discharge this open-ended commitment on the other hand.

At the very least, budget-holding practices will be subject to intense external scrutiny — from FHSAs, DHAs, auditors and, perhaps, their own patients.

(c) *from the consumer's point of view*:

- the cheapest service may not be the best one;
- general practice may for the first time become cash-limited — a worrying development given its open-access nature;
- the existence of two types of practice could create a two-tier system — those with greater purchasing power might have more influence;
- there must be some doubt that GPs will prove themselves competent as managers since their experience and training are limited; doctors' attention may be deflected

from the clinical role for which they have been trained; they are not likely to have the resources to hire high-quality management teams.

Practical considerations

The GMSC suggests that on a practical level participants will need to:

1 Evolve a detailed business plan, identifying:
   (a) the hospital-based needs of existing and potential patients;
   (b) the likely timing of their needs and the provision;
   (c) the costs of these hospital services (including the possibility that some patients will develop complications);
   (d) the prescribing needs of existing and potential patients;
   (e) seasonal trends and their effects on cash flow;
   (f) prescribing policies;
   (g) likely staffing needs (including pay increases, training and redundancy costs).

2 Negotiate the budget with the funding agents.

3 Cost all decisions.

4 Manage cash flow, pay creditors, check costs, payment dates etc.

5 Control the budget, comparing actual against budgeted expenses, with detailed, regular and prompt reporting systems.

This is all but impractical unless practices have a computer system.

The effect of practice size on practice matters

There is no ideal size for a practice but the character, facilities and organization are strongly influenced by the number of principals. In Table 1.5 a large group practice (four or more doctors) is compared with a single-handed practice to illustrate this.

Dispensing

Eligibility to dispense

1 When the drug/appliance is supplied and personally administered by the prescribing doctor. This includes:
   (a) emergency injections;
   (b) anaesthetics;
   (c) diagnostic reagents;
   (d) Intrauterine devices, caps and diaphragms;
   (e) vaccinations;
   (f) certain pessaries and suture materials.
   (Separate regulations for oxygen.)

2 For patients (or temporary residents) who live more than a mile away from the nearest chemist. These patients form the dispensing list. (Note that it is feasible, indeed common, to dispense to patients on the dispensing list from surgery premises less than a mile from the nearest chemist: it is the distance from the patient's *home* that matters!)

Table 1.5 The effect of practice size on practice matters. (Figures from Cartwright & Anderson's 1967 study.)

Aspect	Group practice (≥4 doctors)	Single-handed practice
Patient care	1 More equipment and facilities, e.g.: • ECG machine (60% cf. 13%) • peak flow meter (81% cf. 64%) • treatment room (92% cf. 47%) 2 More services (e.g. diabetic and well-woman clinics) 3 From the patient's point of view, more choice of doctor	1 Personal care of patients with: • good rapport; • better knowledge of the patient; • consistent advice 2 From the doctor's point of view patients who know where they are and who they will see; who cannot 'shop around' and abuse the system
Doctors	1 On call less often (1.4 nights/week cf. 3.8/week)—less personal and family strain; less use of deputizing services 2 Fewer problems covering in sickness and holidays, or coping with epidemics 3 More opportunity for research, audit, teaching, study leave and sabbaticals (44% train, cf. 20% of single-handers)	1 Own boss. No one else to get on with 2 Fewer problems with communications and organization and no decision-making by committee 3 Other problems can be avoided (e.g. shared rota with another practice)
Staff	1 More likely to have attached staff, e.g.: • district nurse (71% cf. 27%); • health visitor (96% cf. 74%); • social worker, community psychiatric nurse, etc. 2 More likely to employ: • practice nurse (56% cf., 27%) • practice manager, caretaker, etc.	
Financial	1 Capital costs of the building are shared 2 In receipt of a Group Practice Allowance 3 More contributors to the pool when expensive practice equipment is bought (e.g. a computer)	1 No dilution of the profit when capital appreciation occurs

Scale of payments

Dispensers receive:

1 The *basic price* of the drug or appliance (as defined in the Drug Tariff, and less a *discount* laid out in Para. 44/Schedule 1 of the Red Book);

2 An *on-cost allowance* of 10–15% of the basic (prediscount) price;

3 A *container allowance* (currently 3.8 p per script);

4 A *dispensing fee* (laid out in Para. 44/Schedule 2 of the Red Book — it depends on the volume of dispensing);

5 A *VAT allowance*.

Claims

All prescriptions, for dispensing and administering doctors, must be noted and sent with a complete FP 34D to the Prescription Pricing Authority (not later than the 5th day of the month following issue of the prescription).

Benefits

1   GPs make a profit on the basic cost of the drug by bulk purchase and also pocket the container fee and dispensing allowance, so dispensing is fairly lucrative and compensates rural practices for their lower lists and higher travel costs. (Profits on dispensing range from about 10 to 17% of the gross turnover of the dispensary.)

2   It also provides a good service to patients, who can find doctor and drugs under a single roof and do not have to make a separate visit to the chemist. Doctors visiting rural patients, the elderly and infirm can dispense the prescription in the same visit — a valuable service.

3   It imposes the discipline of limited list prescribing on the principals and forces them to examine carefully their prescribing habits and rationale. It also brings home the real cost of their prescribing.

4   It is an interesting and stimulating exercise.

5   Dispensing doctors can offer a wider range of drugs out of hours.

Costs

1   Inevitably choice will be limited. It is not possible to stock every prescribable item. Practical problems are more likely to arise for prescriptions arising through hospital directives.

2   It involves extra security precautions, as the dispensary may attract would-be burglars.

3   Other costs include:

(a) insurance of drug stock;

(b) a capital cost to incoming partners (who must purchase a share of this stock);

(c) a small capital risk (investment in drugs that may be discredited/withdrawn from use);

(d) the extra administrative burden, extra commitment of staff time and extra staff responsibilities.

Many dispensing practices employ a pharmacist (qualified dispensers are reimbursed at the higher clerical officer rate in the Whitley Council scale of salaries). There is no legal obligation to employ a qualified dispenser. Nevertheless the legal obligations to dispense accurately, safely and in accordance with the various Drug Acts still apply and so responsibility for the service rests with the dispensing doctor.

Income

The three broad categories of a GP's income are:

1 Private medical work.
2 Income from the NHS.
3 Personal (non-medical) income.

Private income

Income from private medical work depends on the level of commitment to extra-practice activities, the opportunity for private work and the practice's policy towards private patients.

Sources of private income are numerous and include:

● insurance exams and reports;
● other private medical exams and certificates (fitness to start a job, HGV licence applications, fitness to deep-sea-dive, etc.);
● solicitors' reports; court witness;
● cremation fees;
● industrial appointments;
● local authority appointments, e.g. police duties, developmental or family planning clinics; school medical officers;
● hospital appointments (assistantships or practitioner posts);
● lecturing.

Income from the NHS

Income from the NHS comes in the form of:

1 Practice allowances (fixed sum payments and fees based on type or place of practice);
2 Capitation fees (based on number of patients);
3 Item-of-service payments (based on services provided);
4 Fees based on qualifications;
5 Reimbursements and grants.

Table 1.6 summarizes the main allowances and reimbursements. In April 1990 a major overhaul of this complex remunerative system led to key changes, as discussed in Section 1.7.

Outgoings

There are two broad categories of expense:

1 Running costs.
2 Capital expenses.

Running costs

The major running costs are as follows:

1 Cost of premises (including rent, rate, repairs, insurance).
2 Staff costs (including wages, NI contributions and pension payments).
3 Service costs (including heat and lighting, stationery and postage, telephones).

Table 1.6 Income from the NHS.

Category of fee	Red Book reference (para.)	Qualifications
Practice allowances		
1 Basic practice allowance	12.1	Paid to each principal with more than 1200 NHS patients on his list who fulfils the availability requirement of his terms of service (see Table 7.2). In a partnership the *average* must exceed 1200; for doctors with fewer patients pro rata payments are made
2 Designated area allowance	14.1	Paid to encourage doctors to practise in an under-doctored area. Two scales of payment, depending on the average number of patients on the doctor's NHS list. (Very few designated areas now exist)
3 Initial practice allowance (types 1 and 2)	41.1	Paid to doctors setting up practice or joining a partnership in a designated area for an initial period of up to 4 years
4 Inducement allowance	45.1	Paid to doctors practising in sparsely populated areas as a remuneration to offset losses due to their small list size. GPs in England and Wales must have fewer than 1200 patients. They will also receive full seniority and locum sickness allowances
5 Rural practice payments	43.1	Paid to doctors in rural areas where $\geq$10% of patients live $\geq$3 miles from the main surgery. Units are credited, not just on the basis of numbers, but also distance and difficulty of access. (Rural practice units are therefore subdivided into distance units, blocked route units, special district units and difficult walking units!)
6 Assistant's allowance	18.1	Paid to GPs employing assistants when their list size exceeds certain limits (for a full-rate allowance 3000 for a single-hander, or in a partnership 3000 patients for the first doctor and 2500 on average for the rest). Assistants must spend at least 25% of their time on NHS work
7 Associate's allowance	19.1	A scheme allowing two or sometimes three single-handed GPs to employ a doctor between them to allow time off for training. GPs must receive rural practice payments, receive an inducement payment or live >10 miles from the nearest surgery or district general hospital, and not employ assistants
Capitation fees		
1 Basic capitation fees	21.1	The basic fee that each patient on a doctor's list attracts in terms of income. Counted quarterly and paid on three scales depending on age: under 65s; 65–74; 75 and over (ages are those on 1 July)

Table 1.6 *Contd*

Category of fee	Red Book reference (para.)	Qualifications
2 Temporary resident's fee (form FP 19)	32.1	Paid for treatment or advice given to visitors to the practice area seeking medical assistance and staying more than 24 h but less than 3 months. Two scales — one for up to 15 days and a higher one for more than 15 days. (Temporary residents requiring a night visit attract two fees; those requiring only an item-of-service attract only one — *either* the temporary resident fee *or* the item-of-service fee, so claim the larger one!)
3 Deprivation payments	20.1	Additional capitation fees for those patients living in areas of deprivation as identified by the Secretary of State (see Table 5.5 — the Jarman Index)
4 Child health surveillance fee	22.1	Paid to GPs on the FHSA (or health board) child health surveillance list for each under-5 receiving a locally agreed programme of surveillance
5 Registration fee (form FP/RW)	23.1	Paid to GPs carrying out the scheduled registration medical (see Table 8.2) within 3 months of a patient joining the list. No fee if: • the patient is under 5; • the patient was on a partner's list and had a similar medical in the last 12 months
Item-of-service payments **1** Emergency treatment (form FP 32)	33.1	For people in the practice area for less than 24 h (i.e. not eligible to register as temporary residents) and in need of immediate and necessary treatment. (Attracts a higher fee than the temporary resident fee)
2 Immediately necessary treatment (form FP 106)	36.1	Immediately necessary treatment or advice given to a patient permanently residing in the practice area whom the GP is unwilling to accept as a list patient or temporary resident (and who stays in the area too long to qualify for the emergency treatment fee)
3 Anaesthetic fee (form FP 31)	34.1	Paid when the administration of an anaesthetic requires the services of two practitioners
4 Dental haemorrhage fee (form FP 82)	35.1	For the arrest of a dental haemorrhage or the provision of aftercare
5 Night visit fee (form FP 81)	24.1	Paid for a visit requested and completed between 10 pm and 8 am to a patient on the practice's NHS list or to a temporary resident. The patient may be seen at home, or if appropriate, in the surgery or elsewhere in the practice area. On two scales: a higher rate is paid if the visiting doctor comes from the patient's practice (as his doctor, his doctor's partner, assistant, trainee or locum) or from a local rota of no more than 10 doctors

Table 1.6 *Contd*

Category of fee	Red Book reference (para.)	Qualifications
6 Cervical cytology fee	28.1	Payable on two scales: • for full target payment, 80% of eligible women aged 25–64 (or in Scotland 21–60) must have had an *adequate* smear in the last 5½ years; • for the lower payment, 50% (the time scale of 5½ years is to allow for a 6-month call and recall delay). *Notes* **1** Women with hysterectomies involving complete removal of the cervix are exempt from the target group. **2** Work can be delegated to attached staff. **3** Where smears are taken by other GPs they count towards the target of the woman's registered doctor. **4** The sum actually paid will be adjusted to account for the number of eligible women on the practice list as compared to the average anticipated nationally (500) and the number of adequate smears taken by GPs (rather than by others outside general practice)
7 Contraceptive fees (forms FP 1001, 1002 and 1003)	29.1	An annual fee (paid quarterly) for women on the doctor's NHS contraceptive list. Two scales are payable — for contraceptive advice and Pill-prescribing (FP 1001); and for the fitting of an intrauterine device and follow-up (FP 1002 in the year of fitting, FP 1001 in subsequent years). Temporary residents may also receive advice or treatment (claim on an FP 1003). (N.B.: The FP 1001 fee is payable for advice alone, even if the advice is a sheath or sterilization; however, it is only payable in respect of the woman — to claim, the couple or woman alone must be counselled, not the man alone)
8 Maternity fees (forms FP 24/24A)	31.1	All maternity services are paid on a dual-scale basis — one set of fees for GPs not on the FHSA's obstetric list, and another (more than 40% higher) for those who are. There is hot debate, owing to ambiguity in the Red Book, about whether GPs have *personally* to perform maternity services to claim the fees, or whether they can delegate to a midwife and still claim
(a) antenatal care		Paid on three scales depending on the date in pregnancy on which the patient signs for maternity services: • Scale 1 — within the first 16 weeks; • Scale 2 — between 17th and 30th weeks (a lesser sum); • Scale 3 — on or after the 31st week (lower again)

Table 1.6 *Contd*

Category of fee	Red Book reference (para.)	Qualifications
(b) miscarriage fees		If the patient miscarries before 8 weeks and has not signed up for maternity care, no fee is payable. Otherwise (up to 28 weeks) a miscarriage fee can be claimed
(c) abortions		Termination arrangements are generally excluded unless the patient has previously signed up for maternity services
(d) confinement fee		Paid for intrapartum responsibility. Also payable if a doctor is called to a patient who is in labour but not booked under his own care. (In the case of premature confinements, if a live birth occurs after 28 weeks, the fee is paid as if the delivery were at full term)
(e) postnatal fees		The full fee applies to services to mother and child over the first 14 postnatal days, *plus* a full postnatal examination between 6 and 12 weeks (the patient must leave hospital within 48 h of delivery). Partial fees are paid per visit (maximum five) and for the full postnatal examination (A GP can still claim the postnatal examination fee if he has made reasonable efforts to offer an appointment and the patient has not attended)
9 Minor surgery (form FP/MS)	42.1	Paid to GPs on a minor surgery list for sessions consisting of at least fiive procedures per quarter from those activities itemized in Para. 42/Schedule 1 (Table 1.7). A maximum of three claims per quarter or an average of three per GP per quarter in group practices
10 Health Promotion Clinics (form FP/HPC)	30.1	Paid for FHSA-approved clinics normally lasting at least an hour and involving at least 10 patients per session. These can be delegated and in some cicumstances fewer than 10 patients can be seen at a sitting
11 Immunizations (a) children aged <2 (form FP/TC1)	25.1	Divided into three groups: • Diphtheria, pertussis, tetanus (DPT; all three doses); • Polio (three doses); • Measles or measles, mumps and rubella (MMR; one dose). Two payment scales — the higher if 90% * of the appropriate children have been fully immunized on the first day of the quarter, and a lesser sum if only 70%. *Notes* **1** The actual sum is adjusted according to the number of courses done by GPs (as distinct from those given outside general practice), and

Table 1.6 *Contd*

Category of fee	Red Book reference (para.)	Qualifications
		the number of children on the list compared with the average nationally expected (which is 22).
		2 Courses given by other GPs count towards those of the claiming GP.
		3 The GP who gives the final immunization of a course will be credited with giving the full course (even if earlier doses were given by other doctors)
(b) Preschool boosters (form FP/TPB)	26.1	To achieve the full payment, 90% * of the list 5-year-olds must have received a reinforcing dose of DPT; 70% for the lower target The actual sum paid will be derived in the manner described above
(c) Other domestic vaccinations	27.1	Payments can be claimed when vaccinations are approved according to the schedule set out in Para. 27/Schedule 1. In summary: *Diphtheria, tetanus, MMR, measles* — to children aged >6 who have not had a primary course; *Tetanus boosters* — to those leaving school and every 5 years thereafter; *Polio* — to schoolleavers, as a booster for those under 40 or those whose children are being vaccinated; *Rubella* — to children aged 10–14 with no previous MMR; seronegative women of childbearing age; seronegative men in antenatal clinics; *Vaccinations for special-risk groups* — potentially exposed to smallpox, polio, diphtheria, tetanus, anthrax, typhoid, rabies or infectious hepatitis; *Emergency vaccination programmes* — as recommended by the community physician to contain local disease outbreaks
(d) Foreign travel vaccinations		Approved vaccinations depend on the area to be visited: *Canada, USA, Australia, New Zealand, N. Europe* — no special recommendations (keep domestic vaccinations up to date); *S. Europe* — typhoid and paratyphoid; *Africa and Asia* — smallpox and cholera; *Other places* — typhoid and polio; *Known pockets of infection* — the appropriate vaccine (also when a vaccination certificate is a condition of entry); *Overland in areas of poor sanitation* — infectious hepatitis. Note that vaccines can be given separately or in combination — a fee is payable for each *operation*, not for each vaccine. In a course separate fees are paid for each stage. Vaccinations outside the schedule do not qualify for a fee, though you can ask for one from the patient

Table 1.6 *Contd*

Category of free	Red Book reference (para.)	Qualifications
Fees based on qualifications		
1 Seniority allowance	16.1	Paid in three stages, depending on the length of time the doctor's name has appeared in the medical register, and the length of time with the NHS as a GP principal (Scale 1 — registered 11 years and principal for 7; Scale 2 — registered 18 years and principal for 14; Scale 3 — registered 25 years and principal for 21) For the full allowance GPs must qualify for a full basic practice allowance
2 Postgraduate education allowance	37.1	An annual payment to GPs completing 20 days of accredited postgraduate education over the previous 5 years. Courses must include at least two from the three subject areas of: • health promotion and prevention of illness; • disease management; • service management. Reduced payments are available pro rata for fewer days of accredited education
Reimbursements		
1 Dispensing fees	44.1	Paid to doctors who 'supply and personally administer' injections, vaccines, suture and bandage material; and to doctors who qualify for a dispensing list (who receive the drug tariff cost of the prescription, less a discount, but with certain additions — on-cost allowance, VAT and container allowances, and the dispenser's fee — see p. 49)

2 Ancillary staff reimbursement	52.1	Reimbursable costs include staff wages; employer's NI and superannuation scheme contributions; costs of providing training; redundancy payments.
		    All GPs are eligible. The former quota per principal has been abandoned. Instead FHSAs have the discretion to decide:
		• the percentage of costs to be reimbursed;
		• the date from which reimbursements will be made;
		• the minimum qualifications and experience staff will need to be recognized.
		These decisions, made in the light of local need, budget and priorities, can be reviewed at 3-yearly intervals. There are transitional arrangements for staff in post on 1 April 1990 (see Section 1.2, p. 6)
		    Reimbursements may also be available for relief cover during holidays of reasonable length, sickness or maternity leave and training

Table 1.6 *Contd*

Category of free	Red Book reference (para.)	Qualifications
3 Reimbursement of rent, rates and sewerage charges	51.1	Paid by the FHSA quarterly in arrears. The exact arrangement depends on the ownership of the premises: • in Health Centres the FHSA directly reimburses the DHA and the doctors only pay a separate consolidated service charge; • in approved privately owned or leased premises rent reimbursement is 100% of the District Valuer's 'fair rent' assessment (see Section 1.1, p. 1)
4 Payments for computer systems	58.1	A scheme running from April 1990 to 31 March 1993. It reimburses: • 50% of buying, leasing or upgrading costs; • 50% of maintenance costs; • 70% of initial staff costs (for 1 year only). However, upper limits are prescribed in Para, 58/Schedule 1 on a sliding scale related to list size. All GPs are eligible but the scheme is cash-limited and may be suspended if the money runs out in a given year
Grants **1** Improvement grants	56.1	A grant of one- to two-thirds of the cost of improvements to surgery accommodation, but there are several qualifications on standards, project limits, use of the grant etc. (see Section 1.1 Improvement grants, p. 3)
2 Training grants	38.1	Paid to approved doctors who employ and supervise a trainee GP under the auspices of a training scheme. It comprises: • the trainer's grant; • the salary to be reimbursed to the trainee; • the employer's NI and superannuation contributions for the trainee; • an additional car allowance (to reimburse the trainee's travel expenses) • miscellaneous trainee expenses (phone extensions, defence union payments, removal costs)

It is expected that the average GP's annual new contract income will be made up as follows:

Capitation fees	60%
Allowances	17%
Items of service	15%
Health promotion clinics	4%
Minor surgery	2%
Target-based payments (smears and immunizations)	2%

However, these average figures are likely to disguise wide variations, in particular related to the number of health promotion clinics provided and the degree of success in meeting targets. Practices also vary widely in respect of their non-NHS income.

* This target may be raised to 95% soon, in line with the WHO's declared aims.

Table 1.7 Minor surgery procedures eligible for a fee.

Injections	Intra-articular
	Periarticular
	Varicose veins
	Haemorrhoids
Aspirations	Joints
	Cysts
	Bursae
	Hydroceles
Incisions	Abscesses
	Cysts
	Thrombosed piles
Excisions	Sebaceous cysts
	Lipomas
	Skin lesions (for histology)
	Intradermal naevi, papilloma, dermatofibroma and similar conditions
	Warts
	Removal of the toe nails (partial and complete)
Curette cautery and cryocautery	Warts and verrucae
	Other skin lesions (e.g. molluscum contagiosum)
Other	Removal of foreign bodies
	Nasal cautery

4 Professional fees (including accountancy, subscriptions, bank charges, personal health and professional insurance).
5 Travel expenses (including petrol, road tax and depreciation).

1 and **2** are discussed in more detail in the sections devoted to reimbursements (see Sections 1.1 and 1.2 and Table 1.6). Suffice it to say they are to a large extent reimbursable, while **3** and **4** leave only a limited scope for economy. The running costs associated with a car (**5**) include such items as:
• petrol, oil and antifreeze;
• road fund licence and car insurance;
• servicing, MOT and replacement parts (e.g. tyres);
• AA/RAC membership; cleaning, etc.
These items are tax-deductible but only for the proportion attributable to practice use. A percentage (negotiable with the Inland Revenue) is not allowable, representing private use. Commonly 90% of expenses are allowable for a first car and 50% on a second 'back-up' car. (In addition the Inland Revenue allows GPs an allowance that qualifies for tax relief on the *capital* expense (see below) of their vehicle — 25% of the 'written down' value of the car annually, subject to a maximum allowance of £2000, and with a reduced allowance for a second car.)

Capital expenses
Non-recurring expenditure on buying (or building) something
new is classified as capital expense. Replacement items are included, but repairs are treated as running costs. Examples of
capital expenses include a new computer, electric typewriter, or an
ECG machine. For tax purposes 25% of the 'written down' value is
allowable annually in the same manner as for GPs' cars.

Breakdown of expenses
Prior to recent Red Book amendments, the typical breakdown of
practice expenses was as follows:
Premises — 12%;
Staff — 43%;
Capital allowances — 7%;
Motoring — 10%;
Medical supplies — 15%;
Other (telephone, etc.) — 13%.
    In future it will probably depend on the extent to which staff
salaries are reimbursed. In addition GPs pay 6% of their gross
remuneration (less practice expenses) into the NHS superannuation scheme. *Benefits* from this include:
1   A pension (1.4% of the aggregate, over the whole service
period, of gross remuneration less practice expenses — corrected
to take account of inflation);
2   A retirement lump sum (three times the pension);
3   A widow's pension;
4   An incapacity pension;
5   A death gratuity.

Tax allowances
All running expenses legitimately and wholly incurred in the running of the practice are tax-deductible. The special concessions
related to car use and the tax position on capital expenditure have
been described above. GPs also benefit from two other sources in
addition to the usual practice-based expenses:
1   *Wives as employees.* Most male GPs pay their wife as a receptionist, and claim from the Inland Revenue an annual expense just
short of the amount at which NI contributions are required and
well short of the wife's earned income allowance (after which
income tax is paid). The validity of this claim has been queried by
the Inland Revenue, and some health authorities recommend that
wives perform measurable book-keeping and secretarial duties at
home, and that the transaction is sealed by the transfer of funds
by cheque.
2   *Use of the home for consulting.* Providing a substantial number of
patients are seen at home, the GP can claim tax relief on:
    (a) his mortgage interest payments (unless already tax-allowed);

(b) his rates and water rates;

(c) maintenance, lighting and heating costs.

Normally a proportion of the total expenses (say 20%) is deemed tax-deductible and for business use, and the rest is not deductible, representing private use. The exact proportion is negotiable with the Inland Revenue.

Concern has been expressed that GPs selling their home may then be liable to capital gains tax (CGT) on the part claimed as business property but, providing no particular area of the house has been designated for exclusive use in this way, and the doctor merely changes his primary residence, this attracts 'roll-over relief', and CGT is not payable.

1.7 THE DEVELOPMENT OF GENERAL PRACTICE

The 1966 General Practice Charter represented in its time something of a watershed in the development of modern general practice. Until the middle of the 20th century it was normal for GPs to be single-handed, to work from their own homes, employing their wives as secretaries, and with a minimum of supporting staff; premises were often substandard, gloomy places; and there were no financial incentives for change. Lack of a clear postgraduate training structure and lack of academic prestige also left GPs the poor relations of their hospital colleagues in the glamour specialties, and recruitment to general practice was a problem. The Charter of 1966 made a great impact on this situation. Its principal ingredients were better pay, seniority, group practice and designated area allowances, financial recognition of out-of-hours services, and the reimbursement schemes for staff salaries.

In 1967 the GPFC was founded as a source of loans, and hand in hand with these two changes there emerged an improvement in staffing, premises and general practice recruitment.

Several changes followed that helped to boost professional status and self-esteem:

1 Granting of the Royal status to the College of General Practitioners (1967).

2 The recommendation of a 3-year Vocational Training Scheme by the Royal College on Medical Education (1968), later to become compulsory.

3 Direct access to laboratory facilities, helped by the Report on Organisation of Group Practices (1971).

4 The emergence of general practice as a specialty capable of original research and publication.

5 The building of multidisciplinary Health Centres by DHAs.

Such was the impact of these changes (and the lack of a satisfactory career structure in hospital medicine) that general practice became oversubscribed with a glut of eager well qualified trainees chasing a shortage of principal vacancies!

Surprisingly, however, over the period 1964 to 1977, when Cartwright and Anderson conducted two major general practice surveys, the *patients* became *more* critical of the service, although the overall level of satisfaction was high in both studies. Some significant changes in attitude and service were highlighted, for example:

1 A dramatic swing towards appointment systems.
2 Improved access to hospital facilities.
3 Fewer frustrations concerning lack of leisure and poor pay amongst practitioners.
4 A slight increase in the percentage of practitioners expressing satisfaction with their careers, and a slight decrease in the number reporting frustration with unreasonable patients and trivial consultations.
5 A fourfold increase in the criticisms that patients made concerning doctors' availability to visit.

The rising tide of consumerism which characterized the 1980s, coupled with ballooning health service costs and reported inconsistencies in the standard and delivery of family services led to another major landmark in the development of general practice, presaged by the Government's White Paper *Working for Patients* and crystallized in the NHS Community Care Act 1990 and revised Terms of Service for GPs.

The key changes included:
1 An increase in the proportion of income derived from patient numbers as compared with automatic fixed-item allowances.
2 The setting of strict performance targets.
3 New separate payments to encourage minor surgery, child health surveillance and health promotion, as well as to encourage doctors practising in deprived areas.

In addition the Government sought to encourage:
1 Greater accountability for the spending of public funds, e.g.:
    (a) stricter availability requirements;
    (b) medical and financial audit;
    (c) indicative prescribing budgets;
    (d) the budget-holding scheme;
    (e) compulsory practice reports.
2 More patient choice:
    (a) practice information leaflets and a local directory of family doctors;
    (b) an easier system for changing doctors;
    (c) a revised complaints system.
3 Greater FHSA autonomy (e.g. to set performance standards and to determine staff reimbursement levels).

4 Cost-consciousness and downward pressure on FHSA budgets.

5 The wider use of modern information technology (computers).

A reader approaching this account afresh may wonder why these proposals met with such a hostile reception. Some changes were felt to be regressive, some financially or politically motivated, some of unproven medical value. Concerns were expressed that patient care would suffer; that bureaucracy would increase; that many of the details were ill conceived or impractical, and that at best the workload would mushroom without new funds being made available to compensate.

What happened is now history. A conference of the local medical councils opposed the proposals and recommended a ballot of all GPs. This in turn led to a decisive rejection of the new Terms of Service by the profession. The Health Secretary imposed a contract amidst calls for legal or industrial action, even resignation. The popularity of general practice as a career option slumped dramatically in the initial aftermath.

Even now there are rumours of further radical change (including greater emphasis on 'core pay' for 'core duties' with income topped-up through locally negotiated incentive targets and cost-of-living allowances). It is still too early to say how this latest twist in the fortunes of the profession will develop. However, some practices have reacted to change with tremendous energy and vigour, and there is enough vitality and talent around to have confidence that general practice will emerge from this period of transition with its fundamental values unscathed.

2 The Consultation

According to Stott and Davis (1979) the potential exists within the consultation to address several issues:

1 The management of presenting problems.
2 The management of continuing problems.
3 The modification of health-seeking behaviour (education).
4 Opportunistic health promotion (education, screening and preventive activities).

Research into the consultation has examined the extent to which this potential is realized. Studies have attempted to define process (what the doctor and patient do) and its relationship to outcome (what happens to the patient afterwards). This chapter considers processes and outcomes, the methods used to examine them, the extent to which the consultation realizes its potential, and how consultation techniques can be improved. The chapter concludes with sections on prescribing and the referral of patients for secondary care.

2.1 CONSULTING

Studying processes

Studies from other fields suggest that social skills and social competence have a great impact on overall effectiveness in dealing with people. Thus, Argyle (1972) found a variation up to 16-fold in absenteeism and labour turnover in industrial workforces led by supervisors with different styles. There is evidence that this competence consists of a repertoire of learned behaviours that may be identified and taught to less adept people. This approach has proved successful in training sales staff and American medical students, and has stimulated a great deal of interest in general practice processes and how to improve them.

The methods used to observe the consultation include:

- audiotaping;
- videotaping;
- the use of two-way mirrors;
- sitting in on colleagues' consultations;
- role-play.

No single method has proved entirely satisfactory: audiotapes miss important non-verbal information and contain uninterpretable pauses; role-play is to some extent artificial; and the presence of a video camera, or a second doctor, or the knowledge that there are eavesdroppers may modify the behaviour of doctor or patient or both. Despite these problems much useful descriptive information has been obtained. Taped consultations may be replayed and subjected to peer review and small group analysis, or dissected into their various social, linguistic and psychological components.

Analysis of this sort has led to several complex models of the doctor–patient relationship:

1   *The sociological model* — doctors and patients have beliefs based on the norms and values of their peers; their behaviour is consistent with the rules of these roles.

2   *The anthropological model* (e.g. Hellman 1981) — illness behaviour is promoted by the attempt to answer questions like 'What has happened?', 'Why now, and why to me?', 'What would happen if I did nothing?' Patients form a theory based on their experience, imagination and peer group views, to answer these questions, and this colours the consultation.

3   *The transactional model* (e.g. Berne 1964) — at any one point in time, three states of mind (ego states) operate in doctor and patient: parent, adult or child. Correct combinations communicate in transactions occurring in a predictable way and leading to a predictable outcome (rituals). Sometimes transactions are *crossed* (when for example the doctor talks like a parent and the patient adopts the role of subservient child), or *oblique* (when an ulterior message is aimed at another ego state in the recipient). A familiar example is the 'Why don't you? — Yes but . . .' ritual in which the doctor plays the parent ('I can make you grateful for my help, whether you want it or not') and the patient plays the child who always wins ('You go ahead and try . . .').

4   *The psychological model* (e.g. Rosenstock 1966) — patients vary in their health motivation, perceived vulnerability, the perceived seriousness of a problem, and the perceived costs and benefits; they behave rationally and consistently in the light of their own beliefs, which are fostered by a variety of cues, and modified by different outcomes.

One variation of this model (Rotter 1966) proposes that patients can be subdivided into those who explain what happens to them in terms of their own actions (i.e. have an internal locus of control) and those who explain everything as if they have little control (i.e. have an external locus of control). This aspect of the patient's psychological make-up influences outcome — thus, internal controllers are more likely to accept advice, keep appointments and take their prescriptions.

5   *The verbal model* — doctors develop a style, vocabulary, fluency and familiarity that control the relationship and structures it predictably. Byrne and Long (1976) analysed 2500 audiotaped consultations and defined various characteristic phases (phase 1 — relationship established by doctor; phase 2 — reason for consultation established by doctor; phase 3 — examination conducted by doctor, etc.); about 75% of the medical content of the

consultation was doctor-initiated. Workers have observed that doctors develop a style and vocabulary early in their careers that subsequently varies little from one consultation to another.

6   *The non-verbal model* — more information is conveyed by non-verbal cues than by speech; doctors and patients read one another's non-verbal messages and sometimes acknowledge and act on them, but non-verbal messages that are inconsistent with spoken ones hinder communication.

7   *The Balint model* — Balint (1957) pioneered a school of thinking altogether more sensitive to the nuances of the consultation. The main themes of his philosophy were:

(a) that patients' problems cannot be divided into physical and pyschological categories: the two always coexist to a greater or lesser extent. Psychological problems often manifest physically, and physical diseases usually have psychological sequelae;

(b) that doctors have feelings and these have a function in the consultation;

(c) that doctors vary in their awareness of (a) and (b), but they can be trained to improve their awareness level.

Valuable though these models are, they often suffer the short-coming of failing to relate process to outcome.

Studying outcomes

Measures of outcome are imperfect: it is extremely difficult, for example, to measure the average health, medical knowledge or prognosis of a doctor's list and to relate it to variations in his consultative approach. Three important outcomes that can be counted are patient satisfaction, patient recollection and patient compliance. When the consultation is judged according to these criteria it is clear that its potential is often not fully realized.

Are patients satisfied?

Communication is an aspect of care in which patients are most *dissatisfied*.

1   In one hospital study (McGhee 1961):

(a) less than 40% were dissatisfied with medical care, food, amenities;

(b) 65% were dissatisfied with communication and 21% sat-isfied only with reservations.

2   In general practice surveys (e.g. Kincey *et al.* 1975):

only about 50% expressed complete satisfaction with communications.

3   In outpatient surveys (e.g. Reader *et al.* 1957):

(a) 67% of patients wanted more information;

(b) 75% wanted to know 'as much as possible';

(c) 40% wanted the results and implications of *all* tests conducted.

What do patients remember?
1 Many studies suggest that more than 50% of information has been forgotten when patients are interviewed within a few minutes of leaving the surgery.
2 The characteristics of *memorable* information are that:
   (a) the patient believes it to be important (often diagnosis rather than treatment);
   (b) the patient understands it;
   (c) the information is given early in the consultation;
   (d) not too much is given at once.

How good is patient compliance?
Compliance is assessed in a variety of ways (by biological methods, subjective ratings, self-report, pill counts and direct observation). Whatever the method of evaluation, non-compliance rates are high — varying from 12 to 70% (e.g. Davis 1968) — and it seems likely that 50% or so of medical advice is not taken. Richard Podell (1975) proposed the 'rule of threes':
- one-third follow advice closely enough to make it effective;
- one-third follow *some* advice, though *not* closely enough to make it effective;
- one-third do not accept or follow advice at all.

Other studies on outcome
Two other types of outcome sometimes studied are patient well-being and the ability of doctors to make true and accurate diagnoses.
1 Egbert *et al.* (1964) demonstrated that patients counselled prior to surgery on the likely postoperative course experienced less pain and required less analgesia postoperatively than others who were unprepared. This is an example of the beneficial effect that process can have on the outcome of well-being.
2 Shepherd *et al.* (1966) reported wide variations between London GPs in the level of psychiatric illness they detected — from 38 per 1000 up to 323 per 1000, which is a ninefold discrepancy. Goldberg (1981) has identified certain patterns of behaviour practised by GPs adept at identifying mental ill-health:
   (a) empathy;
   (b) early eye contact;
   (c) directive rather than closed questioning;
   (d) clarification of the complaint at an early stage.

Improving consultation techniques

Consultation analysis has suggested various explanations for the relative failure in communication observed in doctor–patient studies:

1   *Patient factors*:

(a) limited knowledge of illness (many misconceptions and folk-models of illness);

(b) diffidence in asking for clarification. This is class-related. Only 45% of hospital patients obtain the information they want by asking, but 65% of class 1 ask, while only 40% of class 5 do (Cartwright 1964);

(c) the negative effect of anxiety;

(d) the 'hidden agenda' — Patients often legitimize their desire to consult over one matter by presenting with another one that they think is a more respectable reason in the eyes of their doctor. If their complaint is taken at face value, the 'hidden agenda' may remain hidden and the patient leaves the room dissatisfied.

2   *Doctor factors*:

(a) professional and personal attitudes. Doctors vary at the extremes from autocratic, high-status information-withholders to egalitarian sharers of information who place emphasis on the patient's role;

(b) medical uncertainty and doubt — which doctors prefer to hide;

(c) inappropriately technical language;

(d) too much information too quickly;

(e) failure to establish what concerns the *patient*;

(f) non-verbal cues of uncertainty or doubt, at variance with what is said.

3   *Doctor–patient relationship factors*:

(a) communication and compliance are better if there is doctor–patient rapport (usually a doctor who is perceived to be empathetic and a patient who conforms to the doctor's idea of a model patient!);

(b) class differences between doctor and patient are important. There appear to be linguistic and other social factors that produce better communication if doctor and patient come from a similar background. Thus, Cartwright and O'Brien (1976) found that middle-class patients, on average, spend longer in consultation, raise more questions and cover more problems with their doctor than working-class patients do.

Consideration of these factors suggests that various techniques can be employed to improve such outcomes as diagnostic accuracy, patient satisfaction, communication and compliance. Thus, Ley *et al.* (1976) and others have stressed the need for:

- a good relationship (caring and confiding; Korsch & Negrete 1972);
- establishing and giving due weight to the patient's concerns, beliefs and expectations;
- giving information *early* in a consultation;
- keeping the message simple and clear (and not imparting too much in one session);
- repeating the message and stressing its importance;
- providing *specific* information and *concrete* examples;
- giving written instructions as a reminder.

In addition:
- according to Bertakis (1977), recall and satisfaction are both enhanced when patients are asked to repeat and give feedback on the instructions they are given;
- Francis *et al.* (1969) have shown that compliance and satisfaction are enhanced when explanations are spontaneously volunteered by the physician;
- outcome is improved by the correct use of non-verbal cues (e.g. body posture can communicate concern; several studies have shown that good communicators smile more, look at the interlocutor more and have a different intonation when compared with less successful colleagues);
- the structure of the consulting environment affects the amount of information exchanged (e.g. seating arrangements can reduce or enhance exchanges by a factor of six; Pietroni 1976).

One interesting paper has looked at the doctor himself as a therapeutic instrument in the consultation, and the extent to which this is enhanced by a positive, assertive approach. Thomas (1987) found that in the 40–60% of consultations where no firm diagnosis can be made, patients feel better in the hands of a positive physician.

The difficult patient

In the MRCGP exam (and in real life), there is a special interest in how to handle the difficult patient, the non-compliant 'troublemaker', the addict who will not relinquish his tranquillizer, the liberated rebel, giving birth in an unheated caravan, contraceptive and ethical conundrums, problem families and so on. Such characters feature prominently in the MEQ part of the exam, and are thick on the ground in the viva too!

At the simplest level the courses of action open, given a contentious request are: to agree, to disagree, or to refer/bargain/educate/counsel — and each will have predictable implications.

At a slightly more sophisticated level, there have been several attempts to classify the so-called 'heart-sink' patient (Cohen 1986).

Table 2.1 Types of 'difficult' patient.

Class	Features
1 The dependent clinger	Expresses excessive gratitude for doctor's actions, but seeks regular reassurance over minor problems
2 The entitled demander	Frequently complains about imagined shortcomings in the service received
3 The manipulative help-rejector	Presents a series of symptoms the doctor is powerless to improve
4 The self-destructive denier	The patient who refuses to accept his behaviour affects his disease and will not modify self-harming habits

Table 2.2 International comparison of prescribing rates.

Country	Scripts/patient/year
USA	16.6
Italy	11.3
West Germany	11.2
France	10.1
Spain	9.6
New Zealand	8.5
Australia	7.7
UK	**7.0**
Sweden	4.7

Table 2.3 Health care spending — international comparisons.

	Health care and drug spending as a percentage of GNP (1985)	Spending per head on private health care (£)
Sweden	8.4	1172
France	6.7	1072
West Germany	6.3	983
UK	**5.2**	**627**

Groves (1951) has defined four categories of difficult patient (Table 2.1).

Gerrard and Riddell (1988) define 10 categories of patient, from 'black holes' to 'secrets'. Others have found heart-sink patients to be a disparate group of individuals, defying obvious classification and sharing in common only the ability to 'exasperate, defeat and overwhelm' (O'Dowd 1988).

The common response to such patients is unnecessary investigation or inappropriate referral, arising from a need to escape for a time from contact with the patient.

Coping strategies include:

1 Recognition by the doctor of his true feelings.

2 Help from counsellors and psychologists (for the patient, or doctor, or both!).

3 Alternative sources of therapy — the extended family network, religious organizations, self-help groups.

4 The work of Balint groups.

5 Peer group meetings — for support, information-sharing and to formulate multidisciplinary management plans.

Problem patients will occupy a disproportionate amount of our time, both within exams and outside them, and this is an area worthy of special exam preparation.

The consultation is *the* central process in the practice of medicine. It is not surprising therefore that attempts at raising standards have placed such an emphasis on consultation techniques. This chapter is a simple résumé of a large and complex body of literature. For a more comprehensive review the interested reader is referred to *Doctor–Patient Communication* by Pendleton and Hasler (see Further Reading).

2.2 PRESCRIBING

Is it all necessary?
At least 50% of all consultations end with a prescription being written, amounting to 13 000 scripts per GP per year. The cost is considerable: The number of prescriptions dispensed in the UK almost doubled from 240 million to 413 million between 1964 and 1987; 2.3 billion pounds was spent, amounting to £70 000 per annum per GP, and an average of seven prescriptions per head of the population.

Though large in absolute terms, these figures stand up well to international comparison (Tables 2.2 and 2.3). Yet we are all familiar with examples of unnecessary prescribing; for example, when:

- diagnosis is still in doubt;
- ingredients are probably ineffective;
- combinations and formulations are irrational;
- the value of treatment is debatable (in obviously self-limiting illness).

The variation in prescribing habits between doctors is often highlighted. In prescribing surveys net ingredient cost per item may vary more than threefold and prescribing rates from 24.5 to 160.9 items per 1000 patients per month within a single FHSA area (Troup 1989).

There is a lack of hard data relating prescribing practices to outcome, and without this it is difficult to judge performance and cost-effectiveness. However, a public enquiry by Sainsbury (1967) into more than 2200 prescribed drugs concluded:

1 50% were effective;
2 8% were rational combinations;
3 35% were undesirable (obsolete, ineffective or irrational).

This raises important issues, such as:

1 Why are these drugs made?
2 Why are they allowed?
3 Why are they prescribed?

The first two questions are really political and economic: drug companies, operating within legal guidelines and the international codes of pharmaceutical practice, produce drugs for which they claim there is a market (proven by doctors' willingness to prescribe them and patients' willingness to take them). They make profits, some of which are ploughed back into research and development, they pay a large amount in taxes, and their employment record is good. A lot of money is spent on drug promotion and on political lobbying, and some drugs are of undisputed importance.

The Government seeks to maintain a delicate balance: it must appear a neutral watchdog and must maintain the faith of doctors and drug companies, but also has to control its own budget. To curb drug company profits on non-essential drugs might affect research into future winners; to regulate too strictly could alienate drug companies and doctors alike and produce adverse political propaganda. Previous Government strategies focused on education:

1 Free prescribing information for doctors (the *British National Formulary, Prescriber's Journal, Drugs and Therapeutic Bulletin.*
2 Feedback from the Prescription Pricing Authority in the form of brief annual analyses (PD2s), detailed analyses on requests (PD8s), and visits from the Regional Medical Officer (to doctors who deviated markedly from the norm in their prescribing habits).
3 Attempts to control costs by negotiating with drug companies to limit prices and profits (various voluntary price-regulation schemes have been tried).
4 Voluntary initiatives have also been encouraged — many on an intraprofessional basis with the Royal College and leading academic practices taking a prominent role.

However, beginning with the Limited List (1985), the Government sought a more direct control over prescribing costs.
5 The Limited List scheme was based on successful precedents in NHS hospitals and in other countries like Norway and New Zealand, and apparently saved the NHS 75 million pounds in its first full year of operation.

Two other initiatives are noteworthy:

6   The Prescribing Analysis and Cost (PACT) package.
7   The so-called Indicative Prescribing Scheme.

The PACT scheme

The PACT scheme comprises a series of quarterly prescribing reports for GPs in England (in Wales and Scotland there are parallel systems). Prescribing and dispensing reports relate to principals and partnerships and information is fed back at three possible levels (Table 2.4).

Table 2.4 The PACT scheme.

PACT level	Format	Availability
1	The simplest level. A four-page report with basic information: • quarterly prescribing costs; • average costs per item; • relationship to list size; • subdivision by therapeutic group; • comparison with practice, local and national averages	All GPs receive this overview
2	More detailed information with special emphasis on the most expensive sections	On request. Also sent automatically to high-cost practices*
3	Full reports running to more than 100 pages with an index and technical guide	Only on request

* Practices whose total costs exceed FHSA averages by at least 25% or where costs in one of the six major therapeutic categories is at least 75% above average.

(Several authors have pointed out limitations to the system and also explored its value in review, audit, personal and trainee education. PACT results, like other counting exercises, need to be related to outcome, dealing as they do in quantity but not quality.)

The Indicative Prescribing Scheme

Indicative prescribing amounts are to be set by each FHSA through its Prescribing Medical Adviser in discussion with practices. The amount is determined individually, but based on:
• historic prescribing patterns;
• average prescribing costs locally;
• list size and age profile (a key determinant);
• special factors not previously recognized but identified by the practice;

● with time and experience, special factors identified by 'improved NHS management systems'.

This amount should cover a year's prescribing, including that by deputies and locums on the practice's behalf. Once the amount is set for the financial year practices are required to monitor their prescribing profiles on a monthly basis, to ensure that their year-end target is met. They are assisted by:

● quarterly PACT reports;

● an indicative prescribing statement and monthly budget information (including a year-end projection);

● an annual summary return;

● more detailed breakdowns from the Prescription Pricing Authority on request.

In addition a number of new bodies and posts are being established to assist the effort (Table 2.5).

Table 2.5 New bodies and posts created to improve prescribing practices.

The National Medicines Resource Centre	Centrally funded. Located in the Merseyside Regional Health Authority. Staffed by drug information pharmacists. Produces a monthly bulletin
Prescribing Unit, Department of General Practice, Leeds University	To investigate the range of normal prescribing and to assist research
Medical prescribing advisers	Doctors appointed at FHSA level to establish, monitor and advise on indicative prescribing
Medical Audit Advisory Groups	Established at local level to assist GPs' efforts at audit

A sanctions procedure may be evoked where there is clear evidence of overspending. An overspend triggers an FHSA enquiry carried out by their prescribing medical adviser. If the overspend can be justified no further action follows; if not, the adviser will discuss with the practice ways of containing their prescribing costs. Ultimately the FHSA can apply for a formal investigation by a specially constituted professional committee.

(Note that overspending FHSAs and regional health authorities must similarly justify their position, taking all necessary remedial action to meet future budgetary targets; they will receive analogous monthly and annual returns from the Prescription Pricing Authority and FHSAs will be encouraged to develop voluntary formularies to meet local needs.)

A number of local voluntary incentive schemes are also planned whereby FHSAs and local medical councils can nominate a target saving, half of which may be made available for agreed primary care projects. Thus, a range of initiatives at local, regional and national levels are envisaged.

There are significant implications for medical practitioners. In future they will be forced to consider the cost of their prescribing policies; more than ever they will have to justify their actions, and they will need tighter management controls and ways to identify exceptional costs as they arise. The adoption of a formulary is likely to be one of the central administrative tools in this process.

What is rational prescribing?

Though it is relatively simple to collect prescribing statistics, it is not simple to interpret them. For example, it has been pointed out (Stott 1989) that doctors with above-average prescribing costs may:
- have expensive patients (for example, those on growth hormone, or domiciliary oxygen, or fertility treatment);
- do more good (be more aware of the therapeutic possibilities; keep patients out of expensive hospital beds; keep them productive and at work etc.);
- be more efficient in screening for (and then treating) latent problems like hypertension or hyperlipidaemia.

The implicit assumption that above-average prescribing is 'bad medicine' and below-average is 'good medicine' has been challenged, since process has not been related to outcome.

The Government has made regional health authorities responsible for the first time for both hospital and family practitioner services, and hopes thereby to compare the relative costs of alternative approaches, but information is not presently available at this level of sophistication. How then are we to define rational prescribing?

One serviceable definition would be that prescribing conforms to consensus opinion of the best current practice.

How to prescribe rationally

The choice of a drug is influenced by several considerations:
1 Is the diagnosis known?
2 Is a drug required?
3 Will it work?
4 Will it harm?
5 How much will it cost?
6 Have all the alternatives been considered?
7 Is the likely benefit:risk ratio acceptable?

What to look for in a prescriber

The responsible prescriber has several duties:
1 To ensure the diagnosis is right.
2 To make a positive and correct decision that a drug is needed.
3 To choose a drug appropriate to the patient's needs.

4 To consult the patient, and to ensure there is informed consent.
5 To explain the patient's role and to secure his cooperation.
6 To keep accurate prescribing records.
7 To oversee the course of treatment.
8 To terminate it when it is no longer needed.

Social reasons for prescribing

However doctors often prescribe without proof of efficacy. Why should this be? Contributing factors include:

1 True variations in medical opinion (in Germany in 1974 doctors issued 154 000 hypertensive scripts per million populus; in the UK the figure was 200 per million).
2 The pressure of pharmaceutical advertising.
3 Habit, peer group recommendation and ignorance.
4 Patients' demands (there is evidence that this is overestimated and that a larger percentage leave a consultation with a prescription than those expecting one beforehand. Indeed, up to 20% of patients do not even have their scripts dispensed!).
5 Attempts at placebo prescribing (see below).
6 A variety of social reasons:
   (a) to play for time until the true picture becomes clearer or natural recovery occurs;
   (b) to cover uncertainty, rather than admit it;
   (c) because of medicolegal worries;
   (d) to keep faith with patients, to justify their efforts and to demonstrate concern;
   (e) to hasten the conclusion of a consultation;
   (f) to avoid confrontation;
   (g) to keep faith with your partners (hence the 'Friday afternoon antibiotic');
   (h) personal experience: we like to think we are scientific but often base our prescribing on limited and subjective experiences with our own small patient samples.

Many patients are adept at securing social prescriptions and use well recognized ploys to obtain what they want (e.g. insistence, flattery, bargaining, comparison with other doctors).

Placebo prescribing

The response rate to placebos is high, of the order of 30–40%. According to some sources there are particular personality traits (e.g. extroversion, sociability, neuroticism, awareness of autonomic function) that identify the placebo responder. However other studies suggest no clear correlation and show that most people can respond given the correct situation.

Many conditions can be helped (Table 2.6). Note that the

Table 2.6 Some conditions susceptible to the placebo response.

Angina	Enuresis	Insomnia
Anxiety and depression	Hayfever	Peptic ulcer
Arthritis	Headaches	Postoperative pain
Asthma	Hyperglycaemia	Premenstrual tension
Blood pressure	Hyperlipidaemia	Social problems

response is not entirely psychological: physiological changes have been observed, suggesting a 'real' effect, e.g. placebos have:
- reversed the motility effects of ipecacuanha;
- lowered blood sugars;
- lowered blood pressure;
- reduced cholesterol (and mortality from ischaemic heart disease according to one study).

The time-response of placebo treatment also mimics the pharmacokinetics of active drugs.

Up to 40% of patients experience placebo side-effects including: headache; anorexia; diarrhoea; nausea and vomiting; dry mouth; vertigo; lassitude; palpitations; dermatitis; even addiction!

Factors affecting the placebo response include:

1 Pain levels — the more severe, the more likely is a placebo response.

2 Anxiety levels.

3 Tablet size, appearance and formulation: to be effective tablets should be:

(a) very small or very large;

(b) unlike an everyday medicine in appearance;

(c) capsules or injections rather than tablets;

(d) bitter to taste.

Colour is also important (see Table 2.7).

Table 2.7 The effect of tablet colour on placebo response.

Colour	Best response in:
Blue or green	Creams/ointments
Green	Anxiety
Red	Analgesia
Red or brown	Elixirs
Yellow	Depression

4 Patient expectation.

5 High technology: attendance at outpatient clinics, X-rays, and especially invasive investigations have a therapeutic effect.

The conviction of the prescriber, his charisma and the doctor–patient relationship probably also contribute. Male patients tend to respond more frequently than females, and higher social classes are especially prone.

Ethical problems

Proponents of the placebo argue that:

1   It is effective (what does the mechanism matter if the result is satisfactory?).

2   It is reassuring, and helps morale in chronic/incurable disease.

3   It fulfils patient expectations.

4   There is no significant toxicity.

5   There is evidence of an underlying physical basis (e.g. naloxone has been shown to reverse placebo pain relief suggesting a possible endorphin-based mechanism).

Those against placebo prescribing argue that:

1   It is deception and an abuse of a relationship of mutual trust.

2   It may generate hurt and ill-feeling if the deception is uncovered.

3   It delays true diagnosis.

4   It reinforces the sick role.

Whatever the rights and wrongs, placebo prescribing is widely practised, and (if we admit it to ourselves) so is the habit of prescribing for largely social reasons.

Generic versus branded prescribing

In all, 35% of prescriptions are generic, the rest are by brand name. Health officials have counselled the use of generic alternatives, suggesting that the taxpayer should not pay for expensive brands when there are cheaper alternatives. The two sides of the argument have been well expressed by Collier (1988) and Cruickshank (1988). Table 2.8 illustrates that the matter is not as clear cut as might be supposed.

Practice formularies

Every doctor, consciously or unconsciously, uses a personal drug formulary for his routine prescribing needs — often on the basis of familiarity, previous training, habit, the preference of colleagues or local consultants, and so on. However, many authors argue that this piecemeal approach is no longer sustainable — legally, administratively, contractually or ethically. The Government has strongly advocated the development of local prescribing formularies. Others too have made the case.

Advantages

1   In writing practice formularies doctors are forced to look critically at their personal prescribing habits, and to make choices which are hopefully safer, better, cheaper, more rational and more cost-effective.

Table 2.8 Generic versus named-brand prescribing.

Supporting more generic prescribing (Collier 1988)	Defending brand prescribing (Cruickshank 1988)
1 There are fewer generic names, making learning and teaching simpler	1 There are more than 40 generic versions of propranolol alone: changes in tablet size, colour and taste confuse patients and may prejudice compliance
2 Generic names are international and used routinely in scientific publications: this allows clear exchange of information. Generic names convey an indication of chemical class, facilitating an understanding of their uses	2 Generic names are often long and confusing. Brand names are shorter, simpler and more memorable
3 Stocking a smaller line of drugs would be simpler and more efficient for the chemist, who could achieve savings through bulk purchase	3 Chemists, reimbursed on a fixed-price basis, have an incentive to purchase only the cheaper generics; in the case of overseas sources quality may be suspect
4 The NHS drug bill may be reduced by up to 100 million pounds per annum	4 Relatively small savings to the NHS (in percentage terms) represent punitive losses to research drug houses who need reserves to develop new drugs
5 Under the Medicines Act the licensing authority and its inspectorate guarantee comparability of quality between like products	5 (a) There have been examples of clinical inequivalence between generic versions in some studies; (b) therapeutic data are not always required by the authorities and no data on efficacy/side-effects; (c) ingredients other than the active agent (up to 95% of the tablet) can differ from the original product; (d) ultimately, if the manufacturer of a generic cannot be identified, product liability may fall on the supplier (doctor or pharmacist)

2   There has been a fourfold increase in the number of available medicines over the last 30 years, producing a mountain of product information too large for anyone to assimilate. If prescribers are to keep abreast of current knowledge they must by necessity read and choose selectively.

3   Drug formularies can reduce practice prescribing costs (Beardon *et al.* 1987). Doctors with formularies can justify their spending (see **The Indicative Prescribing Scheme**, above), and their efforts are more accessible to audit.

Home-produced versus standard formularies

Several excellent formularies already exist, including a respected version by the Royal College of General Practitioners' Northern Ireland Faculty. There are advantages to adopting one of these standard formularies:

- the hard work of preparation has already been done;
- such sources will be periodically updated;
- they provide an accepted standard of excellence.

Alternatively doctors can produce their own practice formulary. This has the advantage that they will learn a lot of therapeutics and pharmacology along the way, and can adapt to local needs and hospital colleagues' known preferences.

Disadvantages include:

- the considerable effort required;
- the need for regular updating;
- possible medicolegal problems arising from errors and omissions.

In writing a practice formulary, several practical steps need to be taken:

1 Secure the agreement and involvement of all the partners.

2 Divide the work up between them (different doctors may choose different therapeutic groups).

3 Get each person to research his topic, and then select and justify an appropriate list of drugs.

4 Meet and agree a first-draft formulary. If necessary seek arbitration (e.g. from the head of the local drug information service).

5 Agree circumstances under which deviation from the formulary is permissible.

6 Check and countercheck all prescribing information before producing a final version, which should include information on side-effects and drug interactions.

7 Agree policies for:

(a) initiating drug treatment;

(b) drug treatment started by hospital colleagues and other GPs;

(c) reviewing maintenance therapy.

8 Review in the light of new developments and information.

Local prescribing groups may make lighter work of the task, and the Family Health Service Authorities' medical prescribing adviser should prove a useful source of advice.

2.3 REFERRING

Questions have arisen recently concerning the general practice referral system — its effectiveness, strengths and weaknesses;

consumer choice and the equitable rationing of health care services; how to refer rationally and how to identify rational referrals.

The rationale for the present system
The present referral system from generalist to specialist arose historically from mid 19th-century demarcation disputes between apothecaries, physicians and surgeons. Although this restrictive practice was intended to protect the livelihood of doctors, it has since been justified as a rational and effective basis for allocating health care resources.

Patients can only bypass the gatekeeper system in the case of urgent personal need (casualty), or public interest (sexually transmitted disease services). It is argued that the generalist can, from this position:
* ration access according to need;
* target care more specifically;
* protect against over-investigation and over-medicalization;
* prevent the misuse of expensive high-technology facilities, and needless trafficking between specialisms.

He is also best placed to appreciate the whole picture, and the patient benefits from two complementary views — personal and technical.

Criticisms of the present system
Although there are obvious arguments in favour of this approach, critics have pointed out that:
* GPs exercise a virtual monopoly in their control of access to secondary care in the UK;
* other countries' health care systems function without such a restriction of choice;
* therer is unacceptable variation in the performance standards of the gatekeepers, with expensive and potentially unfair consequences.

To what extent are these criticisms justified?

A restrictive practice?
The referral system was granted special dispensation from the Restrictive Practices Act 1976 because of its perceived advantages to the public. However, this is a topic on which the Monopolies and Mergers Commission has been seeking a review, and doctors cannot assume that the status quo will remain unchallenged. Marinker (1988) considers that doctors will need to take active steps to fight their corner.

Quality and quantity of GP referrals
Descriptive studies have established a variation in referral and investigation rates not accounted for by characteristics of the

population studied. At extremes they varied from 2.9 per 100 consultations to 11.8 per 100 consultations in one study (Wilkin & Smith 1987); and in another study from 5 per 1000 per month to 115 per 1000 per month (Last 1967). A 20-fold variation in referral rates seems stunning. Is it an indictment of standards within the profession?

Variations can arise through errors of counting, random fluctuation of demand, true differences in demand or different referral thresholds between physicians. There is some evidence that a combination of these factors contributes. Thus:

1 There is scope for error in:

(a) not counting private referrals (in some practices a substantial percentage of the total);

(b) relating referral rates to personal list size rather than workload and consultation rates in practices with shared-list systems.

2 There is also doubt as to which denominator (list size, episodes of illness, number of consultations, category of disease) best measures the rate in question.

3 Using too short a study time may lead to random peaks and troughs in demand. Moore and Roland (1989) point to the many factors influencing referral rates and suggest that a significant part of the variation may be due to the fairly small number of referrals in most studies and the effect of chance. They conclude however that 'there remains a substantial part of the variation that cannot be accounted for'.

Two points are worth noting:

1 Variations in referral rates do *not* seem to correlate with the age of doctors, their use of investigations, postgraduate qualifications or experience in a specialty (which actually *increases* referrals to that specialty; Morrell *et al*. 1971).

2 High referrers are not necessarily profligate or inadequate: they may be more aware of the diagnostic and therapeutic possibilities and offer a better service. It requires a better measurement of outcome to make this judgement.

Referral thresholds

Nevertheless, there are a number of criteria — not all medical — that doctors apply by common agreement in making their referral decisions, and other circumstances that doubtless sway them (Table 2.9). Differences in subjective judgement inevitably arise.

One study has focused on doctors' capacity to cope with uncertainty, comparing the referral thresholds of Dutch, Belgian and British GPs (Grol *et al*. 1990). There was a marked difference in their comfort with a wait-and-see policy: all doctors dislike uncertainty but some can live with it better than others.

In principle risk-taking can be quantified through a closer

Table 2.9 Factors influencing referral decisions.

1 Distance from local hospitals
2 Availability of public transport
3 Family and social expectations
4 Community support services
5 Quality and quantity of available hospital services
6 Variations in morbidity, age–sex structure and other environmental factors within the population
7 The training, interests and experience of the GP
8 The GP's ability to abide uncertainty

understanding of the sensitivity, specificity and positive predictive value of clinical symptoms and signs in the community: doctors with desk-top computers should 'learn the language of probability' and its application in improving the assessment of referral need, according to a leading editorial (*Lancet* 1990). Perhaps this day will come.

3 Prevention and Screening

3.1 PRINCIPLES

Definitions

There is some confusion over the use of the terms primary, secondary and tertiary prevention. One school of thought defines the three degrees of prevention as follows:

1° *(primary) prevention*: Removing the causal agent, e.g. sanitation measures of the 19th century;

2° *(secondary) prevention*: Identifying presymptomatic disease (or disease risk factors) before significant damage is done, e.g. screening for hypertension;

3° *(tertiary) prevention*: Limiting complications/disability in patients with established disease by regular surveillance, e.g. trying to prevent diabetic problems by good control, regular fundoscopy, foot care, etc.

According to this definition *screening* is a form of secondary prevention. It can be defined as the application of sorting procedures to populations by doctor initiative with the aim of identifying asymptomatic disease or people at particular risk from it.

Others have taken primary prevention to mean measures taken *before* an event (e.g. in trying to prevent a myocardial infarction), and secondary prevention to mean those measures taken *after* an event to limit damage or prevent recurrence.

Anticipatory care

Anticipatory care is an approach to medicine that concentrates attention on anticipating and precluding problems. It is in fact an effort to offer all appropriate forms of prevention (however defined) within the consultation and the organizational framework of primary care.

Methods of screening

Methods of screening follow two broad lines:

1 *Case finding (opportunistic or anticipatory care)* — This means taking the opportunity when the patient attends on another matter to screen him for the desired characteristic. This method is simple, involves no extra administration or expense and reaches 70% of the practice population in 1 year and 90% in 5 years.

2 *True screening* — The active pursuit of cases by questionnaire, letter, home visit, purpose-designed clinic or whatever. This involves more administrative work and the expense (partly offset by item-of-service payments where applicable) is borne by the GP.

Table 3.1 Pros and cons of opportunistic versus formal screening.

	Pros	Cons
Opportunistic screening	Simple, cheap to administer	Requires organization, time and commitment
	Does not depend on patient compliance	Does not offer 100% coverage to the target group
	Reaches a section of the public who will not attend for preventive advice alone	The time used is not 'protected': more urgent demands may take precedence
	Can be made relevant to the circumstances of attendance	Patients seen when ill may be less receptive to health education
Formal screening approaches	'Protected' time for discussion	Requires organization, time and commitment
	Purpose of attendance understood by all parties	Important non-attendance problem, wasting health care resources
	Attenders are (by definition) motivated and more receptive to advice they have personally solicited	Users are often those least in need of the service
	Comprehensive coverage of related health areas can be planned	Administrative obstacles are considerable
	Financial incentives now favour the formal health promotion clinic	

The major disadvantage is that patients do not always share their doctor's passion for screening and there is often a significant non-attendance rate. The advantages and disadvantages of these two approaches are compared in Table 3.1.

Requirements of a screening programme
Wilson (1966) proposed these criteria:
1 The condition must be:
   (a) common;
   (b) important;
   (c) diagnosable by acceptable methods.
2 There must be a latent interval in which effective interventional treatment is possible.
3 Screening must be:
   (a) simple and cheap, if possible, and in any case cost-effective;
   (b) continuous;
   (c) on a group agreed by policy to be at high risk.
   To this we can add the requirements that the disease is readily treatable and that screening tests are highly sensitive (few false

Table 3.2 Sensitivity, specificity and positive predictive value of screening tests.

---

1 In order to assess a new screening test comparison is made with a reference method (which is the best currently available)
2 Cases and non-cases are identified by applying both tests and a 2×2 contingency table constructed:

	Reference method		Totals
	+ve	−ve	
New screening test			
+ve	*a*	*b*	*a + b*
−ve	*c*	*d*	*c + d*
Totals	*a + c*	*b + d*	*a + b + c + d*

3 If it is assumed that the reference test is always correct,
- *a* cases are true positives
- *d* cases are true negatives
- *c* cases are classified falsely negative
- *b* cases are classified falsely positive

4 The *sensitivity* of a test is the proportion of true positives detected as positive by the test, i.e.:

$$\text{sensitivity} = (a/(a + c)) \times 100 \ (\%)$$

In a highly sensitive test *c* is very low, i.e. there are few false negatives
5 The *specificity* of a test is the proportion of true negatives detected as negative by the test, i.e.:

$$\text{sensitivity} = (d/(d + b)) \times 100 \ (\%)$$

In a highly specific test *b* is very low, i.e. there are few false positives.
6 The *positive predictive value* of a test is the proportion of those detected as positive by the test who truly *are* positive, i.e.:

$$\text{positive predictive value} = (a/(a + b)) \times 100 \ (\%)$$

More simply, it is the likelihood that the test is right in an individual whom the test declares positive

---

negatives), highly specific (few false positives), safe, non-invasive, acceptable to the patient and easy to interpret. If used in mass screening programmes a test should have a high positive predictive value (Table 3.2).

Relatively few conditions exist for which all criteria could be said to be met. It is certainly true, since screening is doctor-initiated, that benefits should outweigh costs.

Weighing costs and benefits
Several theoretical and practical considerations have a bearing on the cost–benefit equation:
1 There is always a trade-off between sensitivity and specificity in a screening test — that is, the looser the definition of a case, the fewer the number of borderline cases missed, but the larger the number of false positives.

2   Even tests of high specificity and sensitivity may have a low predictive value in populations where the prevalence of a condition is low (odd but true).

3   Screening tests often unearth disease at an earlier stage in its genesis; this may lead to the spurious belief that survival has been prolonged, when in truth treatment has been ineffective and the true time course is unaltered (Fig. 3.1). Overall mortality and morbidity are the final arbiter.

4   Decisions about the target population (e.g. age group) and recall frequency are often arbitrary and based on imperfect ideas of natural history.

| Clinical case: | A ───────────────→ B ──────────────→ C |
| Screened case: | A ──────→ B ─────────────────────→ C |

A = Start of the disease process
B = Point of awareness (presentation as a case or detected during screening)
C = Death

In this case the time course of the disease (A–C) has not changed, although earlier detection has created the impression that survival time (B–C) has improved.

Fig. 3.1 Spurious effects on survival produced by an earlier diagnosis (lead-time bias).

Costs and benefits are not easy to establish.

Benefits
1   Improvement in mortality and morbidity needs if possible to be confirmed by randomized trials.
2   The possible economic saving on future treatment is particularly hard to quantify.

Costs
1   Costs to patients:
    (a) unnecessary anxiety or even psychological harm;
    (b) false reassurance (some of the time);
    (c) economic costs (e.g. time off work).
2   Costs to doctors: time and resource costs (test and follow-up).
3   Costs to the NHS:
    (a) costs of the test (direct and indirect);
    (b) costs of follow-up, further investigation or treatment.
    Financial cost–benefit assessments have been attempted, as shown below, but these estimates remain tentative.
1   Cervical cytology — 40 000 smears, 200 excision biopsies and up to £300 000 per life saved.
2   Mammography — £3000–5000 per quality-adjusted life year saved.
3   Hypertension — £1700 per quality-adjusted life year saved.
    Psychological costs are well described:

1 Telling patients they have hypertension has led to absenteeism, lower self-esteem and poor marital relationships (Haynes *et al.* 1978).

2 Unfortunately, the damage once done is not easily undone:

(a) Bloom and Monterossa (1981) followed up people who had been told they were hypertensive, and who were later assured it was a false alarm: they had more depression and a lower state of general health than matched controls initially told they were normotensive;

(b) other studies (e.g. on maternal alpha-fetoprotein levels and neonatal thyroxine levels) confirm that once the seeds of doubt have been sown by a false-positive result, people suffer lasting unease.

3 There are also concerns that the communication of a negative result may be harmful. It may, for example, reinforce an unhealthy lifestyle or make participants less likely to return for repeat tests.

Marteau (1989) suggests that sensitive pretest counselling is necessary in anticipation of these problems, and that the long-term behavioural outcomes of widespread screening initiatives need to be fully assessed. Others too see this as an ethical imperative, as in many instances the efficacy of intervention and cost-effectiveness of screening initiatives can be questioned.

Possible screening activities

Despite the failure in some cases to demonstrate objective benefit, a range of screening activities have been suggested as appropriate to primary care and approved as ingredients of remunerated health promotion clinics (Table 3.3, p. 89).

Obstacles to prevention

Patient-related obstacles

Patients weigh costs against benefits and often perceive costs to be high. Taking smoking as an example, the costs of giving up include:

1 Sacrifice of physical pleasure — the anxiolytic pharmacological action of cigarettes.

2 Sacrifice of the psychological and social benefits — smoking is:

(a) a social activity that binds groups;

(b) a relaxation ritual;

(c) a conversation filler;

(d) a risk-taking, and hence exciting exploit;

(e) in adolescence, a form of rebellion.

Hence people rationalize or ignore:

1 'It won't happen to me' (the ostrich approach).

2 'I don't believe they know the true facts' (the sceptic's approach).

Table 3.3 Possible preventive activities.

Screening
Hypertension screening, detection and follow-up
Cervical cytology
Developmental surveillance
Well-woman and well-man clinics
Visiting the elderly at home
Mammography
Blood fat estimation
Faecal occult bloods
Screening for psychiatric illness/alcohol abuse
Well-person periodic medicals

Preventive interventions
Immunizations/vaccinations
? Post-menopausal hormone replacement
? Calcium supplements
? Lifestyle counselling
Advice on smoking
Keep-fit and aerobic programmes
Weight-watching

3 'You go when it's your turn and you can't change that' (the fatalist's approach).

Sometimes people are genuinely ignorant of relative risks ('Life's a risk — you're just as likely to be knocked over crossing the road. . . .').

Doctor-related obstacles
Costs to the doctor include:
1 Time and resources.
2 Frustration (if returns are low).

There are also barriers of organization and enthusiasm, problems with effective, clear communication (see Section 2.1) and in some areas medical debate and uncertainty that make advice-giving harder. In group practices commitment to preventive activities often varies between the partners, and this produces a source of potential friction and a check on the effectiveness of the service.

Overcoming patient-related obstacles
Fowler, Gray and others have suggested the following plan:
1 Point out the debits (seriousness and magnitude of risk).
2 Point out the benefits (social and financial as well as physical; positive as well as negative).
3 Anticipate and be prepared to discuss difficulties.
4 Suggest coping strategies.
5 Give simple advice and supplement it with written information.

The application of this approach to smoking is discussed in Section 6.1 and the subject of improving patient compliance is discussed in Section 2.1.

Setting up a screening programme

Zander (1982) has pointed out the major differences between preventive and routine care:

Routine care	*Preventive care*
(a) Patient-initiated, i.e. demand is unpredictable	Doctor-initiated, i.e. the demand should be predictable
(b) Immediate-type demand	Non-urgent
(c) Usually involving the doctor	Easily delegated to other primary health care team members
(d) Focused on individuals	Focused on high-risk groups
(e) Good records are a help but audit is difficult	Good records are essential; audit is usually straightforward

In general terms the stages involved in setting up a screening programme are:

1 Identifying a problem which meets the Wilson criteria and which the practice agrees is a priority.

2 Auditing the records to establish the baseline performance of the practice, and then deciding whether to proceed.

3 Counting numbers — How big is the undertaking? Do you know the names of the high-risk group? (age–sex register is obviously important here).

4 Defining *objectives* (e.g. to measure the blood pressure of all males over 40 years old).

5 Defining *methods*:
   (a) opportunistic?
   (b) by patient invitation?
   (c) by patient visiting?

6 Defining the *participants* (e.g. practice nurse in hypertension screening and well-woman clinics; geriatric health visitor in over-75s home surveillance).

7 Participants may need training and/or equipment and need to have a protocol. They also need time to do the job.

8 Review after a trial period. Has the performance improved? Are objectives being met? Are teething problems disturbing the balance and effectiveness of the practice in other respects? Then decide whether to continue and what refinements are needed.

These are the principles involved, but the MRCGP candidate might well be expected to discuss screening with reference to

specific examples as they exist (or might exist) in his own practice.
The remainder of this chapter is therefore devoted to some topical
examples of how screening services could be organized. The principles involved are really the same in each case, but they are
described in full so that each topic can be read on its own if
required. (Note that the methods suggested are *not* the only way
to deliver the service but merely examples of the type of approach
commonly employed.)

3.2 CERVICAL SCREENING

Background and rationale
A total of 2.5–3.0 million smears are performed annually. Despite
this:
- 2000 deaths occur each year in the UK (not much change since
1968);
- the death rate is rising amongst young women.

This represents a poor result compared with the smear campaigns of the USA and Finland, where death rates have fallen by
50% in 10 years.

The current campaign is based on evidence that the natural
history of cervical cancer involves several premalignant stages
(grades of dysplasia and carcinoma *in situ*) detectable by regular
cervical screening several years in advance of frank carcinoma:

	?		10%		20%		50%	
Normal	⇌	Dysplasia	⇌	Carcinoma *in situ*	→	Invasive cancer	→	Death
	40%		25%					
Time	0		5 years		15 years		25 years	

Certain *high-risk* groups have been described:
- low socioeconomic class;
- early age of first sexual intercourse;
- early age of first pregnancy;
- multiple sexual partners;
- frequent pregnancies;
- venereal disease.

Limitations to cervical cytology
1 A false-negative rate of about 10% for carcinoma *in situ* (even
necrotic tumours can give a negative result).
2 A false-positive rate of about 5% (smears showing mild
dysplasias).
3 Sampling problems: the squamocolumnar junction is not
always accessible.
4 Other technical problems which upset interpretation (e.g.

delayed application of fixative; menstruation; pregnancy and the Pill; intrauterine devices and polyps).

5 Limitations of the *cervical smear campaign*:

(a) DSS guidelines are complex, inconsistent and often lagging behind current research (e.g. most authorities now recommend 3-yearly smearing of all sexually active women, but official guidelines and item-of-service payments do not recognize this);

(b) the number of smears taken is probably inadequate;

(c) the right women are probably not being screened: in particular the high-risk groups from low social classes use the service least but need it most (the inverse care principle);

(d) funding is inadequate. Some laboratories have had to place temporary embargoes on smear-taking to cope with the workload, and others have complained that if all women requiring a smear had one, the system would be overloaded;

(e) organization is generally inadequate:

● the old DHSS recall system was disbanded and computerized District Health Authority systems have been slow to replace it;

● they in turn have been loaded with inaccurate age–sex data from Family Health Service Authorities' (FHSA) registers, so that in some inner-city studies nearly 70% of invitation letters have been inaccurate or inappropriate (Beardow *et al.* 1989);

● many practices have not bridged the gap with systems of their own, with coverage apparently varying from more than 80% down to 10–20%;

● a study by Elwood *et al.* in Nottingham (1984) found that only 59% of positive smears were properly followed up;

● Ellman and Chamberlain (1984) reviewing 100 cervical cancer deaths in Sutton found that:

68 had never been screened;

10 had negative smears, but over 5 years previously;

13 suspicious smears were not followed up.

In other words, 91 deaths were potentially preventable but the patients slipped through the net because of shortcomings in organization. Recently a target-based system of fees has been introduced, encouraging GPs undertaking this work to organize themselves more efficiently.

How to set up a cervical screening and recall system

The steps involved (which will become familiar by the end of this chapter!) are as follows:

1 *Define objectives and priorities*, e.g.:

(a) decide whether you want to screen every 3 years or every 5;

(b) should you screen every sexually active woman or just the over 25s and antenatal patients?

(c) consider your priorities (older women are least likely to have had a smear, so some practices start with them first;

others have a policy for high-risk groups and make extra efforts here).

2 *Count numbers and obtain names*. Identify the desired population using the age–sex register.

3 *Define methods*, e.g.:
(a) opportunistic smears;
(b) a cervical smear/well-woman clinic;
(c) a combined approach;
participants, e.g.:
(d) all the partners;
(e) family-planning trained nurse or health visitor;
(f) clerk to operate the recall system;
resources, e.g.:
(g) allocate consulting time.

4 *Establish a recall system*:
(a) examine the notes and establish cervical smear status and next due date; tag examined notes;
(b) set up a card-index system (e.g. for each record examined note on a card the patient's details and next due date; arrange the cards in the desired order of recall and file them in a box under the month/year of the next due screening);
(c) when a smear is performed and the result seen, move the patient's card in the box index to the new 'next due' date;
(d) periodically examine the index and collect the names of people who missed their smear on the due date: they can then be contacted individually (make one person responsible);
(e) it may be advisable to have a separate index for the very important group of positive smears, and possibly for high-risk patients;
(f) a computer system will do all these things more efficiently. It can generate word-processed letters of invitation and monitor progress towards targets.

5 *Implement the screening*, e.g.:
(a) draw up a list of immediately due smears;
(b) devise a plan to clear the backlog (e.g. temporary extra clinics);
(c) if an opportunistic approach is favoured, mark the notes as a reminder ('smear due next time'); otherwise draft carefully worded letters of invitation and offer smear appointments.

6 *Review*. Periodically count numbers:
(a) what percentage of the target group is having smears taken?
(b) what is the success rate of an opportunistic approach?
(c) what is the take-up rate if appointments are offered?
(d) can the figures be improved (e.g. by offering smears with the nurse, smears at more flexible times or educational information)?

Dealing with smear results
It is important to establish a secure system that ensures patients know their smear result. Patient initiative may not be sufficient (as a tragic case in Oxfordshire has made clear) and various approaches have been adopted: at one extreme there are doctors who take the view that the patient should have responsibility for her own health and should therefore make her own arrangements to contact the surgery; at the other extreme there are doctors who adopt the practice (expensive in time and administration) of writing to every patient. The middle-ground approach concentrates on positive smear results: some doctors write to all of these patients, others keep ledgers or leave the result out, and contact patients who do not enquire after a defined interval. The important point is that there is a system and that it is fail-safe and subject to regular review.

3.3 WELL-PERSON ASSESSMENTS

The well-woman clinic
The well-woman clinic has its origin in the old cervical cytology clinics run through local authority services, where it became recognized that women in need of cervical smears also appreciated the opportunity to discuss other problems in a setting specifically tailored for them. The potential to offer health education to women who are in a receptive frame of mind is considerable, and these clinics have therefore become popular.

Advantages
1 These clinics may attract women who might not otherwise come to the surgery, who are inhibited about seeing a doctor and using up his time unless ill.
2 Patients attending such clinics are in a health-conscious and receptive frame of mind.
3 It is often possible to offer more time and a more informal atmosphere.
4 There is greater scope in this elective setting to offer the woman a doctor of the sex she prefers than in the higher-pressure, immediate-demand setting of routine surgeries.
5 A separate clinic also avoids the real pitfall of opportunistic screening, that it is often inconvenient (the surgery is running late; the patient is having a period, etc.).
6 Separate clinics are often more convenient if different members of the team (e.g. doctor, health visitor and nurse) all wish to attend: they can arrange their timetables to suit.
7 There is a large potential for health promotion and educating towards self-help for common, minor problems (perhaps reducing

demand on consulting time in the long run, and helping to relieve health-related anxieties in those with neurotic illness).

8 Income may be boosted (e.g. increased item-of-service work, higher list sizes because a well received competitive range of services is on offer).

9 Greater satisfaction for the patient and doctor, and an extended (more satisfying) role for the practice nurse.

Disadvantages

1 The obvious costs of:
(a) time and energy;
(b) administrative effort and overheads.

2 These clinics may still reach the *most* motivated people, when the need is to reach the *least*.

3 There are dangers that:
(a) it will degenerate into a sick-woman clinic through patient misuse;
(b) a poor uptake will affect morale and enthusiasm, and moreover, unaccepted invitations will squander consulting time. At the very least, demand may be unpredictable.

How to set up a well-woman clinic

1 *Define objectives and priorities*, e.g.:
(a) to screen for cervical cancer;
(b) to screen for breast cancer;
(c) to screen for hypertension;
(d) to screen for gynaecological problems;
(e) to promote family planning;
(f) to give preconceptual counselling;
(g) to teach self-examination of the breasts;
(h) to give health education and advice (self-help for thrush and cystitis; facts about premenstrual syndrome; psychosexual counselling; encouragement to lose weight, stop smoking, eat a healthier diet, etc.);
(i) to˙develop self-help groups (weight-watchers, toddler groups, etc.).

2 *Count numbers and obtain names* — using the age–sex register.

3 *Define methods*, e.g.:
(a) is the format of the clinic letter invitation, or open access or a mixture of the two?
(b) will there be a follow-up for non-attenders?
(c) what is the recall frequency?
(d) should invitations be issued according to priority?
participants, e.g.:
(e) interested female partner (taken on for this purpose?);
(f) health visitor;
(g) practice nurse;

resources, e.g.:

(h) a slot in the timetable; training of staff as required;

(i) letters of invitation and posters advertising the service.

4 *Establish a recall system*, e.g.:

(a) a card index of the target population arranged in the order they are to be recalled (used like the cervical smear system described in the preceding section);

(b) make someone responsible for upkeep of the index and periodically examine it for defaulters.

5 Ensure the protocol is approved for FHSA remuneration.

6 *Review*. Periodically consider:

(a) how many attenders (and defaulters) there are;

(b) how many new cervical smears have been done;

(c) whether patients are satisfied;

(d) whether it has affected the pattern of normal surgeries.

Demand can be measured readily, but satisfaction and understanding are harder to quantify.

Well-man clinics

Less common, but growing in popularity, are the well-man clinics, which are aimed in particular at the overweight and overstressed businessman, and the male smoker from the lower social classes.

Aims may include:

- screening for hypertension and alcohol abuse;
- advice on weight reduction, safe levels of drinking, giving up smoking, a more healthy diet, exercise and fitness;
- optional activities like urinalysis and lipid estimations.

Costs and benefits of well-person screening

GPs' new Terms of Service require well-person health assessments on those registering with their practice for the first time, and those not seen by a doctor within the previous 3 years. The content of this new medical assessment is detailed in Table 8.2, p. 235. It includes some measures whose strict scientific value has been questioned, in particular:

1 There is no evidence that the routine measurement of height and weight is of benefit.

2 Non-selective routine urinalysis has a low yield.

3 The cost-effectiveness of inviting infrequent attenders to attend for a health check has been challenged — Thompson (1990) scrutinized 1488 records: out of 114 patients who had not attended in the last 3 years, 17 were eventually persuaded to attend. Thirteen needed anti-tetanus injections but five refused and five failed to return for immunization; three needed a repeat smear, but all failed to return for it, and one case of mild hypertension was discovered at an estimated cost of 28 h of staff time and 15 h of doctor time.

4 Multi-phasic screening of asymptomatic patients has been 97
a notable disappointment (Oboler & LaForce 1989; South East *Chapter 3*
London Screening Study Group 1977). *Prevention and*

(These arguments appear to be carrying some weight, and it is
rumoured that the 3-yearly medical will soon be abandoned.)

3.4 DIABETIC CARE

The problem

The prevalence of diabetes in the population is about 1–2%. The
incidence is about 1–2 new cases per GP per year. On average
each GP has about 30–40 diabetic patients: three-quarters of these
are non-insulin-dependent, leaving about 8–10 insulin-dependent
diabetics. However, 'the rule of halves' is thought to apply, i.e.:
• half of a practice's diabetics are unknown;
• half of the known diabetics are not followed up,
• leaving one-quarter of the total followed up (often
haphazardly).
    There are two important aspects to diabetic care:
1 Case finding or screening.
2 The follow-up of known diabetics.
    These will be considered separately.

Screening for new diabetics

Since the prevalence is 1–2%, routine urinalysis as a screening
procedure would have a small but definite yield. This could be
improved by considering the at-risk factors, and therefore screening high-risk groups, e.g.:
• the obese;
• those with a family history of diabetes;
• those with big babies (birth weight 10 lb or 4.5 kg);
• those with a history of gestational diabetes (the risk of full
diabetes is about 20% at 5 years).

Follow-up care

Should GPs run separate diabetic clinics?
Potential *advantages* include:
1 It avoids the drawbacks of hospital clinics, namely that they
are:
    (a) overcrowded;
    (b) impersonal;
    (c) staffed by a succession of changing junior doctors;
    (d) care is more haphazard, access more restricted and waiting
    time longer than in a well run surgery clinic.
2 Patients prefer the convenience of a trip to their own surgery
and the security of seeing a familiar doctor who knows their
personal problems.

3 There is also an opportunity to improve doctor–patient rapport.

4 More time can be offered for counselling and advice than at busy hospital clinics.

5 It is more convenient for the GP, e.g.:
(a) time has been calculated and set aside to do the job properly (this cannot be guaranteed in the unpredictable hurly-burly of the routine surgery);
(b) the relevant staff and equipment are to hand;
(c) delegation is then possible;
(d) with only one subject to concentrate on, a more systematic and thorough approach is possible.

6 If diabetic patients are followed up methodically rather than haphazardly, there should be better control, which may mean:
(a) fewer complications;
(b) earlier referrals;
(c) fewer out-of-hours calls.

7 There is greater professional satisfaction if the primary health care team can offer a good service to a group of its own patients with a common chronic condition.

8 Although strictly speaking a tertiary prevention activity (some would say a treatment service), supervision of diabetics qualifies for the health promotion fee if organized into a recognizable clinic.

Potential *disadvantages* include:

1 The extra time and effort involved.

2 Administrative costs — now offset in part by the health promotion fee.

3 It needs interest, enthusiasm and commitment to the subject (not always heart-felt!). There is, for example, an onus to keep abreast of current thinking on the subject and, as with all preventive exercises, enthusiasm may need to be maintained in the face of an apathetic and frustrating response.

4 Doctors may feel underqualified and that patients would do better under the care of a specialist.

Shared care or full care?
Assuming a practice wishes to proceed with a diabetic clinic, two further questions spring to mind:

1 Which patients are suitable?

2 Should we operate a shared-care or full-care system?

Diabetics suitable for exclusively practice-based care would probably include:

● stable, complication-free diabetics treated by diet, tablets or insulin (perhaps 75% of the total);

Specialist input (shared care) is almost certainly required in the case of:

● children;

- pregnant women;
- patients with known complications;
- the unstable insulin-dependent diabetic.

Some practices operate shared-care liaison schemes with interested local physicians which include:
- a cooperation card;
- occasional consultant visits at the surgery;
- a visiting dietician, chiropodist and/or diabetic liaison sister;
- extra laboratory facilities.

There are clear advantages to this system:
- high patient convenience;
- a specialist input which benefits patients and educates GPs;
- extra services on tap;
- a saving to the NHS over seeing the same patients in hospital.

How to set up a diabetic clinic

1 *Define objectives and priorities*, e.g.:

(a) decide on baseline observations (blood sugar, glycosylated haemoglobin, blood pressure, lipids, urinalysis, full history and examination or whatever);

(b) decide on the follow-up parameters and recall frequency (e.g. a 6-monthly check on weight, blood sugar, glycosylated haemoglobin, fundi, feet and pulses, visual acuity, etc.);

(c) decide on the desired level of control;

(d) decide on an advice package (advice on monitoring, hypos, foot care, smoking, etc.).

2 *Count numbers and obtain names*. If the practice has a morbidity index, the job is done. If not, produce one using:

(a) the memories of partners and reception staff;

(b) repeat prescription cards;

(c) hospital correspondence;

(d) opportunistic or systematic review of patient records.

3 *Define methods*, e.g.:

(a) the format of the invitation;

(b) the format of the clinic;

(c) whether shared care or full care;

(d) how the protocol can be streamlined and administered (would a flow chart in the notes or a patient education leaflet speed things along?);

participants, e.g.:

(e) interested partner(s);

(f) practice nurse;

(g) clerk operating the recall system;

(h) empathetic local consultant (sound him out);

resources, e.g.:

(i) a slot in the timetable; training of staff as required;

(j) a practice glucometer;

(k) sound out the local physician on available back-up (visiting dietician, chiropodist, diabetic liaison sister, etc.);

(l) a practice brochure and display posters to advertise the service.

4 *Establish a recall system*, e.g.:

(a) produce a full index of known diabetics, tag their notes and establish when desired checks are next due;

(b) file the names in order of recall against the proposed month/year;

(c) issue an appointment, and after attendance move the patient's name forward to the new recall date;

(d) periodically check the index and appointment sheets to identify defaulters;

(e) make someone responsible for maintaining and examining the index, and have a system for adding new names as newly diagnosed diabetics appear;

(f) have a practice policy on how to handle defaulters.

5 Ensure FHSA approval of the protocol — to qualify for payment.

6 *Implement the system*: should extra clinics be laid on temporarily to clear the backlog of patients whose check-ups are urgently overdue?

7 *Review*, e.g.:

(a) what is the attendance/default rate?

(b) has diabetic control improved?

(c) what percentage of diabetics are now seen on a regular basis?

(d) have emergency out-of-hours calls from diabetics become less frequent?

3.5 HYPERTENSION SCREENING AND FOLLOW-UP

The problem

Dilemmas in the diagnosis and management of hypertension are fully discussed in Section 4.1. To summarize briefly, problems have been caused by:

• the arbitrary nature of treatment values;

• the validity of measuring techniques;

• doubts regarding natural history, especially in relation to the elderly;

• the size, cost and logistic (organizational) problems of the undertaking;

• conflicting trial results and differing opinions on cost versus benefit.

If the active treatment of mild hypertension is pursued, this could involve 15–20% of the population.

Despite these problems hypertension is perceived to be *par excellence* a condition that should be managed in general practice. According to a survey by Fulton *et al.* (1979), two-thirds of GPs feel general practice is the ideal place for *screening* in particular. There is, however, a big gap between expectations and performance, e.g.:

- in one central London general practice survey only 24% of the population had their blood pressure recorded in the last 5 years, and only 39% of hypertensives so found were followed up (Fulton *et al.* 1979);
- apparently hospitals are no better: in one study only 32% of new outpatients had their blood pressure recorded, and only 38% of hypertensives so detected were followed up.

The 'rule of halves' is believed to operate:
- half the hypertensives are unknown;
- half the known ones are not treated;
- half those treated are not controlled;
- hence, only one-eighth of the hypertensive population receive satisfactory care.

Is screening feasible?
D'Souza *et al.* (1976) found that 93% of patients with a diastolic blood pressure above 95 mmHg visited their GP in a 5-year period. A strong case can therefore be made that opportunistic screening is entirely feasible and has a high yield. Fowler estimates that for a 5-yearly blood pressure check on all the patients of an average list, only 1–2 extra measurements would be required each day (and, of course, there is no need for the doctor to do this task personally — it can easily be delegated).

How to set up a screening and treatment service
1 *Define objectives and priorities*, e.g.:
    (a) the age group to be screened (e.g. over 20s or over 40s?; all women on the Pill);
    (b) the frequency of screening (e.g. 5-yearly);
    (c) devise a protocol which standardizes recording methods, treatment values, baseline investigations, recall frequency, drug policy, etc.;
    (d) fix a target blood pressure so that quality of control can be assessed;
    (e) compile a morbidity index and tag the notes in every case.
2 *Define methods*, e.g.:
    (a) opportunistic screening or a separate clinic (hypertension, well-woman or well-man clinics), or a walk-in service operated by the nurse;
    participants, e.g.:
    (b) all the partners;

(c) the practice nurse;

(d) the clerk who maintains the recall system;

resources, e.g.:

(e) coloured stickers to tag the notes;

(f) a flow diagram sheet for the notes;

(g) prominent posters advertising the service.

3   *Establish a recall system*, e.g.:

(a) identify all known hypertensives (from memory, repeat prescription cards, correspondence, summary notes and surveying the records) then compile a morbidity index; tag the notes;

(b) file the patients in the index in order of proposed recall — against the proposed screening date;

(c) when patients have been screened refile their name in the index against the next proposed screening date;

(d) periodically check the index for defaulters who can be followed up individually; make someone responsible for maintaining the register, and adding and deleting names as required.

Some practices operate the so-called 'three box' method. They divide the patients into three groups on the basis of their blood pressure readings:

- a treatment group;
- a borderline group;
- 'normals'.

The patients are then filed in three separate box indexes. The argument is that the three groups need a different recall frequency:

- the treatment group may need to be seen every 4 months, say;
- the borderline group annually;
- the majority with normal blood pressure only 5-yearly.

For a list of 2500 patients there will be roughly 70 hypertensives under treatment, and up to 150–200 'mild' hypertensives needing annual monitoring.

4   *Review*, e.g.:

(a) what is the percentage of the target population being screened?

(b) what percentage of the known hypertensives have been seen in the last 6 months?

(c) have the chosen investigations produced a reasonable yield? (if not, the protocol could be simplified.)

3.6 GERIATRIC SCREENING

At present 15–17% of the population are over 65 years old, but the proportion of the elderly is increasing, and the proportion of the very elderly is increasing even more. By the year 2000 the ranks of the over-75s may have swelled by 20–35%, and the over-85s by 45%.

Of all non-psychiatric NHS beds, 50% are already occupied by the over-65s, so concern has been expressed that hospital services will not be able to cope. The answer to this dilemma could lie in prevention and in identifying disability before it becomes severe. Another good reason to think preventively is to try and raise the quality of life in old age.

Preventive measures
Preventive measures that may help include advice on:
- the avoidance of smoking and obesity;
- increasing dietary fibre;
- keep-fit activities (and vigorous rehabilitation after acute illness);
- mental recreation;
- avoiding the typical negative attitudes associated with ageing.

Regular attention from the chiropodist, optician and dentist may be beneficial.

Is screening worthwhile?
Screening studies on the elderly show a high prevalence of un-reported problems, so it might be supposed that they would benefit from the regular attention of a screening physician. In fact, only a minority of practices displayed an interest in geriatric screening before it became a condition of service. This is explained in part by doubts repeatedly cast on its feasibility and effective-ness, e.g.:
- Wallis and Barber (1982) estimated that to screen all patients over 75 years of age in their Glasgow practice needed 18 h of health visitor time per week for the first year, and 11 h per week in subsequent years;
- Tulloch and Moore (1979) found that screening produced an increased use of health care and social *facilities*, but not a great change in *health*;
- Hendriksen *et al.* (1984) found a reduction in hospital admis-sions but no reduction in the number of nursing home admissions.
- Coleman (1989) identified in a practice list of 11 000 patients 132 elderly people who had not been seen in the last 2 years: 22% could not be contacted, 51% did not welcome the approach, and in the 36 who were finally seen eight remediable but minor prob-lems were detected at a direct cost of £3400 and at a time cost of 425 h (only 5% spent with patients);
- Epstein *et al.* (1990) conducted a large-scale US study in which patients were randomly allocated between usual and intensive specialist care (geriatrician, geriatric nurse, geriatric social worker):

at 3 and 12 months the health differences between the groups were marginal.

It has been argued by some that most newly diagnosed problems in the elderly are trivial or irreversible, so health spin-offs are small.

Advantages of screening

Proponents of geriatric surveillance point out:

1 That some spin-offs (morale, self-esteem and satisfaction) are immeasurable and come forth when it is shown that someone cares;

2 That today's trivial problem (e.g. uncorrected presbycusis or loose doormat) is tomorrow's major one (e.g. fractured neck of femur);

3 That some worthwhile diagnoses *can* be made (up to one in five over 75s are said to suffer some degree of depression; 6–12% have some degree of dementia, with carers stressed and unsupported).

It has also been suggested:

1 That an opportunistic approach is also feasible, since 90% of the over-75s see the primary health care team anyway over a 1-year period.

2 That *selective* screening of high-risk patients (e.g. the very old; the recently bereaved; the socially isolated; the immobile; the recently discharged) is a more realistic proposition with a higher yield in prospect.

One study on selective screening showed that out of every 12 screened patients:

- three could be helped;
- four needed no help;
- five had irremediable problems.

Other studies have also raised question marks over the discriminating power of the commonly suggested high-risk criteria.

Although lingering doubts remain regarding the cost-effectiveness of screening, this is now a condition of service and doctors have been forced to face head-on the logistic problems entailed.

How to set up a geriatric screening service

1 *Define objectives and priorities*, e.g.:
   (a) who to screen (everyone over 75; perhaps high-risk groups over 65);
   (b) what to screen for (the minimum standard is determined by Schedule — see Table 8.2, p. 235).

2 *Define methods*, e.g.:
   (a) opportunistic?
   (b) home visiting? (must be offered annually to the over-75s)

(c) a combination of these?
(d) a questionnaire pro-forma (locally or nationally agreed? FHSA-approved?)
participants, e.g.:
(e) district nurse;
(f) health visitor;
(g) doctor;
(h) volunteer (e.g. local Age Concern group);
(The obligation to screen can be delegated within the primary care team.)
resources, e.g.:
(i) equip and train the screening personnel.
3 *Identify the patients at risk*, e.g.:
(a) using the records and age–sex register;
(b) construct an at-risk register.
4 *Implement the screen* — after first making contact with the elderly person to establish his interest.
5 *Review*:
(a) feedback on problems discovered;
(b) deal with them;
(c) review the progress (and benefits of screening);
(d) ensure proper records are kept to demonstrate compliance with Terms of Service.

3.7 IMPROVING IMMUNIZATION RATES

In primary immunization, according to national figures published in *Social Trends* (1984):
- 84% complete a course of diphtheria, tetanus and polio;
- 52% complete a course of pertussis vaccination;
- 56% are immunized against measles.

Immunization rates are clearly affected by media publicity (as indicated by the fluctuation in pertussis vaccination rates after various media scares), but within this variation some practices achieve rates worse than average and some achieve rates of nearly 100%.

Recall schemes run by FHSA computer and rubella vaccinations offered through the school health system have ensured a reasonable level of coverage, but there are shortcomings that primary care can redress.

Ultimately the success of immunization programmes depends on the compliance and commitment of parents and the efficient organization of the vaccinating service. A characteristic of practices with high vaccination rates appears to be a clear predetermined practice policy, discussed, agreed and understood by all health care team workers. Particular attention to methods of recall, screening and advertising is needed. A plan might include:

1   Discussion with parents at all available opportunities (for example, in the antenatal period, again at birth, when the health visitor calls, and at the 6-week postnatal check — all times when mothers are likely to be receptive).

2   Further education of parents via surgery posters and notices, a lending library of tapes or review articles (especially on the controversial vaccines).

3   A reminder to doctors in the form of:
(a) immunization record cards;
(b) a box on the antenatal/postnatal record card (to be completed when immunization advice is given);
(c) the tagging of records and age–sex register when vaccinations are completed;

4   A recall system run using the age–sex register and vaccination summary cards, especially to recall:
(a) girls for rubella vaccination (some practices send a reminder in the form of a 10th birthday card);
(b) teenagers (15–19 years old) for tetanus and polio;

5   Opportunistic approaches:
(a) checking tetanus status every time a patient attends with minor trauma;
(b) employing an immunization clerk who checks the notes for surgery and marks them if a booster is due (in some very efficient practices the check is also performed when a repeat script is issued and a reminder attached to the prescription);
(c) offering polio boosters to parents when their children are vaccinated;
(d) checking rubella antibodies when women are first offered contraceptive care and tagging the notes to indicate a satisfactory result.

6   A practice immunization protocol (updated so everyone knows the latest recommendations and gives the same advice).

High immunization rates have virtually eradicated serious infective illnesses like diphtheria, polio and tetanus but epidemics of whooping cough and measles, and the preventable misery they involve, underline the scope for improvement. In addition to improving the well-being of the population, immunizations generate income in the form of item-of-service payments and these payments are contingent on meeting taxing coverage targets.

3.8 PAEDIATRIC SURVEILLANCE

Infant mortality rates have been dropping in all countries, but not as fast in England as some others, notably Japan and France. This has led to the critical examination of the preventive serivices for children. Developmental surveillance has been practised in some form for at least 50 years. Until quite recently one out of every 10 GPs participated in this process with much regional variation. Amendments to the remunerative system may in future encourage more family doctors to participate. However doubts still exist about its value and about how, where and by whom it should be done.

Is it worthwhile?
The early detection of remediable conditions, notably congenital dislocation of the hip, squint and undescended testes, is the main value of the exercise.

1 In one study in 1978 it was found that 232 children out of 2157 needed specialist agency referral.

2 In Glasgow problems requiring treatment or follow-up were encountered in 23% of preschool children, and 15% had a previously unrecognized physical abnormality.

3 Another London study involving preschool children followed for the first 5 years of life found a significant health problem in 20% *at each age*.

Other apparent benefits include a better relationship with children and their parents, opportunity to educate and to offer self-help advice, and perhaps better compliance. However, as Bain (1989) points out, there are costs:

● time and resources are limited;

● non-attendance figures at clinics may be as high as 40%, especially amongst low socioeconomic groups with the greatest need;

● the number of major abnormalities detected will be relatively small in relation to the effort and expense.

Several screening programmes have been evaluated. It is true, on average, that 5–10% of children screened are referred for assessment, but more *severe* abnormalities freshly detected by this route amount to less than 1% of all those seen. Large-scale studies in Sweden have found only a marginal direct impact on health, while the British Paediatric Association has cautioned that a number of routine tests are unreliable, invalid or poorly performed. So, there is uncertainty over the value of routine mass screening.

Should it be scheduled or opportunistic?
Houston and Davis (1985) and others have suggested that children attend sufficiently often to adopt an opportunistic approach to screening. This has the advantage of simplicity and convenience and does not depend on patient response. However Walker (1986) has highlighted some of the pitfalls in this approach:

1 Attendance for medical care falls off sharply after the first year of life.

2 If visits are not planned, children may appear at times that are inappropriate for the assessment of key milestones.
3 Interpretation of screening efforts would be difficult because of background illness.
4 Communities that habitually bypass general practice services might never be considered.

The positive benefits of a separate clinic have also been stressed. Thus:
1 Time is specifically allocated to that purpose and the relevant personnel and equipment are to hand. It is easy to see how the best intentions of opportunists may be spoiled by the pressures of a busy surgery.
2 There is a value to meeting children when they are well.
3 A clearly defined service is appreciated by parents and has benefits for the doctor–patient relationship.
4 A new item-of-service payment encourages GPs to organize their child health work into identifiable clinics.

Who should do the work?
It has been argued that it is artificial and unsatisfactory to divide the responsibilities for surveillance and care in illness, and that general practice is the natural setting for screening. Recent movements to promote its wider practice by GPs include:
1 The Sheldon (1967) and Court (1976) reports.
2 The Conference of Local Medical Councils (1977).
3 The publication of the Royal College of General Practitioners' Working Party *Healthier Children — Thinking Prevention* (1982);
4 Its subsequent joint publication with the GMSC; *Handbook of Preventive Care for Pre-school Children* (1984).
5 Remuneration in the form of the child health surveillance fee.

Traditionally most of the work has been done by clinical medical officers and health visitors who have been adequately trained and have the necessary time and experience. Now GPs are showing a greater interest, but several possible question marks hang over GPs as an alternative or supplement to this service.

Do they have the experience?
Court (1976) argued that GPs need a specialist skill, should spend up to 70% of their time working with children and should train formally as GP paediatricians. The proposal of specialists within primary care was rejected by the GMSC and GPs as a whole who felt the necessary skills were already present. In 1982 the Royal College proposed compulsory paediatric training for new GPs or the creation of a Paediatric List, reluctantly echoing the two-tier proposal of Court. In effect this proposal has now been adopted: to be paid for developmental screening, doctors must be registered on their FHSA's approved list and must be appropriately

qualified. The issue of experience remains controversial, as the required standard has not been centrally defined, leaving FHSAs to formulate their own criteria under the influence of the various interested pressure groups.

Do they have the time?
The Royal College has calculated on the basis of five recommended examinations over a 5-year period that the average GP would see 7–8 extra children per week, so the time involved would be covered by a weekly session of about 2½ h.

Do they have the incentive?
Until 1989 no form of extra remuneration was provided to doctors undertaking this work. Those who adopted it as a matter of good practice were, in fact, penalized by higher overheads. The new paediatric surveillance fee was introduced to rectify this position and to encourage more participants. However, the fee for this work is modest, and still does not provide an attractive financial incentive. Some doctors however find their clinics useful loss-leaders in the push to achieve lucrative child immunization targets; others never viewed the clinics in financial terms anyway, believing in their implicit value to patients, and for them some element of recognition has been welcome.

Screening schedules
The Royal College of General Practitioners in its 1982 report confined its recommendations to feasible, simple, scientifically well validated procedures that did not require elaborate equipment (Table 3.4).

Five examination schedules were proposed and endorsed by the GMSC:
1   At birth.
2   At 6 weeks.
3   At 7 months.

Table 3.4 Screening objectives recommended in the Royal College of General Practitioners report (1982).

Adults	Newborn	Preschool children
Contraception	Chemical screening (e.g.	Immunization
Prenatal and antenatal	phenylketonuria,	(polio, tetanus,
care	hypothyroidism)	diphtheria,
Promotion of breast-	Testes (for descent)	pertussis, measles)
feeding	Hips (to exclude	Hearing
Anti-smoking	congenital dislocation)	Visual acuity
education		Squints
		Colour vision

4 At 2–2½ years.

5 At 4½ years.

Each examination was proposed to include:

(a) a brief physical examination;

(b) a developmental screening examination (gross and fine motor function, social skills and language development);

(c) a check on immunization status;

(d) a general assessment;

(e) a reminder concerning the next examination.

Significant findings (based on the Royal College recommendations) are summarized in Table 3.5 and important developmental milestones in Table 8.1, p. 233.

Table 3.5 Significant findings in deveopmental examinations (adapted from *Handbook of Preventive Care for Pre-school Children*, GMSC & RCGP 1984).

Schedule	Findings
Birth	Low Apgar score Congenital abnormality (e.g. cataract, coloboma, cleft lip/ palate, imperforate anus, extra digits, abnormal genitalia) Congenital dislocation of the hips Chemical evidence of phenylketonuria or hypothyroidism
6 weeks	Major maternal anxiety Restricted hip abduction Unusually small or large head Excessive head lag Asymmetry of tone Delayed visual response
7 months	Major maternal anxiety Restricted hip abduction A head circumference more than 2 s.d. from the mean Abnormal posture Squint Nystagmus Failure to fixate Failed hearing test Delayed social/language development
2–2½ years	Major maternal anxiety Failure to achieve sphincter control Abnormal gait Squint Inability to produce words and simple sentences Unusual skin bruises
4½ years	Major maternal anxiety Clumsiness Visual problems Speech problems Behavioural problems

The principles follow the usual five-point plan suggested throughout this chapter.

1 *Define objectives and priorities*, e.g. follow the recommendations
of the 1982 Royal College of General Practitioners' Working Party,
or aim to complete the schedules in the 1984 GMSC and Royal
College of General Practitioners handbook for all the practice's
preschool children.

2 *Count numbers and obtain names* — using the age–sex register,
health visitor's records or computer.

3 *Define methods*:
  (a) opportunistic or separate scheduled clinics?
  (b) recall frequency and approach to the follow-up of
  non-attenders;
  (c) liaison with health visitors;
  participants, e.g.:
  (d) health visitor;
  (e) interested GPs;
  resources, e.g.:
  (f) a slot in the timetable;
  (g) separate record cards for the notes, mother or both;
  (h) simple screening equipment;
  (i) an FHSA-approved protocol, qualifying for remuneration.

4 *Establish a recall system*, e.g.:
  (a) a card index of the target population filed in order of recall;
  (b) a practice computer;
  (c) make someone responsible for updating the system and
  checking for defaulters.

5 *Review*, e.g.:
  (a) how much time is involved?
  (b) what is the yield?
  (c) what is the uptake?
  (d) should the service be advertised by booklet or poster?

3.9 SCREENING FOR BREAST CANCER

The size of the problem

1 Breast cancer is *the* major form of cancer among women in the
UK. It accounts for:
- 15 000 deaths per annum;
- 20% of all female cancer deaths.
  It is the most common cause of death in women aged 35–54.

2 The UK has a high breast cancer mortality rate compared to
other developed countries.

3 There has been a slight increase in incidence and mortality over

the past 30 years. Treatment has not obviously improved the prognosis over this time.

Risk factors

1 Factors known to increase the risk of breast cancer include:
  (a) increasing age;
  (b) late childbearing (first child after the age of 30);
  (c) nulliparity;
  (d) early menarche;
  (e) late menopause;
  (f) family history (first-degree relative);
  (g) obesity;
  (h) ionizing radiation.
2 Other factors (e.g. high-fat diets, hormone therapy and the Pill) are still being evaluated.

Prognosis

On average two-thirds of all women with breast cancer are alive 5 years after diagnosis. However, those with early local disease fare better than those with metastatic spread (Table 3.6).

Table 3.6 Survival rate at 5 years according to stage of breast cancer.

Stage	Features at diagnosis	5-year survival rate (%)
I	Small mobile tumour confined to the breast; no nodes	84
II	As for stage I plus nodes	71
III	Locally advanced tumour attached to chest musculature	48
IV	Distant metastases	18

Screening by mammography

1 Mammography involves low-level X-ray exposure on one or two planes. The amount of radiation involved is small (1 rad).
2 The tissue of young womens' breasts is dense, resulting in practical difficulties in interpretation. Perimenopausal thinning makes the task easier, so screening is restricted to older (50+) women.
3 The sensitivity of modern mammography is about 80%, and the specificity is 95%. (Clinical examination picks up 50–60% of abnormalities.)
4 Estimates of positive predictive value vary from 9 to 60%, with

the Forrest report (1987) suggesting a 2:1 ratio of benign to malignant biopsies.

5   A programme of screening by mammography is necessarily complex, requiring:

(a) a sophisticated call–recall system;

(b) a relatively expensive test;

(c) interpretation by a trained radiologist;

(d) (in suspect cases) biopsy by a skilled surgeon;

(e) interpretation of biopsies by a skilled histopathologist;

(f) treatment where cancer is found.

There are potential pitfalls at every stage — failure of uptake; loss to follow-up; technical problems; errors of interpretation; treatment failures.

Benefits

It might be supposed, these problems not withstanding, that mammography is bound to be of benefit: after all, it detects breast lumps too small to be palpated, and 5-year survival figures are better for early disease. In fact, as Figure 3.1 illustrates, earlier diagnosis can result in longer survival times from diagnosis without altering the time-course of a disease at all.

Several major trials have considered whether there is a true benefit (Table 3.7). Early results appeared to show a 30% improvement in mortality, but more recent studies have tended to contradict this conclusion.

Costs

Costs are tangible:

1   A typical mammography screening unit comprises a radiologist, radiographer, histopathologist, surgeon, receptionist, nurse and administrator. The capital cost of equipment is high, as is the replacement and maintainance bill. The Forrest report (1987) estimated the financial cost to be £3000 pounds per life-year saved, but other estimates place it much higher.

2   There is also an opportunity cost, as skilled personnel and capital funds could be deployed elsewhere.

3   A low positive predictive value implies over-diagnosis, over-investigation and over-treatment of some false positives, with all the heartache this entails.

4   All women experience anxiety awaiting and undergoing tests, and awaiting results; some experience indignity; some may become phobic.

The UK National Breast Screening Programme

In 1988 health authorities began phasing in a programme of screening recommended by the Forrest report (1987). The target population has been defined as all women aged 50–64 years. A

Table 3.7 Some important trials of breast cancer screening.

Study	Design	Screening method	Age group studied (years)	Screening interval (years)	Reduction in mortality (%)	Comments*
Shapiro et al. (1982) Health Insurance Plan, New York	Randomized control trial	Clinical examination + two-view mammography	40–60	1	30	$P < 0.05$
Tabar et al. (1985) Sweden	Randomized control trial	One-view mammography	40–74	2–3	31	$P = 0.013$ High compliance (up to 90%) Reliable population lists from tax office
Andersson et al. (1988) Malmö, Sweden	Randomized control trial	Two-view mammography	>45	1.5–2	No significant difference between screened and control groups overall	In over-55s a 20% reduction in mortality Relative risk 0.79 Confidence intervals 0.51–1.24 74% response rate
Verbeck et al. (1984) Nijmegen	Case control trial	One-view mammography	≥35	2	52	Odds ratio, screened vs unscreened = 0.48, but wide 95% confidence intervals (0.23–1.00) compatible with 'no effect' Low attendance rates in older groups

| Roberts *et al.* (1990) | Controlled trial | Two-view mammography + clinical examination | 45–64 | 1–2 | 17% (at 7-year follow-up) | Odds ratio = 0.83, but wide 95% confidence intervals (0.58–1.18) compatible with 'no effect' Low attendance rates |
| UK Trial of Early Detection of Breast Cancer Group (1988) | Controlled trial (eight locations in the UK) | Two centres: clinical + two-view mammography (46 000 women) Two centres: breast self-examination (64 000 women) Four centres: controls (127 000 women) | 45–64 | 1–2 | 14% | Odds ratio = 0.86, but wide confidence intervals (0.69–1.08) compatible with 'no effect' |

*The significance of *P* values, relative risk, odds ratios and confidence intervals is explained more fully in Chapter 11.

single oblique mammogram is planned at 3-yearly intervals, with the call and recall procedure organized as follows:

1 The screening office identifies groups of eligible women.

2 The FHSA produces a 'prior notification' list for each GP.

3 GPs amend the list (correcting errors) and then return it.

4 Women are invited and attend for mammography.

5 The results are conveyed to women and their doctors, and follow-up arranged where appropriate.

6 A recall procedure is established.

A 70% uptake is anticipated. It has been estimated that, of those screened:

- 7% will be recalled for investigation;
- 1.5% will have a biopsy;
- 0.65% will have a confirmed cancer.

However, Roberts (1989) points out that those screened are a minority of those who will develop a cancer. For example, in Scotland in any given year only one-third of those developing the disease are in the age group to be screened; in a 3-year rolling programme one-third of these would be invited to attend; if, say, two-thirds did attend and there was a one-third improvement in mortality, at best only 2.5% could benefit.

The role of the GP

Austoker (1990) suggests that GPs can make an important practical contribution to the campaign, improving uptake and acceptability by:

- checking prior notification lists to ensure data are accurate;
- allaying fears;
- providing information and counselling;
- following up the non-attenders.

Breast self-examination (BSE)

There is a long-held view that BSE is a worthwhile preventive exercise, to be taught at every available opportunity. However, the evidence for this view is shaky. Hill *et al.* (1988) reviewed 12 trials: six of them purported to show some benefit as judged by the stage of disease at diagnosis. However, as already discussed, earlier diagnosis does not necessarily confer benefit.

In the UK Trial of Early Detection of Breast Cancer those invited to classes to learn BSE (after 400 000 women-years of observation) actually had a higher death rate than women in control districts!

The *disadvantages* of BSE include inconvenience, embarrassment, anxiety and the risk of false-positive cases. Furthermore guilt may be engendered in those patients with cancer who did not self-examine before diagnosis.

Some doctors have suggested that it is unethical to offer a test that may harm without clearer evidence of benefit. It is not surprising, given the debate concerning mammography, that a less sensitive screening test should be challenged in this way.

117

Chapter 3
Prevention and
Screening

3.10 LIPID SCREENING

Who should be screened?
The case for measuring serum cholesterol is built on several tiers of evidence:

1 Substantial epidemiological data that raised serum cholesterol concentrations are associated with more coronary heart disease.

2 Experiments in animals showing that dietary manipulations that alter serum cholesterol can accelerate or retard atherosclerosis.

3 Evidence from human primary and secondary intervention studies that those who lower their cholesterol level suffer fewer coronary heart disease events.

In the USA in 1985 a consensus of experts agreed that all American adults should have their cholesterol measured at least once; similar views have been expressed by the European Atherosclerosis Society and the American National Heart, Lung and Blood Institute. However, many others take a contrary view on who should be screened, and as Leitch (1989) points out, there is no consensus expert opinion on which GPs can advise and act. Recommendations range from no screening at all to screening everyone before the age of 30 years (Tables 3.8 and 3.9). It is instructive to consider why this should be so.

Does a low-fat diet prolong life?
Many trials have confirmed a reduction in coronary heart disease *events* with low-fat diets and lipid-lowering drugs. None, however, has confirmed a reduction in *overall mortality*. The reason appears to be that too low a cholesterol can also harm. Thus, Isles *et al.* (1989) identified in men a strong correlation between low cholesterol and lung cancer, and a U-shaped association with colorectal cancer, also true for women. There are 21 reports, of which 13 identified a link with cancer and low cholesterol, and eight showed no relationship. An increased incidence of cholelithiasis has also been reported, as well as a number of other effects, including a puzzling increase in deaths from violence and suicide. It seems that the coronary benefit may be offset by other factors. If true, we may enjoy maximum life expectancy with a mean cholesterol.

Table 3.8 Recommendations on who should have their serum cholesterol concentration measured.

Source	Main recommendations
Working group on cardiovascular disease of the Faculty of Community Medicine, 1989	Screening of the population not recommended
Study group of the European Atherosclerosis Society, 1987	General screening to be carried out only if provisions have been made for treatment and follow-up by medical practitioners; screening of specified high-risk groups; screening of patients opportune during routine medical contact (examples given)
British Heart Foundation, 1987	Screening of people with a family history of coronary heart disease
Coronary Prevention Group, 1987	Screening of specified high-risk groups*
Journal of the Royal College of General Practitioners (editorial), 1986	Screening of specified high-risk groups*
Journal of the Royal College of General Practitioners (editorial), 1988	Screening of specified high-risk groups* if screening all adults not practical
Royal College of General Practitioners, 1988	Ideally screening of all adults aged 20–70 or, if this is not possible, of specified high-risk groups*
Drugs and Therapeutics Bulletin, 1987	Ideally screening of all adults or, if this is not possible, of specified high-risk groups*
British Hyperlipidaemia Association, 1987	Screening of all adults, preferably before age 30

*See Table 3.9.
Adapted from Leitch (1989) with permission.

The practical problems

1 *The cholesterol screening* test. Several practical considerations apply:

(a) the test is not perfect: it has a sensitivity of 38% and a specificity of 75%;

(b) serum cholesterol is not static: it varies up to 20% in the course of a day, and rises with age until the fifth or sixth decades;

(c) the range of values is a continuum without a sharp cut-off point between health and disease for most of the population;

(d) high cholesterol is not in itself a diagnosis: it may be primary or secondary, and if primary, one of a complex group of disorders.

This leads to a situation that has an analogy in the problems of defining hypertension:

(a) strictly speaking we should take the mean of several readings before confirming an abnormality;

Table 3.9 Advice on screening high-risk groups. Adapted from Leitch (1989) with permission.

Source	High-risk groups								
	People with family history of coronary heart disease	People with family history of hyperlipidaemia	People with personal history of coronary heart disease	People with physical signs of hyperlipidaemia — for example, arcus xanthoma, xanthelasma	People with hypertension	Diabetics	Obese people	People with a history of gout	Smokers
Study group of the European Atherosclerosis Society, 1987	Yes, especially if history is in relative <50	Yes		Yes (specified)	Yes	Yes	Yes	Yes	Yes
Coronary Prevention Group, 1987	Yes (age unspecified)	Yes	Yes	Yes (specified)	Yes	Yes			
Journal of the Royal College of General Practitioners (editorial), 1986	Yes, if patient is <60		Yes		Yes	Yes			Possibly
Journal of the Royal College of General Practitioners (editorial) 1988	Yes (age unspecified)		Yes	Yes (specified)		Yes	Yes (gross)		
Royal College of General Practitioners, 1988	Yes, if history is in relative <60	Yes	Yes	Yes (specified)	Yes	Yes			
Drugs and Therapeutics Bulletin, 1987	Yes, especially if history is in relative <50	Yes		Yes (specified)	Yes	Yes	Yes		

(b) then proceed to a range of supplementary tests;

(c) then take an arbitrary decision, based on actuarial risk, as to who should be treated.

2 *The size of the problem.* The mean cholesterol level in the UK is 6.3 mmol/l. Many authorities believe dietary advice, further investigations and individual intervention become appropriate at or around this value — that is to say, for nearly half the population!

(a) An American study has estimated (after assuming a 10% decline in serum cholesterol with appropriate dieting) that 7% of men and 4% of women would need drug treatment, 41% lipoprotein analysis, and 84 million people would need interventionist treatment costing several billion dollars (Sempos *et al.* 1989; Wilson *et al.* 1989);

(b) A British study estimated that even more people would need drug treatment. Assuming 100% compliance and no harmful effects from this, over 4000 people would have to be treated to save one life every 5 years. Twice the number of coronary events might be saved by devoting the effort instead to reducing the mean population cholesterol by 0.5 mmol/l by public health measures.

3 *The compliance problem.* It has been pointed out that:

(a) only a proportion of those screened and found to be at increased risk will return for follow-up counselling;

(b) only some of these will receive and remember accurate dietary advice;

(c) only some of those remembering advice will take it;

(d) only some of those will comply enough to influence their serum cholesterol.

Even if compliance at each step is reasonable, the cumulative effect of drop-outs over the various stages will considerably detract from the potential benefit inherent in the initial screening (Table 3.10).

Table 3.10 Compliance at each stage of a high-risk strategy cholesterol screening campaign.

Study	% of those with high cholesterol returning to their doctor	% of those returning who report receiving dietary advice
Kinlay and Heller (1990), Australia*	82	82
Heart health programme (1988), Minnesota	58 (>6.9 mmol/l)	73
Wynder *et al.* (1986), New York	33 (>5.7 mml/l)	36

*In Kinlay and Heller's study, three-quarters of those who reported receiving dietary advice acted on it. However, this represented only 0.82 × 0.82 × 0.75 — 50% of those found in screening to be at greater risk.

4 *The negative effect of a normal cholesterol level.* Communication of a normal result could engender unwarranted complacency in the recipient. Indeed, there is some evidence on re-testing that serum cholesterols are higher the second time around!

Furthermore, the Multiple Risk Factor Intervention Cohort Study (of 300 000 men over a 6-year follow-up) found that 30% of deaths occurred in those with cholesterols <5.2 mmol/l, and 60% in those with cholesterols <6.5 mmol/l. These are people who might well assume, on the basis of their blood test, that their diet was satisfactory. It is important not to obscure the community message — that we should all consume less fat.

Selective versus general screening

Many authorities argue that selective testing is more cost-effective than whole-population screening. The pragmatists identify the foregoing problems, which are considerable; the theorists invoke the findings of the Multiple Risk Factors Intervention Trial, in which subjects were grouped according to age, sex and smoking habits, and banded into fifths according to blood pressure and serum cholesterol. It was possible to calculate, by subtraction between groups, the maximum theoretical benefit on mortality when moving from the top fifth to the bottom fifth of the population's cholesterol league-table, for any given combination of other risk factors. This so-called cholesterol-attributive risk was found to vary enormously depending on the size of other risk factors: in men aged 35–45 who had a normal blood pressure and did not smoke, the extra risk from a high cholesterol was minute, whereas in the presence of other risk factors the risk was multiplied manyfold.

All authorities agree that assessment of coronary heart disease risk must be multifactorial: some have argued on the basis of these findings that cholesterol screening can be reserved selectively for those in whom other significant risk factors have been identified.

3.11 SCREENING FOR BOWEL CANCER

Doctors will doubtless be considering what ingredients to include in their well-person screening programmes. Some enthusiasts advocate screening for bowel cancer using faecal occult blood-testing kits.

The *advantages* are obvious. The technique is:
- non-invasive;
- cheap;
- simple to administer.
  Disadvantages include:
- inconvenience;

- relative insensitivity (occult blood is not uniformly distributed in faeces, and some lesions bleed intermittently);
- relative non-specificity (lesions other than cancer can generate positive tests);
- poor compliance (around 50–70% with wide variation);
- technical interference (from red meat and vegetables rich in peroxidase).

How good is the test in practice?

1 If asymptomatic individuals are screened, about 2% come out positive.

2 If the test is positive there is a one in 10 chance of cancer and a one in three chance of an adenoma; over half of the detected tumours are Duke A at presentation (five times more than in the unscreened group).

3 If the test is negative there is still a one in 200 chance of a cancer and a one in 50 chance of an adenoma in the next 4 years.

4 Overall, 3–20 malignancies are detected per 10 000 screened, but faecal occult bloods are only positive in 50–60% of cases.

Almost all of the reported screening studies have been uncontrolled, and the benefit of detection again remains unproven because of the possibility of lead-time bias artificially inflating survival intervals (Fig. 3.1).

The bulk of the *cost* in faecal occult blood testing lies in investigating the false positives.

Do realistic alternatives exist?

Alternative screening strategies (endoscopy, radiology) are expensive and invasive. Flexible sigmoidoscopy would miss one-third of significant lesions; even total colonoscopy is not 100% effective and carries a distinct morbidity (1/1000 perforate); and resources are not adequate to cope with mass screening.

Some authors advocate endoscopic screening of high-risk groups (e.g. those with a personal or family history of bowel cancer or polyp), but even here the recall interval remains undefined. Further progress in the field probably depends on the new developing generation of circulating tumour markers and gene probes.

3.12 PREVENTING OSTEOPOROSIS

The size of the problem

Around 45 000 people in England and Wales suffer a fractured neck of femur annually. Two-thirds are elderly women.

Treatment costs run into hundreds of millions of pounds a year. The major contributory factor is osteoporosis — one-tenth of women in their 60s and one-half in their 70s suffer an osteoporosis-related fracture.

Preventive strategies

At present there is no satisfactory treatment for the condition and thoughts turn naturally to prevention. Five initiatives may confer benefit:

1 *Regular exercise* — highly effective in preventing bone loss. (Ideally exercise should start well before and continue through middle age.)

2 *An adequate diet* — there is debate concerning the role of dietary calcium, but it would be prudent to ensure an intake of 1400 mg per day (many adolescent girls risk a suboptimal intake).

3 *Enough sunlight* — 15 min per day may be enough to allow skin synthesis of vitamin D.

4 *Hormone therapy* — oestrogen is effective in reducing bone loss (hormone replacement therapy can halve the risk of a fracture if given perimenopausally). Treatment should probably be long-term (more than 10 years) with a mixed oestrogen/progestogen regimen for those who have not had a hysterectomy. (This mitigates against the risk of endometrial cancer. The risk of breast cancer remains unclear. That of coronary heart disease is reduced by oestrogen, and probably broadly neutral in combined preparations.)

5 *Giving up smoking* — smoking lowers circulating oestrogen levels.

Osteoporosis is a common and important condition, deserving closer attention that it presently receives from GPs.

4 Clinical Dilemmas

Few topics in general practice (as in medicine as a whole) are straightforward. Usually there is room for debate — definite clinical uncertainty. Sometimes areas of clinical debate are the same as in medicine as a whole (does strict control of diabetes prevent complications? when to treat hypertension?) and sometimes there is an important or unique general practice bias — the management of the sore throat, earache or backache; home care for coronaries or maternity cases.

Of course the debate in general practice does not stop with purely clinical issues; it encompasses the fields of administration, legal and ethical dilemmas, finance and priority allocation. The remit is wide: how to run a business; how to maximize resources; how to handle sensitive issues; how to manage tonsillitis; how best to do X, Y or Z.

A large part of this book is devoted to the non-clinical issues: appointment system; deputizing services; computers; personal lists. This chapter reviews some of the clinical dilemmas and is meant to illustrate how debatable most of our actions are.

Note that in many cases totally opposite points of view are defensible or at least merit consideration. This is important in an examination like the MRCGP where you are expected to be sensitive to the debate, to be aware of the breadth of opinion, to avoid dogmatism and admit contrary possibilities.

For the examination you are expected to marshal facts into an argument, so some facts are marshalled into arguments in this chapter but remember that as the debate unfolds these 'facts' may change, so keep up to date! Try to supplement this chapter with a list of your own topics because the arena of debate in general practice is now very wide. This is important exam preparation which should pay off in the viva.

4.1 WHEN TO TREAT HYPERTENSION?

The treatment of hypertension is an area that can be broken down into a series of dilemmas.

The dilemma of definition
1 Systolic and diastolic blood pressures (BPs) are continuous variables with a 'normal' distribution in the population and no clear cut-off point between disease and health.
2 Actuarial tables (produced for insurance purposes) show a direct relationship between height of BP and longevity for all

values, so everything is relative: all other things being equal a person with a BP of 135/90 mmHg will not live as long as another with a BP of 120/80 mmHg. Clearly the cut-off point for treatment is *arbitrary* and depends on your views about costs and benefits.

The dilemma of measurement
1 Everyone's BP *fluctuates* (e.g. with posture, level of arousal). This can lead to a significant over-diagnosis of hypertension in borderline cases. The recent development of non-invasive techniques for constant measurement of BP has allowed ambulatory BPs to be compared with the traditional cuff method in the surgery: they are often lower.
(a) Pickering *et al.* (1988) described so-called 'white-coat hypertension' in 22% of 292 patients with borderline high BPs;
(b) In a retrospective study of 638 patients with hypertension in a cardiology unit, 89% satisfied the World Health Organization hypertension criteria on resting measurements, but about half that number were judged hypertensive on ambulatory monitoring (Kenny *et al.* 1987).
2 Other sources of variation include:
(a) measuring technique (size of cuff; observer bias; inaccurate machines);
(b) different end-points (phase V in most trials but phase IV in most surgeries).
Which measurements are representative of true health risk? We should remember that traditional guidelines (e.g. three readings on separate occasions) are *arbitrary*. A solitary raised reading from the actuarial point of view means a shorter life on average.

The dilemma of natural history
In Fry's (1979) untreated group of 1000 hypertensives over a 15-year period:
• diastolic BP decreased spontaneously in 30%;
• diastolic BP remained unchanged in 20%;
• diastolic BP increased in 50%.
It appears there is almost a one in three chance that diastolic BP will fall spontaneously in follow-up.
There is also a dilemma of *heterogeneity*: hypertensives are not a uniform group; they vary in their associated cardiovascular risk factors and hence in the likely natural history. Treating these different groups at the same BP level is an oversimplification.

Dilemmas in the elderly
1 In Fry's study of untreated hypertensives the standardized mortality ratio falls with age and after 60 years is not more than expected.
2 In another study death-rate clearly increased with systolic BP below age 70 years but there was no correlation above this.

The natural history of untreated hypertension in the elderly is a matter of lively debate and cost–benefit assessments are difficult to make.

Logistic dilemmas

As Fry has observed, there are 5–7 million hypertensives in Britain (85% of these classified as mild). This is prevalence of 10–15%. If they are all seen 2–4 times per year and given a script worth about £10 each time, the drug bill alone could cost £150 million, and added to this is the use of the resources and time of doctors and nurses on a large scale. This is a sizeable and costly undertaking. As described in Section 3.5 general practice has so far failed to organize itself to meet this challenge; perhaps only one-eighth of all hypertensives are currently well controlled.

The cost–benefit dilemma

Benefits

The benefit of treating severe hypertension is generally un-disputed and so is the effect on longevity of untreated mild/moderate hypertension; the problem arises in demonstrating a benefit from treatment in the milder groups. Several expensive large-scale trials have examined this (Table 4.1) but unfortunately this brings us on to *the dilemma of the muddling trial results*. Contra-dictory methods and findings have left the clinician in a confused position.

Even where there is agreement that treatment is needed the target BP is in doubt. The traditional counsel has been to lower raised BPs to as near normal as possible, but some authorities have recently argued that the relationship between mortality from coronary heart disease and BP achieved after treatment is J-shaped — in other words, lowering BP too far may actually *cause* extra deaths!

Costs

The costs are more readily counted:

1 The *labour* cost (considerable administrative problems; doctors' time, allocated in the face of competing priorities).

2 The *financial* cost (in drug bills and the salaries of medical and paramedical staff).

3 The *iatrogenic* cost (claudication, complete heart block, heart failure, impotence, fatigue, drug interactions, etc.).

4 The *psychological* cost (the illness label which some previously asymptomatic individuals wear around their necks!).

Studies suggest that many vague and non-specific side-effects (headaches, tiredness, light-headed feelings, lack of well-being) are no more common in treated than untreated groups, but some real costs, like impotence in thiazide-treated hypertensives, may

Table 4.1 Some important hypertension trials.

Trial	Groups examined and methods	Results	Possible criticisms
Veterans Administration Cooperative Study, USA (1970) (*Journal of the American Medical Association* 1970; **213**,1143)	380 male 'veterans', average age 50 years, with diastolic BPs averaging 90–115 mmHg. Double-blind randomization between placebo and active treatment	Risk of developing a morbid event over 5 years was 18% in the treated group and 55% in the controls, most impact being in the higher BP patients and for cardiac failure and strokes, rather than coronary artery disease	Veterans were highly selected for their adherence to a drug regimen and the persistence of their hypertension
Hypertension Detection and Follow-up Program, USA (1979) (*Journal of the American Medical Association* 1979; **242**, 2562)	Patients with diastolic BPs in the 90–105 mmHg range. Hospital stepped care was compared with referral back to GP. (Stepped care included systematic follow-up, education and financial assistance)	Deaths from cardiovascular disease were reduced. BP control was better in the stepped-care group	1 There were no controls 2 The stepped-care group also showed a fall in non-cardiovascular deaths (cumulative 5-year mortality 5.9/100 compared with 7.4/100) suggesting better overall care in this group
Australian National Board Hypertension Study, Australia (1980) (*Lancet* 1980; **i**, 1261)	3427 men and women aged 30–69 years with a diastolic BP in the range 95–110 mmHg, randomized in a single-blind fashion between placebo and active drugs. There were 14 000 patient-years of observation	1 A two-thirds reduction in cardiovascular deaths 2 A fall in overall mortality 3 Most effect was seen when diastolic BP was greater than 100 mmHg	1 The trial stopped prematurely because of the results, at a time when they were just marginally significant 2 About one-third of patients prematurely stopped the regimen to which they had been randomized
Multiple Risk Factor Intervention Trial (1982) (*Journal of the American Medical Association* 1982; **248**, 1465–77)	8000 men aged 35–57 with diastolic BPs of 90–114 mmHg randomized between an intensive heart disease prevention programme (addressing diet, smoking habits, hyperlipidaemia and hypertension) and 'usual care'	No reduction in CVAs observed in the treated hypertensive subgroup	The incidence of CVAs in the control group was unusually low, suggesting a high standard of 'usual care' in the control group

Table 4.1 *Contd*

Trial	Groups examined and methods	Results			Possible criticisms
			Deaths per thousand		
			Treated	Untreated	
MRC mild hypertension trial, UK (1985) (*British Medical Journal* 1985; **291**, 97)	A 15-year trial costing £4½ million. 85 570 patient-years of observation by 176 GP groups: 500 000 people screened; 50 000 were eligible but only 17 000 joined the trial. 35- to 64-year-old age group with diastolic BPs of 90–109 mmHg. Single-blind randomization between bendrofluazide, propranolol and placebo	CVAs 1.4	2.6		1 30–40% withdrew from the treated group because of side-effects (but were included in the treatment group when the results were analysed)
		MIs 5.2	5.4		2 Bendrofluazide was used in doses we now fear may exacerbate other cardiovascular risk factors (raising glucose, uric acid and lipids without additional hypotensive benefit)
		Overall 5.8	5.9		
		i.e.: 1 A reduction in CVA rate 2 *No reduction in MIs or overall mortality* 3 One CVA saved per 850 patient-years of treatment			
European Working Party on Hypertension in the Elderly (1985) (*Lancet* 1985; **i**, 1349)	Patients over 60 years. Double-blind randomization between placebo, hydrochlorothiazide and triamterene (with or without methyldopa). Conducted in 18 European collaboration centres over 12 years	1 Deaths reduced from MIs 2 Deaths from CVA *not* reduced 3 Overall mortality *not* reduced			1 Only 840 patients were recruited (on average 4 per centre per year) 2 The trial was so long that only one-third of patients were still in the double-blind part at the end

CVA, cerebrovascular accident; MI, myocardial infarction.

go unrecognized for some time, and the unexpected complications of practolol therapy have made people rightly critical in appraising the need for long-term drug treatment.

Conclusions

In 1989, with no major prospective trials still on the horizon, and recognizing the need for some sort of consensus conclusion, the British Hypertension Society Working Party produced a series of recommendations, summarized in Table 4.2. However, these answers to the cost–benefit dilemma are not definitive, so the clinician faced with real patients will have some hard decisions to make. The element of uncertainty in these decisions should be recognized, as well as possible implications.

Table 4.2 The British Hypertension Society Working Party's recommendations (1989) for treating mild hypertension.

• Treat patients under 80 with diastolic BPs over 100 mmHg for 3–4 months
• Observe patients with pressures of 95–99 mmHg every 3–6 months
• Use either diuretics or beta-blockers as first-line treatment
• Use other agents if these are contraindicated, ineffective, or poorly tolerated
• Warn all patients against smoking and heavy alcohol intake
• Advise weight reduction in obese patients
• Reports of a J-shaped mortality curve do not provide a sufficent basis for advice but, if confirmed, a diastolic BP of 85–90 mmHg would be the aim of therapy
• No firm advice at present on the treatment of isolated systolic hypertension

---

4.2 IS STRICT CONTROL OF DIABETES WORTHWHILE?

Some element of control is indisputably important in diabetes; for example, hypoglycaemic coma is potentially fatal; prior to the development of insulin, diabetes was a rapidly fatal disorder and pregnancy was very dangerous. But good control is bought at a cost, be it the risk of more hypoglycaemic episodes or the disruption of a person's lifestyle. Does strict control prevent complications? Does strict control benefit those who already have complications? And does the benefit outweigh possible risks and costs?

The relationship between diabetic control and vascular complications

Most studies on the relationship between diabetic control and vascular complications founder because of:
1 Problems in accurately assessing control;

2 Other confounding risk factors (e.g. smoking and hypertension) not considered.

Knowles (1970) reviewed 300 studies:
- only 85 had no major design errors;
- 50 of these found a positive correlation between poor control and vascular complications;
- a further 25 found no correlation;
- the remaining 10 were undecided.

Three studies in favour of a correlation are listed in Table 4.3. The dilemma could best be resolved by a prospective study in which newly diagnosed patients were randomly allocated into well and poorly controlled groups, but this approach would take many years to provide an answer and is, of course, unethical.

Table 4.3 Studies supporting an association between diabetic control and vascular complications.

Study	Conclusion
The Bedford study	Retinopathy only develops in patients whose blood glucose exceeds 11.1 mmol/l at 2 h in a glucose tolerance test (GTT)
Epidemiological studies of the Pima Indians of Arizona (50% of whom are diabetic)	Retinopathy and nephropathy were confined to those with fasting sugars over 8 mmol/l or 2-h GTT sugars over 13 mmol/l
Chemical pancreatectomy studies in dogs and rats	High blood sugar levels damage eyes and kidneys in this experimental model of human diabetes. Sugar itself appears to be the toxic agent when present in excess

The relationship between existing complications and strict control

The relationship between existing complications and strict control is also unclear:

1 *Retinopathy* — Initial studies involving sudden normalization of blood sugar levels in patients with existing retinopathy actually provoked deterioration, even progression to a proliferative form. More recent studies suggest this is a transient effect. The situation is now being studied using continuous subcutaneous insulin infusions (CSII) to perfect control:

(a) in the Oslo study (1986) patients did better on CSII — there was no regression of vascular damage, but the rate of deterioration was slowed;

(b) in the Stena study (1983) the most marked deterioration in retinal function was seen in those with the worst and *best* degree of control. This suggests there is an optimal range of glycaemia, and that being too strict may be as harmful as being too lax!

2 *Nephropathy* — A small number of studies have demonstrated a regression in the basement membrane changes of kidneys showing diabetic nephropathy when transplanted into non-diabetic patients.

The hazards of stricter control
The most obvious risk of stricter control is hypoglycaemia (in fact many patients sabotage their control to avoid it). Hypoglycaemia seems to be very common: for example, in a 1-year Nottingham study at least 9% of the insulin-dependent clinic population received hospital treatment for hypoglycaemia. Despite the high frequency, death and measurable brain damage seem rare. Also it is by no means clear that hypoglycaemia is more common in those who strive for stricter control: many authorities believe it is more common in the 'casual' diabetic.

For whom is strict control not suitable?
This is contentious. The decision may be swayed by such factors as:
- the presence of complications;
- the age of the patient;
- the competence of the patient;
- the degree of psychological and social interference stricter control causes.

4.3 SHOULD OBESITY BE TREATED IN GENERAL PRACTICE?

At least 30% of adults are more than 10% above their lean fit weight and 10% of children are said to be overweight, so an average general practice list contains more than 300 patients with a weight problem.

The problems of obesity
The risk to *mortality* from obesity only applies when patients are very obese (e.g. if men are >25% over ideal body weight, or women >30%, the number of deaths from heart disease increases 40%, and the incidence of diabetes fourfold). However, there is a significant *morbidity* to obesity that affects the quality of patients' lives: for example, osteoarthritis — hips, knees, backache; flat-feet; reduced exercise capacity; varicose veins and varicose ulcers; haemorrhoids; gallstones; oesophageal reflux; ventral hernias; increased complications in abdominal surgery and childbirth; reduced fertility; diabetes, gout and coronary heart disease; hypertension; and an increased risk of carcinoma of the colon, breast and uterine body.

There are of course *psychological* problems as well in a society where the obese are often ridiculed or treated as unattractive.

The debate

It is obviously difficult not to be sympathetic when approached for help by patients trying to do something positive to promote their own health. However, many authors have argued that:

1 Obesity is not a *disease* but a social/behavioural problem with medical complications, and hence the solution is not necessarily a medical one; perhaps the onus should not be put on doctors to treat.

2 The risk to mortality is much *less* than previously thought.

3 The condition is so common that an undertaking to treat *all* obesity would be a great drain on medical resources.

4 Many other problems are seen on a large scale, the treatment of which may be more deserving of medical time (e.g. smoking and hypertension, a reduction of which would have a greater impact on morbidity).

5 Long-term results in medical hands are fairly poor (about 1–12% in studies). There is no evidence that doctors achieve better results than self-help groups like Weight-Watchers, and this approach would seem to spare overstretched NHS resources.

There is less debate that obesity should be tackled in the following *medical* conditions:

(a) Maturity-onset diabetes;

(b) Hyperlipidaemia;

(c) Hypertension (a 5 kg weight loss reduces BP by 8–16/4–8 mmHg);

(d) Medical conditions aggravated by obesity, e.g. angina.

(A review of obesity appears in Section 6.3.)

4.4 ANTIBIOTICS FOR SORE THROATS?

On average the practitioner sees about 600 upper respiratory tract infections including 100–150 sore throats each year. Despite the frequency of this condition there is no universally accepted management policy.

Although the presence of palatal petechiae and vesicles is suggestive of viral inflection, and tonsillar exudate in patients under 15 years of age is more likely to be streptococcal, while in those over 15 it is more likely to be glandular fever, it is generally felt that the aetiology cannot be predicted from appearance with any degree of certainty.

When a throat swab is taken from an acute throat the following results are obtained:

- 40% yield no growth;
- 30% grow a beta-haemolytic streptococcus;
- 20% grow a virus;
- other less common growths are *Haemophilus*, *Candida*, pneumococcus, and the organism of Vincent's angina.

symptoms and beta-haemolytic streptococcus can be grown from
asymptomatic throats without any rise in ASOT titre (Haverkorn *Chapter 4*
et al. 1971). *Clinical*
Dilemmas

Hence, the correlation of symptoms, throat appearance and
even throat swab growth with infection is, at best, imperfect.
Prescribing habits, not surprisingly, vary between the extreme
views of 'antibiotics for all' and 'no antibiotics at all' with many
GPs occupying the middle ground and prescribing for various
indications of their own choosing (e.g. fever, malaise) which again
correlate poorly.

Benefits?
1 *Complications*. Although the incidence of rheumatic fever and
post-streptococcal glomerulonephritis has fallen dramatically, the
evidence suggests this has more to do with improved living standards than the widespread prescription of penicillin (the fall
started early in the 20th century, pre-dating the introduction of
antibiotics).
2 *Duration of illness*. Several studies suggest that this is *not* much
affected, e.g. Whitfield and Hughes (1981) found that illness was
not shortened at all, irrespective of whether there was fever,
purulent tonsils or lymphadenitis; Brumfitt and Slater (1957) felt
that duration was shortened by about 24 h.
3 Doctors, however, perceive a pressure to prescribe, which
provides several *social* benefits (see also Section 2.2):
  • it demonstrates concern;
  • it lets the patient down gently, justifying the efforts made
  to attend;
  • it represents an attempt to do something, which patients
  appreciate and expect;
  • it is a quick way to conclude a consultation;
  • the precedent of other doctors' prescriptions often makes it
  hard *not* to prescribe.
In fact doctors perceive more pressure than really exists.
According to Cartwright and Anderson (1981), 41% of patients
entering consultations expect a prescription but 67% leave with
one!

Problems?
1 There is a very small risk of anaphylaxis but a much greater
risk of nuisance side-effects (e.g. gastrointestinal upset, vaginal
candidiasis).
2 Although penicillin is a cheap drug, the cost to the NHS when
prescribed on a huge scale is considerable.
3 Widespread antibiotic prescribing encourages drug resistance.
4 Prescribing fosters a patient's dependence and reinforces the
sick role, teaching him that he needs medical attention with his

next illness episode. Apparently patients only take a sore throat to their doctor on one in 18 occasions (Banks *et al.* 1975), which is fortunate as the system might well be overwhelmed otherwise! It is possible that ready prescribing saves time in the short term but generates more work in the long term.

4.5 MIDDLE EAR PROBLEMS IN CHILDHOOD

Acute otitis media is predominantly a disease of the first 10 years of life, especially the preschool years, and is very common. Thus:
1   The attack rate has been estimated to be between 10 and 15% in the under 10-year-olds.
2   One in four children is affected at some time.
3   On average a GP expects to see about 100 cases per year.
4   This amounts to about 1.5 million episodes annually in England and Wales.

Approximately 40% of children will suffer at least one recurrence in the following year and those with unresolved middle ear effusions from the original attack are particularly prone.

If the middle ear fluid is aspirated and cultured:
1   66% of cases grow bacterial pathogens, usually *Haemophilus influenzae* and *Streptococcus pneumoniae*.
2   25% of aspirates are sterile.
3   Mycoplasma and anaerobes are sometimes grown, and Gram-negative organisms in 10–20% of neonatal cases.
4   Viruses are isolated in 4% of cases (although viral titres are raised in 25%, suggesting that viral infection may precede bacterial infection).

Other predisposing factors include:
1   Persistent eustachian tube dysfunction. This may be:
    (a) functional;
    (b) due to large adenoids;
    (c) due to allergy (there is an increased family history of allergy in recurrent sufferers).
2   Unresolved middle ear effusions (a high percentage of asymptomatic effusions grow bacteria).

The debate
Major issues include:
1   The role of antibiotics in management.
2   The role of alternative treatments in the acute stage and in recurrent disease.
3   The management of the middle ear effusion.
    These will be considered briefly in turn.

Antibiotics or not?
Proponents of antibiotic treatment argue that:

1 It is rational since a bacterial aetiology is likely in most cases (more so than the sore throat).
2 Antibiotics are cheap and generally very safe.
3 There has been a decline in the incidence of serious complications, especially chronic suppurative otitis media and mastoiditis since their widespread use.
4 Clinical experience suggests patients obtain quick pain relief after prescription.
5 Some trials support a prescribing policy, e.g. Laxdal *et al.* (1970) found in a non-double-blind study that children under 3 years of age did better on ampicillin than placebo.

The case against antibiotics runs as follows:
1 Several trials do *not* show an objective advantage for the majority (Table 4.4) — spontaneous resolution occurs in up to 85% of cases without treatment.

Table 4.4 Studies suggesting that antibiotics are not needed routinely in acute otitis media.

Study	Finding
Fry (1958): more than 500 cases	85% resolved completely without antibiotics. At follow-up the degree of hearing loss and frequency of recurrence were no different from the antibiotic group
Halstead *et al.* (1968): 89 cases randomized between antibiotic and placebo	No advantage found in the antibiotic group
Van Buchem *et al.* (1981): 240 cases of acute otitis media randomized between antibiotics, placebo and myringotomy	No significant difference found. Most placebo cases resolved after 24–48 h with analgesia alone

2 There is a low frequency of serious complications. This may not be due to the widespread use of antibiotics but to a decline in the virulence of pathogens or improved herd immunity.
3 Antibiotics prescribed en masse cost the NHS a lot of money.
4 Widespread prescribing may discourage the development of natural immunity, or promote drug-resistant organisms.
5 Ready prescribing may promote dependence on doctors.
6 Up to 29% of treated cases report nuisance side-effects.
7 The rising incidence of glue ear is thought to be iatrogenic, with antibiotics as the culprit.

Alternative treatments?
1 In *acute attacks*:
    (a) myringotomy has not been shown to be beneficial in routine cases;

(b) antihistamine decongestants are prescribed in 50% of cases but there is not much evidence that they affect the outcome.

2 In *prophylaxis*:

(a) antibiotics appear to reduce the recurrence rate in susceptible children;

(b) grommets in some studies reduce recurrence rate to an even greater extent than prophylactic ampicillin;

(c) adenoidectomy and/or tonsillectomy: this is controversial. Maw (1983) found adenoidectomy had a beneficial effect, not enhanced by tonsillectomy, for up to 12 months in 40% of chronic cases with effusion, but other studies have reached different conclusions.

The management of middle ear effusions

Persistent middle ear effusions are a common sequel to acute otitis media. In studies:

- approximately 40% have fluid at 3 months;
- 20% have hearing losses of 20 dB or more 6 months after treatment;
- 17% have hearing losses 5–10 years after an attack.

Referral policy is unclear, but some authorities suggest:

- sustained hearing loss of 30 dB on two or more frequencies or 20 dB throughout the normal frequency range.

The management of the overlapping disorder *glue ear* is also debatable. Here approximately one-third of all children are affected by the 5th year of life for reasons which are unclear, but suggested to be:

- viral or bacterial otitis media modified by immunological factors;
- otitis media modified by antibiotics;
- a catarrhal disorder with eustachian tube dysfunction;
- large adenoids;
- allergy;
- cigarette smoke (case control studies suggest up to one-third of cases may be due to passive smoking).

The natural history is *benign*:

- most children grow out of their catarrhal phase by 7–8 years old;
- no permanent deafness results;
- there is natural self-resolution over a period of years.

Medical (drug) treatment includes antibiotics, antihistamines and decongestants. Efficacy is not proven.

Surgical treatment is by myringotomy and the insertion of a grommet which aerates the middle ear and corrects hearing loss. After eventual extrusion of the grommet 70% of children remain trouble-free, but the remainder have recurrence and a further grommet is often necessary; thus very young patients may be submitted to several procedures. Various concerns have been raised about this operation which has been performed with much greater frequency over the last decade:

1 It is used to treat a condition that is common and benign.
2 Although glue ear does not cause permanent deafness, an operative complication may do so.
3 Surgery can cause permanent effects such as scarring of the drums.

The serious complication rate is probably less than 2% however, and the social and educative cost of even temporary hearing loss to the young child is difficult to determine and perhaps considerable.

4.6 ARE NEBULIZERS SAFE IN PRACTICE?

A nebulizer is a device that delivers a drug in aqueous solution as a mist of very small particles. Ultrasonic energy or compressed gas is used to break up the liquid into the correct particle size. The latter may come from a cylinder, electrical compressor or foot-pump.

Uses
Uses commonly proposed include:
1 Acute severe asthma.
2 Chronic asthma — not controllable by any other method (except long-term steroids).
3 Bronchospasm in children and young infants.
4 Bronchospasm in other patients who cannot use inhalers (or other devices like spacers, nebuhalers and rotahalers).
5 Prophylactic drug administration (e.g. nebulized sodium cromoglycate).

Advantages
The advantages of nebulization are:
1 Better compliance.
2 A possibly beneficial effect from the aqueous vehicle itself.
3 The use of much larger drug doses, perhaps equivalent to 25 puffs of an inhaler. (In both inhaler and nebulizer only about 12% of the drug reaches the small airways, but a nebulizer is not just an inhaler with more puffs; with an inhaler the poorly targeted drug tends to deposit in the mouth and is swallowed; with the nebulizer it tends to disperse in the air allowing large doses to be used with a greater safety margin.)

Concerns
1 *A high-risk group.* Patients given home nebulizers are usually a highly selected group with worse-than-average asthma — the very

patients most at risk of sudden death. Should they treat their asthma alone at home?

2 *Does it breed overconfidence?* There are really two concerns here: first that patients may delay in seeking medical advice and second that doctors will be falsely reassured by initial improvement (bronchospasm is only one element of airflow obstruction; oedema and hyperviscous mucus persist after nebulization so relapse after apparent improvement is not uncommon).

3 *The risks of bronchodilators.* There is a theoretical risk that patients with ischaemic heart disease can suffer *arrhythmias* or *angina* on a nebulized beta-agonist. Increased *hypoxaemia* has also occasionally followed the use of bronchodilators. Because of the latter risk it has been recommended that oxygen (rather than air) should be the driving gas, but this poses practical difficulties for home nebulization in the emergency situation.

4 It is well recognized that patients become *psychologically dependent* on their nebulizers.

These reservations notwithstanding, nebulizers have considerably helped the management of asthma in the community and are very valuable in the administration of prophylactic drugs and in the control of severe chronic asthma where the alternative is oral steroids. They have not, however, reduced the death rate from asthma, which is perhaps food for thought.

4.7 THE MANAGEMENT OF BACKACHE

The scale of the problem
There are about 25 new cases per 1000 patients each year (i.e. 1 million new cases per year and 10–15 million working days lost per year). A GP with an average list sees about 50 acute backs per year (but many sufferers do not consult).

The natural history
- 80% recover in 3–4 weeks without treatment;
- in 80% of cases no specific diagnosis is made;
- however, nearly 50% of patients suffer recurrence within the following 4 years.

Should cases be referred?
Of the 1.1 million people who consult with backache annually:
- 0.3 million (about one-third) are referred for an opinion;
- 30 000 people are admitted and 5000 undergo surgery (less than one in 200 of the original sufferers, and one in 60 of the referrals).

Naturally many patients are referred for primarily social reasons: patient insistence on a second opinion; to reassure the patient that all possible avenues have been explored; to demonstrate continuing concern; or to reassure the doctor that no serious pathology has been missed. However, since relatively few cases are amenable to specialist help this represents a questionable use of orthopaedic resources.

The element of referral due to medical ignorance could be reduced by clear departmental guidelines by local specialists (for example, to see patients where there is a past history of malignancy or tuberculosis, systemic symptoms and weight loss, a high erythrocyte sedimentation rate, progressive neurological signs, unremitting and uncontrollable pain, and persistent rest pain). The element of referral due to social factors is more difficult to tackle, although counselling may help once it is acknowledged for what it is.

Should X-rays be used?
The yield from lumbosacral X-rays is low. Thus:
- in one district general hospital where there were 3000 such X-rays per year, 30–40% were reported normal and about 40% showed degenerative changes only;
- many large studies have found a very poor correlation between degenerative changes and symptoms;
- Nachemson (1976) estimated that a routine lumbosacral X-ray in the absence of suspicious features reveals unexpected disease on only one occasion in 2500.

Despite these drawbacks surveys indicate that a high percentage of backache sufferers eventually present to the X-ray department, e.g.:
- 20% of all American sufferers (according to the National Ambulatory Medical Care Survey 1980);
- in the UK there are half a million lumbar spine X-rays annually.

Why then are so many patients referred for X-rays at great cost in terms of personnel, money and convenience? In general many of the social reasons for referral are mirrored in the use of X-rays and other investigative procedures. Important factors include:
1   The insistence of poorly counselled or impatient patients.
2   Impatience or ignorance on the part of the doctor.
3   The fear that something important may be missed.
4   The psychological benefit that patients (and doctors) gain from a normal X-ray report.

What treatment should be given?
Rest
Rest probably should be prescribed, e.g.:
- 60% of patients have an attack lasting less than 2 weeks if they rest;
- studies suggest that patients who rest reduce their time off work by 50% (Dillane *et al.* 1966; Wiesel *et al.* 1980).

Manipulation

1 Some studies have found short-term benefits, not sustained at 3–7 days (e.g. Glover *et al.* 1974).

2 In one study Doran and Newell (1975) randomly allocated 450 patients between manipulation, physiotherapy, corset and rest/analgesia groups and found no difference in outcome.

3 A more recent study (Mead *et al.* 1990) has claimed significant benefit from chiropracter manipulation, but its methods and conclusions have been challenged.

4 Manipulation requires some expertise and is potentially harmful in the presence of neurological complications and certain pathological conditions (fractures, metastases, osteoporosis).

5 However some patients derive comfort from manipulation and believe in it.

Is education helpful?

In cases and ex-cases

1 In one study patients attended four lectures on back anatomy and function, and received instruction in lifting and exercising. Recovery was hastened but no difference was observed in the likelihood of recurrence.

2 Another study prescribed regular exercise programmes but found no difference in the duration of recurrences (Berquist-Ullman & Larsen 1977).

3 However, in a randomized controlled trial used to evaluate an educational booklet in general practice, significantly fewer of the counselled group consulted with back pain in the following year; fewer were referred and admitted; but there was no significant change in certified absence from work with back problems (Roland & Dixon 1989).

In non-cases (primary prevention)

1 A number of studies in industry have shown initial benefits from lifting training programmes, but the benefit generally diminishes with time.

2 Routine radiographs have not proved effective in screening out workers who are at increased risk of back injury prior to employment in heavy industries (e.g. coal mining).

The economic consequences of backache

Each year about 12 million working days are lost by 0.3 million people because of backache. This represents a total annual cost of more than £1000 million. Some 80 000 people are permanently crippled through chronic backache and many are in receipt of welfare benefits. Lumbar spine X-rays form 4 to 5% of the average X-ray department's workload and about 20% of all new orthopaedic referrals are for backache. At least one out of every two people in western society suffers from back trouble at some time, and on a world scale the annual toll runs into billions of pounds.

141
Chapter 4
Clinical
Dilemmas

4.8 MATERNITY CARE

Obstetric standards have improved over the last few decades, e.g.:
1   There has been a fall in the perinatal mortality (PNM) rate (from 38 per 1000 total births in 1949 to 15 per 1000 in 1980).
2   A 10-fold decrease has occurred in maternal mortality (from more than 90 per 100 000 in 1949 to 10 per 100 000 births recently).
   Several other trends have emerged over the same period:
1   The transfer of childbirth from home to hospital maternity units (66% of births were in hospital in 1960, but more than 95% in 1980).
2   A steady fall in maternity beds available to GPs as a percentage of the whole (now down to 18%).
3   A change in the disposition and deployment of maternity staff (more consultants and hospital midwives; fewer community midwives).
   It is clear that childbirth has become hospitalized and removed from community hands (the average community midwife now attends no more than three home deliveries per year, and a GP one every 6–7 years). Antenatal care by contrast is still shared to a large extent. Trends to hospitalize childbirth have not been entirely unopposed.
   Important debating points include:
●   the place of birth (home confinements or not?);
●   the cost-effectiveness of GP maternity units;
●   the antenatal routine (is it streamlined and efficient, or a waste of available resources?).

Home confinements or not?
There has been a tendency to explain the decline in PNM in terms of more and safer hospital confinements. A 1980 report found that PNM was respectively:
●   6 per 1000 in GP maternity units (low-risk cases);
●   18 per 1000 in consultant units (higher-risk cases);
●   23 per 1000 at home.
   It was recommended that home deliveries should be phased out even more. This can be contrasted with the experience in the Netherlands (the only country in Western Europe where home confinement is still common — 34% in 1981):
●   the percentage of instrumental deliveries is the lowest in Europe;
●   the morbidity and mortality figures are *lower* amongst the home group, and amongst the lowest in the world.
   Proponents of home confinement argue that:

1 Continental experience proves alternatives are safe and feasible.

2 A less interventionist policy (fewer inductions, less instrumentation and technology, fewer caesarean sections) should be promoted:

(a) childbirth is a unique emotional experience and should not be spoiled;

(b) the differing caesarean section rates of countries like the UK and USA argue that childbirth approaches are influenced more by expediency and opinion than necessity.

3 People have the right to a free choice.

Opponents of home confinement say:

1 7% of so-called low-risk pregnancies produce potentially life-threatening situations (neonatal asphyxia; postpartum haemorrhage).

2 GPs see insufficient intrapartum work to maintain their expertise with, for example, obstetric forceps. (This is really a false argument since it applies only for the time that home confinement is rare!)

'Active birth' movements appear to be on the increase so this debate may assume more importance in the future.

GP maternity units or not?

There are at least three aspects to this: costs, standards (PNM) and patient preference.

Costs

In 1981 the average GP unit delivery cost £395 and the average consultant unit delivery £485. Of course this does not compare like with like (as the higher-risk consultant patients are offered a high-technology service) but the question is, would a lower-technology service suffice and save money? At present the specialist hospital sector receives more than 80% of the total maternity budget. It has been estimated that savings of 40% could be made simply by postnatal transfer to cheaper GP units. In 1981 a Joint Working Committee of the Royal College of Obstetricians and Gynaecologists and the Royal College of General Practitioners recommended expanding the GP units attached to specialist hospital units.

PNM

This is lower (6 per 1000) amongst the selected low-risk cases in GP units than the higher-risk cases of consultant units (18 per 1000) suggesting that, given proper selection, standards are acceptable.

Patient preference

A 1985 Oxford study found that patients booked for delivery in a GP unit:

• saw their GPs more often in the antenatal period;

• saw fewer midwives;

- received less conflicting information;
- were admitted a little later in labour;
- more often had their GP present at their birth;
- were more likely to breast-feed immediately after birth.

However, a high level of satisfaction was expressed with the care received in both types of unit.

Is antenatal care a waste of resources?

Two particular areas have come under scrutiny recently: the role of midwives and the antenatal routine.

The role of midwives

Concern has been expressed over a needless duplication of resources in the antenatal routine. Nearly two-thirds of midwives work in clinics where GPs carry out an abdominal examination, even when this has already been done by a midwife. This is part of a more general complaint, namely that the skills of midwives are underused: they tend to assemble information, not to make decisions they are well qualified to make.

The antenatal routine: dogma or necessity?

According to a survey by Hall *et al.* (1980), the productivity of routine antenatal visits with respect to detecting new obstetric problems is very low, e.g.:
- the rate of first detection of growth retardation varies from 0.2 to 0.7%;
- the rate of detection of breech presentation after 32 weeks is 0.1–0.9%;
- the rate of detection of hypertension only exceeds 1% after 34 weeks.

Marsh (1985) examined his antenatal routine and found it was possible to reduce the number of antenatal attendances for low-risk primiparae from 15 to eight, and for low-risk parous women from 15 to six without problems. Indeed, benefits counted include:
- more time per patient and a pleasanter working atmosphere;
- more opportunity for patients to ask questions, and hence more satisfied customers.

Few of our routines (or those of hospitals) have been subjected to critical review. It is quite likely that antenatal care is not the only area subject to arbitrary and wasteful policies.

4.9 THE MANAGEMENT OF CORONARY CASES IN GENERAL PRACTICE

Background

In the UK there are 108 000 deaths per year from myocardial infarction. On the average GP's list this means about 9 cases per year, of whom:

- 2–3 will die within the first 30 min;
- 2–3 will have myocardial infarctions in public places (where-upon ambulances are usually called);
- a management decision has to be made on only 3–5 cases per year.

Most deaths occur within the first hour (some 60% of all deaths) but 60–75% of cases are visited after this high-risk time (the mean delay before medical assessment is 3 h, largely because of patients' diffidence). In other words, GPs generally see a sub-group of likely survivors. In view of this, and the small number of cases involved, the question of home care has been examined.

Advantages
Possible advantages of home care include:
1 Avoidance of transport risks (there is some evidence that tachycardia, arrhythmias and hypotension are more common in transit).
2 Continuity of care.
3 Comfort and familiarity of the home environment.
4 Psychological benefits to the spouse, who is a carer and not a helpless onlooker.
5 Improved compliance in rehabilitation.
6 Financial savings for the NHS (home care is much cheaper than high-technology coronary care units).
7 It is good for the professional morale of GPs and district nurses.
8 It is possibly less stressful for the patient (one study suggested a disproportionate number of deaths after ward rounds!).

Disadvantages
Possible disadvantages of home care include:
1 80% of patients have arrhythmias — some suffer ventricular fibrillation and are potentially retrievable with immediate care — preventable deaths. The cause of home deaths is often unknown, so it is difficult to know how many deaths could have been prevented.
2 Home care is inappropriate for patients with complications: left ventricular failure, shock, persistent chest pain, bradycardia, etc.
3 Not all patients or their spouses can cope with the uncertainty of home care — some like the comfort of high technology around them: the patient's expectations are important.
4 Although the number of cases per year is small, the number of visits per patient is high.
5 Home care may deny patients the opportunity to receive modern thrombolytic therapy (see below).

Trials on home care: the pre-thrombolytic era
There have been three major UK trials (Table 4.5), all conducted

Table 4.5 Major UK trials on home care after myocardial infarction.

Trial	Results	
	Deaths at home	Deaths in hospital
Bristol study (Mather *et al.* 1976): 455 patients under 70 years seen within 48 h and randomized	12% at 1 month 20% at 1 year	14% at 1 month 27% at 1 year
Teeside study (Colling *et al.* 1976): 2000 patients allocated one-third to home; one-third to a CCU bed; one-third to a general medical bed	8.8% at 1 month	12.9% at 1 month (CCU bed) 18.7% at 1 month (general bed)
Nottingham study (Hill *et al.* 1978): 349 patients assessed by a cardiac team at home. After 2 h stabilization, randomized	13% at 6 weeks	11% at 6 weeks

CCU, coronary care unit.

before the advent of thrombolytic agents. The Bristol study (Mather *et al.* 1976) was criticized by the Royal College of Physicians because only an ill defined minority of cases were randomized. The Nottingham study (Hill *et al.* 1978) also involved stabilization by a cardiac team and the exclusion of 24% of patients from randomization due to complications or social conditions.

However, these studies suggested home care was a credible alternative to hospital referral, and in 1974 the Royal College of General Practitioners published criteria for deciding on home versus hospital care. The situation now needs to be re-thought in the light of new evidence.

Thrombolytic therapy for myocardial infarction
The advantage of these agents has now been confirmed in several large-scale trials (Table 4.6). Streptokinase, the most commonly used agent, can reduce deaths by about 25% in the first 24 h. The best results come from the earliest treatment. Aspirin has a synergistic benefit (a further 20–25%) and must be given routinely in the absence of contraindications.

The major risk of thrombolysis is haemorrhage. Other problems include:
- allergy (streptokinase);
- hypotension;
- prolonged intravenous infusion route (streptokinase);
- cost (the newer agents).

Table 4.6 Important trials of thrombolytic therapy in myocardial infarction (MI).

Trial	Regimen	Patients and controls	Principal results	Comments
ISIS-2 (Second International Study of Infarct Survival) (*Lancet* 1988; **ii**, 349–60)	Streptokinase alone vs aspirin alone vs both vs neither (1.5 million units of streptokinase given i.v. over 1 h; 160 mg aspirin per day)	17 000 patients within 24 h of a suspected MI Placebo controls	At 5 weeks: • Streptokinase reduced mortality by 25% • Aspirin reduced mortality by 23% • Both together reduced mortality by 42% Early improvements were maintained at 15 months	• Streptokinase and aspirin had independent additive effects • The earlier the treatment, the better the outcome (50% reduction in mortality if given within 4 h) • Equally effective in the over-70s
ASSET (Anglo-Scandinavian Study of Early Thrombolysis) (*Lancet* 1988; **ii**, 525–30)	Alteplase (100 mg over 3 h) vs placebo (All received a heparin bolus and infusion)	5011 patients within 5 h of a suspected MI	At 4 weeks: • Treatment reduced mortality by 26% Benefits were maintained at 6 months	• The benefit was confined to those with ECG evidence of infarction
ISAM (Intravenous Streptokinase in Acute Myocardial Infarction) (*New England Journal of Medicine* 1986; **314**, 1465–71)	Streptokinase (1.5 million units i.v. over 1 h) plus heparin infusion vs placebo	17 000 patients within 6 h of a suspected MI Double-blind randomization	At 3 weeks: • Mortality in the streptokinase group was lower, but the difference was not significant	• The ISAM study also assessed infarct size and myocardial function and found a slight improvement in the treated group
GISSI (Gruppo Italiano per lo Studio della Streptochinasi nell'Infarto Miocardico) (*Lancet* 1987; **ii**, 871–4)	Streptokinase vs placebo	11 700 patients within 12 h of a suspected MI Controls were randomized to a 'usual care' group	At 3 weeks: • Mortality in the thrombolytic group was reduced 18% At 12 months the benefit was maintained	• The earlier treatment was given, the greater the benefit

ECG confirmation was sought, except in the ASSET trial where it was non-mandatory. Patients with bleeding tendencies were excluded in all trials.

Table 4.7 Complication rate from thrombolytic therapy (ISIS-2 Trial 1988).

Complications (%)	Streptokinase (1.5 million units i.v. over 1 h)	Placebo controls
Haemorrhage	0.5	0.2
Haemorrhagic strokes*	0.1	0
Embolic strokes*	0.6	0.8
Allergic reactions	4.4	0.9
Transient hypotension	10.0	2.0

* Most of the trials show a small increase in haemorrhagic cerebrovascular accidents (CVAs) with thrombolysis, offset by a fall in embolic CVAs. The overall CVA rates in treated and untreated groups are comparable.

These risks were quantitated in the ISIS-2 study (Table 4.7).

All experts would exclude from treatment those with a predisposition to bleed, e.g.:
* bleeding diathesis;
* haemorrhagic cerebrovascular accident;
* recent haemorrhage;
* recent surgery, subclavian puncture, or other invasive procedure;
* peptic ulcer;
* suspected aortic dissection;
* uncontrolled hypertension.

Many believe, because of the risks to treatment, that all patients should have an ECG first to confirm diagnosis. These studies have important implications for GPs seeing patients prior to hospitalization.

Should GPs give immediate thrombolytic treatment?
Several practical problems arise for the GP:

1 He would need to carry and be able to use an ECG machine, and to read the tracing, and to maintain these skills although only seeing three to five cases a year.

2 He would need to carry a relatively expensive stock of medicine for occasional but vital use.

3 He would obviously prefer to administer a single bolus injection rather than a prolonged infusion. At present this is a more expensive option and the drug of choice is undecided.

4 He would need to ensure skilled after-care and supervision.

5 The benefits of thrombolytic therapy have been tested on hospital inpatients. It is not known whether patients seen at home differ in important (as yet undefined) ways from those on coronary care units.

The British Heart Foundation Working Group (1989) recommends with the present state of knowledge that thrombolytic therapy should be deferred until the patient reaches hospital.

How does this influence the criteria for home management of coronary cases?

The implication is that all patients likely to benefit from treatment (excluding those for whom thrombolysis is contraindicated) should be admitted as soon as possible.

There is evidence that GPs' attitudes to home care have changed in response to this new therapeutic option. Thus, in 1975 21–39% of GPs were prepared to consider home care in an uncomplicated coronary in a 45-year-old man (Hampton *et al.* 1975); in 1990 only 3% would do so (Pell *et al.* 1990).

Attitudes change with the age of the patient. Two-thirds would still manage patients over 80 at home, although there is evidence that age is not a contraindication to therapy, and in fact the greatest benefit is seen in the elderly.

The role of thrombolytic therapy in general practice needs to be clarified and the criteria for home management redefined. A large study is presently being conducted by the Royal College to examine this very issue.

Trials on home treatment cannot of course assure the GP that in the individual case the correct decision is made. GPs who cannot accept the death of a home-managed myocardial infarction case without self-recrimination should not be attempting it, irrespective of these considerations.

4.10 WHO SHOULD TAKE ASPIRIN?

The background

The bleeding tendency induced by aspirin has been recognized for years, and the suggestion that prevention of clotting in the right place (e.g. skin cuts) might be put to advantage in preventing clots in the wrong place (e.g. coronary arteries) was first made in the 1950s by Laurence L. Craven, an American family doctor.

Pharmacologically, aspirin inhibits cyclo-oxygenase, a key enzyme in the conversion of arachidonic acid to prostacyclin and thromboxane. Two opposing effects are induced:
1 In the platelets — reduced thromboxane synthesis, reducing their tendency to aggregate.
2 In the vascular endothelium –– reduced prostaglandin synthesis, encouraging vasoconstriction.

In practice the endothelial effect is thought to be transient and that on the platelets more prolonged. The net result is an antithrombotic predominance.

In the 1960s, following a better understanding of these processes randomized therapeutic trials began and the last decade has proved a most exciting one in the history of this ancient medicine.

The evidence of benefit

In secondary prevention of vascular disease

1   In 1988 the Antiplatelet Trialists' Collaboration published an overview of 25 randomized, placebo-controlled trials of the use of antiplatelet agents in some 29000 patients who had recovered from some vascular event (thrombotic stroke, myocardial infarction or transient ischaemic attack), or who had unstable angina. Most trials were of the aspirin versus placebo type. The collaborators found that allocation to the antiplatelet group:
   • reduced vascular mortality by 15%;
   • reduced non-fatal vascular events (cerebrovascular accidents and myocardial infarctions) by 30%.

The results were similar in all categories of vascular event, and aspirin therapy was especially impressive in unstable angina (reducing deaths and non-fatal myocardial infarctions by 36%). Furthermore, it was highly effective in preventing first myocardial infarctions in those presenting with cerebrovascular accidents and vice versa.

2   The ISIS-2 trial (1988) confirmed that low-dose aspirin given in the early stages of a myocardial infarction reduces the risk of death by about a quarter (Table 4.6).

These trials indicate a strong benefit for aspirin (unless contraindicated) in patients who have had a primary vascular event.

In the primary prevention of vascular disease

Two large, expensive primary prevention studies have reached differing conclusions:

1   A study of 5000 male British doctors, taking 500 mg aspirin daily was negative. Although total mortality was 10% lower in the treatment group the difference was not statistically significant, and the incidences of non-fatal stroke and myocardial infarction were not reduced (Peto *et al.* 1988).

2   The American Physicians' study (1988) also sought to study the effects of beta-carotene on cancer incidence. Thus, 22071 male doctors aged 40–84 were randomized between combinations of aspirin (325 mg), beta-carotene and placebo. The aspirin part of the study was terminated prematurely because of the large reduction in fatal and non-fatal myocardial infarction in those taking aspirin (an overall 47% reduction).

It has proved difficult to reconcile these differences, though they may conceivably be related to a lower dose of aspirin in the American study, or to the use of beta-carotene, although it is not presently known to have an effect on vascular disease.

The potential for harm

1 Aspirin can worsen any bleeding condition. Thus, in patients with a haemorrhagic stroke it has the potential to worsen intracranial bleeding (and this itself poses practical problems as only two-fifths of health districts in England and Wales had a computerized tomography scanner in 1988). If used in primary prevention an increased risk of intracranial bleeding would need to be offset against potential benefits.

2 It can cause gastrointestinal bleeding and induce or worsen peptic ulceration.

3 It can exacerbate asthma and induce allergic reactions.

Who should take aspirin?
Those who have suffered a primary vascular event, including those with:

- a non-haemorrhagic stroke;
- transient ischaemic attacks;
- unstable angina;
- myocardial infarction (at the earliest possible time).

Who should not?
Aspirin is contraindicated in patients with a bleeding tendency, e.g.

- known bleeding diathesis;
- haemorrhagic cerebrovascular accident;
- recent haemorrhage;
- recent surgery, subclavian puncture, or other invasive procedure;
- suspected aortic dissection;
- uncontrolled hypertension.

It should not be used in those with peptic ulcers or a known aspirin sensitivity, and only with extreme caution in those with asthma.

The advantages and disadvantages of treatment may need to be weighed on an individual basis, as a balance of risks is likely to exist.

At the present time the role of aspirin in the primary prevention of vascular disease is uncertain, so a blanket suggestion that we should all take an aspirin a day cannot be supported.

4.11 THE POST-VIRAL SYNDROME

Features
Post-viral syndrome, also called myalgic encephalitis (ME) and epidemic neuromyasthenia, has the following epidemiological and clinical characteristics:

1 *Occurrence* — sporadic and in epidemics.
2 *Sex ratio* — 10 times more common in women than in men.
3 *Social class* — more common in social classes 1 and 2 and especially among medical personnel.
4 *Symptoms* — typically follows an upper respiratory tract infection with incomplete recovery. Symptoms are protean (Table 4.8).
5 *Signs* — usually non-specific.
6 *Laboratory tests* — usually non-specific.
7 *Diagnosis* — by exclusion.
8 *Outcome* — in three camps: full recovery, chronic illness and relapsing and remitting ill health.

Table 4.8 Common symptoms seen in the post-viral syndrome.

Profound muscle fatigue*	Fainting attacks
Myalgia	Poor memory
Headache	Poor concentration
Paraesthesia	Poor sleep
Dizziness	Mild dysphasia
Urinary frequency	Hyperacusis
Cold extremities	Emotional lability
Bouts of sweating	

*Excessive muscle fatigue is generally regarded as the cardinal symptom.

Aetiology
This remains controversial with some evidence supporting a psychogenic origin and some favouring an organic one.
1 Epidemics have occurred with all the characteristics of mass hysteria (e.g. the Royal Free outbreak in 1955). Some of the epidemiological features of the condition (class, sex and professional predilections), and some of the presenting features have been held to support this conclusion. An increased incidence of pre-existing neurosis has been reported in sufferers.
2 However:
(a) some patients do have neurological signs;
(b) some routine laboratory tests have been abnormal;
(c) abnormal lymphocyte function and immunological changes have been described;
(d) muscle biopsies have found necrosis and type II fibre predominance;
(e) abnormal potentials have been described in electromyogram tracings;
(f) nuclear magnetic resonance abnormalities suggest intracellular acidosis at an early stage in exercise;
(g) many viruses have been implicated — varicella, influenza, the Epstein–Barr virus, and especially the coxsackievirus (antibodies to this have been found in 30–70% of studied groups).

There is obviously a problem in lumping together cases with a wide variety of non-specific symptoms and treating them as a homogeneous group with a single disease entity. This problem besets research into the post-viral syndrome, whose very basis and principal defining features remain enshrouded in a degree of mystery.

Experts' views fall into two camps: those who support the psychogenic hypothesis and those who believe the condition to be organic. A half-way house approach holds that there is an organic origin, promoting some psychiatric symptoms, and a degree of hysteria and functional overlay in vulnerable individuals.

Management

This is even more problematic. Patients with genuine psychiatric illness may become mislabelled; other conditions may mimic the protean symptoms; many patients are reluctant to accept psychiatric treatment and worried by the lack of a firm diagnosis. An outbreak of ME is likely to prove a taxing management problem!

A variety of treatments have been attempted, including:
- immunoglobulin G injections;
- oral antifungal agents;
- steroids, azathioprine, interferon, acyclovir;
- carbamazepine (for myalgia);
- pizotifen (for headaches);
- exclusion diets and dietary supplements;
- sulphasalazine.

There is no clear evidence of benefit over placebo treatment.

Rest is regarded as the mainstay of treatment. Otherwise the approach has been symptomatic, with analgesia, anxiolytics, antidepressants and supportive counselling. The latter in particular is necessary as these patients suffer considerable distress.

A self-help group, the Myalgic Encephalomyelitis Association, exists to assist sufferers and to disseminate information and sponsor research. It is hoped with time that a more specific causal agent will be identified. In the meantime, a mixed physical and psychological approach seems appropriate, regardless of aetiology.

4.12 MEASURING QUALITY OF CARE

There exist wide variations in the quality of care and range of services offered in general practice. Thus:
- three large descriptive studies by the Department of General Practice at the University of Manchester (Wilkin *et al.* 1984) established variations in consulting, prescribing, investigating, referral and average consultation time that could not be accounted for by the characteristics of the population studies;

- referral rates between doctors vary from 5 per 1000 per month to 115 per 1000 per month (Last 1967);
- visiting rates may vary by a factor of 32 (Fry 1973);
- the ability to detect psychiatric illness varies by a factor of nine between studied London GPs (Shepherd *et al*. 1966).

Factors contributing to the variation in referral and prescribing rates are reviewed in Chapter 2. Interpretation of such statistics is not straightforward — in particular, 'above average' does not mean 'excessive' or 'profligate', and average is not necessarily the desired endpoint. Costs and effort must be related to outcome, and this is a far harder exercise. However, such variations have generated demands to promote greater consistency in the range and quality of services and several developments and initiatives have followed (some of a legislative nature):

1 The Royal College of General Practitioners was established in 1952 to promote standards within the profession.

2 The postgraduate examination in general practice (MRCGP) followed in the 1960s.

3 In 1973 a system was developed for the selection and reselection of trainers based on the practice visit.

4 Vocational training was introduced in the 1970s and became a 3-year mandatory programme in 1981. Several valuable spin-offs have evolved from this (the development of teaching practices; a clearer definition of the content of general practice; the promotion of small group learning and so on).

5 Over the last 20 years there has been a great deal of fundamental research within primary care.

6 Government requirements (e.g. the introduction of annual reports and indicative prescribing budgets).

7 *College initiatives*. In 1983 the Royal College of General Practitioners launched its 'Quality Initiative' (Royal College of General Practitioners 1983) which encouraged doctors to introduce the principle of quality assessment into their everyday practice. In 1985 they developed the 'What Sort of Doctor?' projects (Royal College of General Practitioners 1985c), a study in which participating practices subjected themselves to voluntary quality assessment in the form of structured practice inspection by a visiting team of peers. A subsequent policy statement, 'Quality in General Practice' (Royal College of General Practitioners 1985d), reiterated the college's ambition to promote quality assessment and professional development from within by voluntary initiative. Other innovative suggestions include:

- the concept of protected time for study;
- further education for young principals in their early years of practice (a voluntary extension of vocational training);
- regular reassessment of established principals.

Admirable though these voluntary initiatives have been (less

palatable some of the legislative ones), there remains a fundamental question that must be asked: what is good quality of care
and how does one measure it?

As Clark and Forbes (1979) point out, this is an emotive subject. Quality of care means different things to different people
at different times. From the patient's perspective it presumably
relates to his personal needs and if his expectations are met he is
more likely to be satisfied, even if from the medical viewpoint the
treatment was inappropriate. From a doctor's perspective, quality
of care relates to accuracy of diagnosis and efficient treatment; and
from the community's viewpoint it must include just and accurate
rationing of resources: a doctor who offers prolonged counselling
to one patient and denies six others an early consultation is offering high-quality care to the former patient at the expense of the
others.

There are other problems: quality assessment is fine as long as
activities can be easily counted (the number of BP checks, the
number of smears, the percentage vaccinated) but a number of
highly desirable qualities are not easily counted, e.g.:
- approachability of staff and doctors;
- a sympathetic ear;
- compassion and dedication;
- the ability to inspire confidence in patients.

Attempts to measure these qualities are beset with difficulties
and open to the charge of subjectivity.

Furthermore, in many circumstances GPs cannot agree on the
best policy anyway; formal protocols may not be flexible enough
to reflect individual circumstances. Even when there is a consensus view on good management, this has seldom been subjected to rigorous validation; there is a danger in identifying
practices which we *think* are beneficial and calling them good
practice without showing objective benefit.

There are problems in conducting research in general practice,
both from the point of view of methods and that of ethics (see
Section 1.3 and Section 7.11). Finally it is important to appreciate
that many practices (inner city ones particularly) function under
difficult circumstances and any system of assessment must recognize this in its accounting methods.

To its credit the Royal College of General Practitioners has
proposed ways in which subjective aspects of good practice can be
measured. Principal amongst these is the concept of peer review,
and although it remains a difficult exercise to measure quality in a
field which is still as much an art as a science, this is not an excuse
for refusing to try.

5 Social Medicine

5.1 SOCIAL CLASS

Definitions

The Registrar General's classification of social class is based on *occupation*:

- for men and single women on their own occupation;
- for married women on their husband's occupation;
- for children on their father's occupation;
- for the retired and unemployed on their last significant period of employment.

This system is widely accepted and is comprehensive for the whole population, although it is clearly not precise to label people on the basis of their job alone, and even less precise to label women on the basis of their spouse's job. The classification has five divisions, as shown in Table 5.1.

Social inequalities related to class

Various studies [e.g. those by the Office of Population Censuses and Surveys (OPCS) and by the Department of Employment and the Royal Commission on the Distribution of Income and Wealth] have highlighted class inequalities in areas like wealth, income, living and working conditions. Typical findings are illustrated in Table 5.2.

If anything, the gap between rich and poor is widening. Thus, according to the 1987 *Social Trends* the income of the bottom two-fifths of households fell from 10 to 6% of the total, while the top one-fifth's share rose from 44 to 49%.

Health inequalities related to class

Unfortunately there is no perfect measure of health: self-reported symptoms are often unreliable and, while death is an unequivocal event, it does not help in the measurement of minor and chronic illness. Field-workers have attempted to circumvent this problem by examining a *variety* of parameters. In fact, as Table 5.3 illustrates, the relationship of health to social class is so clear that it is borne out for *all* the parameters considered.

Inequalities in health through the social classes mirror the social inequalities described above; these inequalities exist whatever the parameter of ill health considered; and, as Table 5.4 shows, there is a clear gradation through the classes, which applies to all ages and both sexes: class 5 has the worst health, class 1 the best, and the other classes are in between, in the exact order that they appear in our class structure.

Table 5.1 Registrar General's five divisions of social class.

Social class	Description	Population (%)
1	Professionals (e.g. doctors, lawyers) Larger employers and businessmen	5
2	'Lesser' professions and trades (e.g. teachers, shopkeepers)	20
3 N	Skilled non-manual (e.g. clerical workers, secretaries)	15
3 M	Skilled manual (e.g. electricians)	33
4	Semi-skilled manual (e.g. machinists, farmhands)	19
5	Unskilled manual (e.g. labourers)	8

On the 10th anniversary of the Black Report commentators pointed out that socioeconomic differences in health, like those in wealth, were widening (Davey *et al.* 1990). Similar patterns can be seen in all industrialized countries collecting relevant data (Lynge 1981).

Two contradictory theories have been proposed to explain these findings:

1 *Health determines social class*: e.g. sickly individuals fail to hold down good jobs, or ill health over several generations produces a similar social drift — there is no great evidence to support this theory.

2 *Social class determines health*: e.g. exposure to disease-producing agents and access to medical resources is class-related. There is some evidence in favour of this model:

(a) lower social classes use the preventive services less than classes 1 and 2;

(b) lower social classes are more likely to indulge in unhealthy habits like smoking;

(c) the lower classes live in less healthy environments and suffer more deprivation.

The distinction between these two theories is of more than academic importance: if social class *does* determine health it suggests that health inequalities are best combated by tackling social inequalities, and this approach would be sociopolitical rather than medical. (Many commentators and epidemiologists indeed believe this to be true.)

Inequalities of access to health care

Tudor Hart (1971) argued that the 'inverse care law' applies in the UK: i.e. the *provision* of health care is inversely related to the *need* for it. He attributes this to market forces in a free economy:

Table 5.2 Social inequalities related to class (from: Royal Commission on the Distribution of Income and Wealth 1980; OPCS 1973; Department of Employment 1977).

Item	Upper classes	Lower classes
Personal wealth	Top 1% own 25% of the total Top 10% own two-thirds	90% are left with the remaining one-third
Income	Top 10% receive 25% of the total	The bottom 50% also receive 25%
Living conditions: 1 Official overcrowding (more than 1.5 persons per room)	Virtually unknown	10% (class 5)
2 No shower/bath	Virtually unknown	10% (class 5)
3 Central heating	80% (class 1)	27% (class 5)
4 Car	90% (class 1)	18% (class 5)
5 Telephone	88% (class 1)	27% (class 5)
6 Home environment	Generally good areas	Close to heavy industry and pollution; more often lacking private garden, etc.
Diet		*Less* fruit and vegetables, meat and dairy products *More* refined products, e.g. bread and sugar
Working conditions: 1 Shift work	Less than 5% (class 1)	25% of all manual workers
2 Holiday	Usually 4–6 weeks	Typically 3–4 weeks
3 Working hours		7 hours/week longer on average
4 Job content		Less varied; closer supervision; more disciplinary activity (e.g. more than 90% 'clock-on')

prosperous areas attract more resources and more highly skilled personnel.

There *is* some evidence in favour of this 'law':

• some depressed areas with high morbidity receive poorer facilities than the so-called affluent areas;

• the higher social classes, who appear to be the least in need of preventive services like cervical screening, are the highest users of the service;

• according to OPCS surveys, the upper social classes are more likely to be referred to hospital than their working-class counterparts in the event of chronic handicapping illness;

Table 5.3 Health inequalities related to social class (OPCS 1978).

Parameter	Social class 1	Social class 5	Approximate relative risk
Stillbirth rate (deaths/1000 total births)	9	17–18	2.0:1.0
Infant mortality rate (deaths in first year/1000 live births)	10–14	27–35	2.5:1.0
Standardized mortality ratio:			
• for 1–14-year age group	74–89	156–162	2.0:1.0
• for 15–64-year age group	77–82	135–137	1.7:1.0
Acute sickness rate (number of restricted activity days/person each year)	11–16	21–22	1.6:1.0
Chronic sickness rate (per 1000 reporting limiting long-standing illness)	80–86	234–299	3.0:1.0
Standardized mortality ratio by specific disease (for males aged 15–64 years):			
1 Lung cancer	65	193	3.0:1.0
2 Bronchitis	36	188	5.0:1.0
3 Motor vehicle accidents	77	174	2.3:1.0
4 Pneumonia	41	195	4.8:1.0

Table 5.4 The relationship of mortality to social class (OPCS 1978).

Social class	Standardized mortality ratio	
	1–14 years	15–64 years
Males		
1	74	77
2	79	81
3 N	95	99
3 M	98	106
4	112	114
5	162	137
Females		
1	89	82
2	84	87
3 N	93	92
3 M	93	115
4	120	119
5	156	135

Standardized mortality ratio is the ratio of observed mortality in a population subgroup to that expected as average for the whole population. It is multiplied by 100, so that a standardized mortality ratio of 100 denotes average risk, less than 100 below-average, and more than 100 above-average risk.

- according to Cartwright and Anderson's survey, practices in middle class areas are more likely to employ doctors with higher qualifications, and less likely to use deputizing arrangements than practices from working-class areas; they are also more likely to have extra equipment like an ECG machine;
- on average, middle-class patients have longer consultations with their GP (6.2 min) than working-class patients (4.7 min); they ask more questions and cover more problems; doctors in working-class areas have heavier surgeries.

Deprived areas

Nowhere is the inequality of access to health care more clearly illustrated than in inner cities, where there are problems in the recruitment of health care personnel because of high overheads, vandalism, vagrant or highly mobile populations and social problems like alcohol and drug addiction. This has also led to GPs who live outside their practice areas, to the heavy use of deputizing services, and to the use of hospital casualty departments by patients for basic primary care problems.

To redress this problem a deprivation payment has recently been introduced for GPs whose areas are officially 'deprived'. These areas are identified using the Jarman Index, a scoring system based on factors identified by a panel of GPs as contributing to increased workloads (Table 5.5) (To obtain the Jarman Index, each factor was weighted according to its perceived impact on workload, and scores were linked to 1981 census data for each electoral ward in England and postcode in Scotland. Deprivation payments are made at three levels according to the score.)

Table 5.5 Factors scored in the Jarman Index of deprivation.

Elderly living alone	Single-parent households
Under-fives	Overcrowded households
Unskilled	House-movers
Unemployed	Residents in ethnic minorities

The need for a deprivation payment has generally been acknowledged. Critics of the current arrangements point out however that:
- the score at which payment is accepted is far higher than Jarman himself intended (with many fewer wards qualifying);
- the Jarman Index is based on 1981 census data, since which major demographic changes in employment and housing have occurred. (The 1991 census will form the basis for revising the index, but the results may not be incorporated until 1993–4.)

5.2 ILLNESS BEHAVIOUR

The clinical iceberg

Many minor conditions are extremely common and it is normal for people to feel ill a lot of the time, e.g.:

- in one survey more than 90% declared themselves to have been ill in the last 2-week period (only 20% consulted their GP);
- another survey found that patients only take about one in 37 symptom episodes to their GP (and only one in 109 gastro-intestinal upsets, one in 184 headaches and one in 456 energy level changes; Banks *et al.* 1975).

The level of self-care is very high. According to a study by Dunnell and Cartwright (1972), in a 2-week period:

- 80% of all adults and 55% of all children had taken at least one medicine;
- the average number of medicines taken was 2.2 for adults, and 1.1 for children (two-thirds were non-prescription medicines).

It is clear from these data that a clinical iceberg exists and the majority of symptom episodes do not reach medical attention.

Social definitions of illness

It is a basic tenet of medical sociology that definitions of illness and health *vary*, depending on socially determined perceptions; for example, whether you regard tension headaches, hyper-tension, alcoholism or premenstrual tension as illnesses depends on your viewpoint: doctor and patient may disagree, and one generation may disagree with the last.

Illness behaviour

Given the foregoing comments it is interesting to consider what prompts a person to consider himself in need of medical advice; a complex decision which sociologists call illness behaviour. Factors shown to be important include:

1 *Culture*: e.g. Italians, Jews and those of Mediterranean origin have been shown to have lower thresholds for reporting pain.

2 *Symptom presentation*: symptoms presenting in a striking way are more readily perceived as illness.

3 *Lay beliefs.*

4 *Sex and social class*: women and social classes 4 and 5 consult more often.

5 *Accessibility of medical care*: e.g. as the distance between home and the surgery increases, the likelihood of consultation decreases.

6 *Learned behaviour*: much anecdotal experience suggests that high usage of medical services runs in families, perhaps because members learn their illness behaviour from one another and pass them on to future generations.

7 *Trigger factors*: Zola (1973) identified five triggers that influenced the *timing* of decisions to consult:

(a) another interpersonal crisis;

(b) perceived interference with personal and social relations;

(c) perceived interference with job or leisure activities;

(d) the pressure of other family or friends (approximately 75% conduct lay consultations prior to the professional one);

(e) the setting of an arbitrary deadline ('If I feel the same next week . . .').

The Health Belief Model, developed by a group of social psychologists in the 1950s, proposes that people vary individually, and for different conditions, in:

• health motivation;
• perceived vulnerability;
• the perceived seriousness of the condition;
• the perceived costs and benefits of obtaining medical care;
• cues for action (new symptoms, TV article, friend's advice, etc.).

The decision to consult does *not* correlate with:

• the true seriousness of the illness;
• the doctor's perception of a need to consult.

In other words, patients are poor judges of illness and take decisions often at variance with what doctors believe to be the correct use of the service. According to Dunnell and Gartwright (1972) 20% of GPs felt half or more of their consultations were trivial, unnecessary or inappropriate. It is, however, fortunate that only one in 37 symptom episodes receives medical attention, as the health service would otherwise surely be overwhelmed!

5.3 STRESS

Stress rating scales

Several attempts have been made to quantify the amount of stress attached to important life events. Holmes and Rahe's Social Readjustment Rating Scale (SRRS) was obtained by asking a large sample of people to score 42 life events, pleasant and unpleasant, according to the amount of readjustment needed (Holmes & Rahe 1967). Taking marriage as the midpoint (50) on a scale of 1–100, typical ratings were:

• death of a spouse   100
• divorce   73
• marriage   50
• major change at work   29
• change of house   20
• holiday   13

Stress and physical illness

The SRRS shows a crude correlation with physical illness, e.g.:

- one study classified doctors into high-, medium- and low-risk groups, based on their stress scores: the ratio of self-reported illness over the next 9 months was approximately five times greater (49%) in the high-risk than in the low-risk group (9%);
- another study found a linear relationship between stress scores and illness in naval personnel (Holmes & Masuda 1974).

Other studies suggest that major life events can affect physical problems like peptic ulceration, urticaria and diabetic control.

Stress and psychiatric illness

There is a relatively poor correlation with the SRRS here, but much empirical experience in general and psychiatric practice indicates that stress is a vital precipitant of psychiatric ill health. The failure of the SRRS has been blamed on the relative crudity of a scale that ascribes the same rating to an event without examining the individual and the context of the event.

Brown and Harris (1978), investigating depression in women, found that stresses mattered only if they were believed to have long-term threatening implications (major loss or potential loss of health, marriage, job, etc.). Painful but self-limiting stresses were less important. The same authors were able to identify predisposing vulnerability factors in the womens' environment or past history, e.g.:

- lack of a confiding relationship at home;
- no employment outside the home;
- three or more children under 15 years old at home;
- loss of mother before age of 11 years.

Studies like this further emphasize the importance of social factors and life events in the course of a mental illness.

Important stress factors

Bereavement

Parkes' studies (Parkes *et al.* 1969) suggest a much higher morbidity and mortality in the recently bereaved, e.g.:

- widowers aged 55 years or over have an increased mortality of about 40% in the first 6 months after their wife's death and there is still an effect at 1 year;
- although deaths from suicide are increased, much of the effect is from cardiovascular disease;
- the risk is greater for men and greater for close relationships than distant ones.

Work

The relationship between health and stress factors at work is unclear. Thus:

- manual workers paid by result have higher catecholamine levels than other workers, and stressed air traffic controllers have high blood pressure on duty, but these findings do not correlate with cardiovascular disease or psychiatric breakdown;
- ambitious, rapidly promoted employees of big companies fail to show an excess of cardiovascular disease despite heavier responsibilities.

Lack of work
Retirement does not appear to be a major stress factor, assuming it is planned; redundancy by contrast is a great source of stress. Thus:
- self-reported illness, including chronic ill health, is more common;
- in the short term, blood pressure and serum cholesterol can be raised;
- loss of work, or threat of it, is associated with markedly higher consultation rates, both for the individual and the spouse (and GPs in areas of high unemployment can therefore expect to have higher caseloads);
- longitudinal mortality studies from 1971 to 1981 showed, after adjustment for social class, an excess of mortality of 20–30% among the unemployed (Moser *et al.* 1987);
- deaths from suicide, lung cancer and ischaemic heart disease are more common; so too are depression and parasuicide.

Unemployment is concentrated in the lower social classes and this may partly account for the observed class inequalities in health.

Marriage
Clearly this can be a positive or a negative force, e.g.:
- the married have a lower mortality rate than the unmarried, widowed or divorced (this effect is greater for men than women);
- however, marital problems are a well recognized precipitant of alcoholism, suicide, accidents and psychiatric illness, and the constrained role of mother and wife, in particular, may cause depression in housewives.

Family problems
Problems within the family are a potent source of stress that can affect more than one generation, e.g.:
- child-battering and alcoholism are often passed from parents to children;
- loss of a parent in childhood by death, divorce or separation has been associated with diverse effects such as suicide, tuberculosis and serious accidents in later life (Chen & Cobb 1960);

- Laing and others have proposed that schizophrenia is a rational response to an abnormal family environment;
- maternal deprivation seeds many emotional disorders of childhood.

Social upheaval

Migrant and other studies suggest major upheaval can predispose to physical and mental ill health.

The role of personality

Friedman and Rosenman (1974) proposed two types of personality related to cardiovascular risk:

1 Type A people show:
    (a) impatience;
    (b) competitiveness;
    (c) a sense of the pressure of time and responsibility.
2 Type B people do not exhibit any of these traits.

Some studies suggest that type A men have twice the risk of heart disease when compared with type B men.

Attempts have been made to link physical illness to personality type for other conditions like peptic ulceration but the results have not been scientifically validated. Vulnerable personalities are certainly a well established concept in psychiatric illness (e.g. the schizoid personality is linked to schizophrenia, and the cyclothymic to bipolar depression).

The value of social support

Social integration

Integration into a social community or family is generally protective, e.g.:

- lower mortality rates in married men;
- lower death rates in Mormons and Seventh Day Adventists.

Family support

Support of a family can:

- reduce the impact of stress (e.g. following enforced redundancies men supported by family and friends experience fewer stress-related symptoms);
- influence the course and outcome of physical illness (e.g. orthopaedic patients rehabilitate more quickly if they are married and have children at home);
- influence the course and outcome of mental illness (e.g. Brown's studies suggest relapse in schizophrenia is higher when patients come from families with high expressed emotion);
- provide vital care for those with chronic illness and handicap [e.g. Harris *et al.* (1971) found 37% of the *very* severely handicapped elderly, often senile, bedfast, or doubly incontinent,

receive only family support and no community service input; other surveys indicate that only one-tenth of the physically disabled in the UK are in homes or hospital].

Families can also constitute a *pathological* influence (as described earlier).

The structure of family life is changing (more divorces, more single-parent families, working women and mobile populations). This threatens to undermine the supporting role of the family, especially with respect to their ageing relatives.

5.4 ETHNIC MINORITIES

Historically much of the immigration to the UK was encouraged by the British Nationality Act 1948, the poverty and poor prospects of the colonies and Britain's demand for labour in the 1950s and early 1960s.

There are two main patterns of migrant-community relationship:
1 'Integrated' or 'assimilated' (e.g. West Indian communities).
2 Culturally separate and isolated (e.g. Asian communities).

There is strong evidence that racial prejudice places immigrant groups in a position of social inequality (Table 5.6).

Table 5.6 The influence of racial factors on social status and employment (adapted from Smith 1976).

Nature of job	Whites	West Indians	Indians
Professional/white collar	40	8	20
Social class 4 and 5 jobs	18	32	36
Professional jobs with equivalent qualifications	79	31	

As in the case of social class, social inequalities are mirrored by inequalities in physical and mental health:
1 *Physical health*. Migrants have:
   (a) lower birthweight babies;
   (b) a higher perinatal mortality rate;
   (c) more anaemia (sometimes dietary, sometimes due to ethnic diseases like sickle cell and thalassaemia);
   (d) more rickets;
   (e) more imported and tropical diseases.
2 *Mental health*. It is sometimes difficult to distinguish between cultural beliefs that seem bizarre to the western mind and true mental illness. However, some studies on West Indian migrants suggest that the stress of social upheaval, alien culture and racial discrimination cause more mental breakdowns.

The inequality in health is in part explained by behavioural traits (e.g. less use of antenatal and postnatal services; restrictive diets), in part by genetic vulnerability, and in part by social disadvantages like employment, housing and discrimination.

Cultural differences also pose problems in the doctor–patient relationship, e.g.:

- language barriers;
- completely different values and beliefs;
- different (culturally determined) patterns of illness behaviour;
- taboos concerning the physical examination of women.

It is therefore difficult to ensure that these patients are not also disadvantaged in the medical care they receive.

5.5 THE ELDERLY

The size of the problem

1   The percentage of the population over 65 years of age is now approximately 15%, comprising:

(a) 9% in the 65–74 years age group;

(b) 6% aged 75 years or over.

2   This represents a considerable growth in the elderly population, e.g.:

(a) the percentage of over-65s was 6% in 1901;

(b) the number of over-65s increased by 2 million between 1961 and 1985.

3   The percentage of very elderly (over 75 years old) is growing faster than that of the elderly as a whole.

4   There are three reasons for this growth:

(a) a slight increase in life expectancy;

(b) a fall in birth rates (which means the young are a relatively smaller percentage of the whole);

(c) a present glut of elderly produced by the dramatic decline in perinatal mortality at the turn of the century.

Characteristics of the elderly

1   More often women than men:

(a) mean life expectancy of men is approximately 6 years less than women;

(b) 80% of the over-85s are women and there are twice as many women as men among the over-75s.

2   Multiple physical problems.

3   Drug problems:

(a) polypharmacy and drug interactions;

(b) impaired drug handling and clearance;

(c) sensitivity to drug effects.

4   Financial status. On the *plus* side the elderly gain:

(a) a statutory retirement pension;

(b) certain exemptions and concessions, e.g. on prescription charges and travel fares.

On the *debit* side of course they lose their earning power. On balance the latter is not compensated for and studies suggest about 50% of the over-65s live below, or occasionally far below, the official poverty level.

Although state benefits may help in part, they are under-claimed because:

(c) the benefits system is complicated and confusing;

(d) the elderly fear the humiliation of means testing and the stigma of 'scrounging';

5   Other problems:

(a) inadequate housing;

(b) subnutrition;

(c) social isolation and apathy;

(d) physical handicap.

A combination of these factors renders the elderly population prone to an increased risk of hypothermia.

Support for the elderly

1   Family trends (fewer children, a more mobile population, more working women) mean fewer carers nowadays. Also society's current values place the elderly in relatively low esteem when compared with the right of other family members to exercise their independence. Studies in London in the 1950s showed that 70% of the elderly received regular family help, and 15% were kept out of hospital only because of it, but in the 1980s more elderly people live alone for the reasons described:

(a) 40% live with an elderly spouse;

(b) 30% live alone;

(c) 12% live with their children;

(d) 12% are in other households;

(e) 6% are in residential care or hospitals.

2   Where family support is provided, there is a cost, e.g.:

(a) loss of paid work, social life and holiday opportunities;

(b) family discord;

(c) impaired health of the carers.

3   Alternative support systems are provided through the Social Services departments:

(a) *Home helps.* For more than 700 000 elderly, who pay accord-ing to their means, home helps perform many important services — cleaning, washing, shopping, collecting prescrip-tions and pensions. They also provide companionship and are an early warning system for the primary health care team.

(b) *Meals on wheels.* Hot meals provided from central kitchens to the home on a subsidized basis. Voluntary organizations also contribute to this service.

(c) *Social Services day centres*. These provide a more stimulating environment and a social outlet for the isolated elderly and day relief for their carers.

4 These support systems are considerably underused in relation to the need; for example, in one study 6% of the 65–75-years age group and 19% of the over-75s used these services, but this supplied only one-quarter of the perceived need for home helps and one-sixteenth of the need for meals on wheels. Similarly there is evidence that aids and adaptations for the home are under-provided, under-used and under-maintained.

Underuse of aids and support services arises because of:
(a) ignorance regarding their availability;
(b) the reluctance of a largely stoical elderly population to ask for help;
(c) the limited provision of resources;
(d) the high level of commitment of many carers, despite personal difficulties and stress.

Institutional care
Options include:
- private nursing homes;
- private residential care;
- Social Services Part 3 accommodation;
- voluntary association non-residential homes;
- local authority sheltered housing (including warden-controlled and other flats for the elderly).

The provision made by local authorities is determined by Part 3 of the National Assistance Act 1948, which imposes a duty to 'provide for those who by reason of age or infirmity need care and attention not otherwise available'. The level of provision is set at 25 per 1000 over-65-year-olds, but standards vary widely. Many homes include a short-stay bed quota for trial periods and relief admissions.

Only 6% of the elderly live in residential or hospital care, and these are divided up as follows:
- 50% in homes for the elderly;
- 17% in geriatric beds;
- 17% in psychogeriatric beds;
- 9% in acute hospital beds;
- 6% in private nursing homes;
- 2% in homes for the handicapped.

Unfortunately there is poor provision for the care of common nursing problems in the elderly, like incontinence, confusion and poor mobility, which often overspill into acute hospital beds (approximately 50% of general beds are occupied by the over-65s). It is feared that this problem will escalate as the numbers increase in line with predictions. The division of resources between NHS,

Social Services and local authorities has also been criticized as a fragmented and poorly coordinated service.

5.6 DISABILITY AND HANDICAP

Problems of the disabled
The disabled encounter various problems which include:
- poor mobility (and hence reduced leisure opportunities);
- difficulties with basic self-care;
- disadvantage in employment and difficulties in education;
- the need for a modified environment at home, at work and in public places;
- poverty;
- the stigma label and other psychological problems.

Mobility and the disabled
Resources that are available include:
- physiotherapy;
- the provision of walking aids;
- home adaptations (handrails, stairlifts, etc.) through the advice of a domiciliary occupational therapist;
- the provision of a wheelchair;
- a mobility allowance;
- sometimes a grant towards a specially adapted car;
- advice, for example from the Directory for the Disabled, on the help that travel agencies, car-hire firms, British Rail and the airlines can provide;
- voluntary or paid visitors, home helps and day centre attendance to combat the problem of isolation.

Employment and the disabled
Unemployment levels are higher amongst the disabled (e.g. in 1981 when the general level of unemployment was 10.1%, unemployment among the disabled was at 15.3%).

Various Disabled Employment Acts have endeavoured to correct the problem, e.g.:
- an employer of more than 20 employees is legally obliged to employ at least 3% of his workforce from those registered disabled under the Act;
- sheltered workshops are provided by local authorities and voluntary bodies;
- under the Sheltered Placement Scheme a host company provides an opportunity for disabled workers to integrate with able-bodied ones: the host company provides tools and training and pays according to output, with the balance of salary provided by an employing sponsor;
- the Government provides Disablement Resettlement Officers

(DROs), Employment Rehabilitation Centres, PACTs (Placement Assessment Counselling Teams) and residential retraining courses to help the disabled find work;
● grants are available for adaptation of premises and equipment to the needs of the disabled, assistance with fares to work (when inability to use public transport incurs extra expense) and a 'job introduction' grant to promote trials of employment;
● a Government-sponsored company, Remploy, provides about 8000 jobs for the disabled;
● certain groups of visually handicapped people can be helped at the cost of engaging a sighted reader at work for their assistance.

Poverty and the disabled
Surveys indicate that the disabled often suffer financial hardship, e.g.:
1 *OPCS survey (1971)*: over 30% of disabled people are on supplementary benefit, while a further 7% are eligible but are not claiming (Harris *et al.* 1971);
2 *General Household Survey (1978)*: approximately 50% of homes where the head was disabled came close to the state definition of poverty (Royal Commission on the Distribution of Income and Wealth 1978).

The *reasons* for greater financial hardship among the disabled include:
● restricted employment;
● extra expenses (special diets, higher fuel bills, transport costs, home adaptations, etc.).

Although welfare benefits are available (see below) they do not adequately compensate because:
● the claim system is complicated and off-putting;
● the rates are not very high (and combinations are not always additive);
● patients miss out through diffidence, embarrassment or ignorance.

Housing and the disabled
The Disabled Persons Act requires local authorities to consider the housing needs of the registered disabled and to provide assistance with structural alterations and adaptations (e.g. ramps, rails, adapted bathrooms, widened doorways).

5.7 WELFARE BENEFITS

Currently about £40 000M is paid out annually in welfare benefits — half of this on pensions for the elderly. The welfare system is very complicated and subject to regular review. Although the details change from time to time, the principles change more slowly, so this discussion will concentrate on principles. The areas of most interest to general practice are those benefits arising from:

1 Sickness.
2 Handicap and disability.
3 Industrial injury and diseases.
    (Other important benefits are summarized in Table 5.7.)

Sickness

The major sickness benefits are:

1 *Statutory Sick Pay (SSP)*. Paid to employees who have made qualifying class 1 National Insurance (NI) contributions and covers them for 28 weeks.
2 *Sickness benefit*. Paid to those who do not qualify for SSP (e.g. the self-employed, unemployed and non-employed) who have made qualifying class 1 or 2 NI contributions. It covers a similar 28-week period.
3 *Invalidity benefit*. Starts at 28 weeks, i.e. when the previous two benefits expire. It consists of:
    (a) an *invalidity pension*;
    (b) a supplement called the *invalidity allowance* for those whose illness began before a certain age (under 60 years for men and 55 years for women).
These benefits all depend on NI contributions.

People who have not made the qualifying contributions (e.g. housewives) are covered by a scheme which parallels invalidity benefit. This was formerly called the non-contributory invalidity pension but is now known as the *severe disablement allowance*. To qualify the claimant must be:

1 Aged 16 years or over;
2 Incapable of work (to a prescribed degree) for at least 28 weeks;
3 Excluded from the contributory benefits already described;
4 At least 80% disabled (if first incapable of work after their 20th birthday).

Handicap and disability

The benefits for the handicapped and disabled are subdivided into:

1 Those received by the patient (patient benefits), e.g.:
    (a) attendance allowance;
    (b) mobility allowance;
    (c) disability living allowance;
    (d) disability working allowance.
2 Those received by the carers (carer benefits), e.g. invalid care allowance.

Patient benefits
1 *Attendance allowance*. To qualify a person must be aged over 65

Table 5.7 Some important welfare benefits.

Category	Benefit	Qualifying conditions
Low income	Income support	Age 18 years or over. Working less than 24 h/week. Low income. Means-tested (savings must not exceed £3000)
	Family credit	People working more than 24 h/week bringing up children on low wages. (Related to family income, number and age of children.) Means-tested (see above)
	Housing benefit	Paid to those finding it hard to pay their rent (rent rebate for those in council housing; a rent allowance for those in private tenancies). Means-tested. Depends on income, family size, savings and level of rent
	Social fund benefits	Exceptional expenses that cannot be met out of income, e.g.: • maternity expenses • funeral expenses • cold weather expenses • budgeting and crisis loans Savings over £500 taken into account. An interest-free repayable loan
Unemployment	Unemployment benefit	Up to 1 year for unemployed people who have made National Insurance (NI) contributions and are available for work
*Maternity**	Statutory maternity pay	Paid by employers who deduct payments from their NI contributions. Women must have worked at least 26 weeks up until the 15th week before birth, and paid NI contributions for 8 weeks before this. Payments are available for 18 weeks. (The self-employed may claim a maternity allowance from the DSS if they have made enough NI contributions. Also paid for 18 weeks)
	Sickness benefit	In the last 6 weeks of pregnancy and for 2 weeks afterwards the maternity certificate is accepted as evidence of incapacity for work, and sickness benefit can be claimed by those who cannot claim statutory maternity pay or the maternity allowance
Children	Child benefit	Tax-free cash payment to anyone who has a child under 16 years, or 16–18 years old in full-time education up to A-level standard. (Not means-related)

Table 5.7 *Contd*

173

Chapter 5
Social
Medicine

Category	Benefit	Qualifying conditions
	Guardian's allowance	Paid when you take an orphaned child into the family. Tax-free
Single parents	One-parent benefit	Paid independent of income and in addition to child benefit
	Tax allowances	Personal allowance may be increased to the value of a married man's allowance
*Widows**	Widow's payment	A lump sum to widows under 60 (or those over 60 whose husbands had not received a retirement pension). Tax-free, but dependent on husband's qualifying NI contributions
	Widowed mother's allowance	Paid to widows who still receive child benefit
	Widow's pension	Age 45 or over when their husband died or their widowed mother's allowance ended. A taxable benefit paid in addition to the husband's pension

* Additional exceptional circumstance payments also possible — see Social fund benefits, above.

and require a lot of supervision or personal care because of severe physical or mental disability. Although normally available only after 6 months of care, an exception is made in the case of those with terminal illness (i.e. those expected to die within 6 months). At two rates: daytime only (lower rate) or day and night (higher rate). Tax-free and can be added to other benefits.

2 *Mobility allowance.* Claimants must be:
(a) aged over 65;
(b) unable (or virtually unable) to walk before age 65 years (and must claim before age 66).
A non-contributory additive benefit.

3 *Disability Living Allowance.* A new allowance replacing **1** and **2** in the under 65s.

4 *Disability Working Allowance.* A new allowance for disabled people in employment but receiving low incomes.

Carer benefits
Invalid care allowance is paid to carers giving up work to look after a handicapped dependant. Carers must be:
• of working age (16–64 years old for men or 16–59 for women);
• looking after someone in receipt of an attendance allowance.

Welfare allowances are not always generous (invalid care allowance, for example, was paid at the rate of £23 per week in July 1986 to those prepared to forgo normal work to care for a dependant). Furthermore the qualifying conditions may be exacting, confusing or non-additive with other benefits. They may also be means-related or limited in supply.

Concessions
Concessions for the disabled are numerous, e.g.:
- road tax exemption;
- community charge relief;
- assistance with travel fares (to hospital and work);
- health benefits (free prescriptions and glasses, free dental treatment, etc.);
- assistance from Social Services (concessionary bus fares, day nurseries, aids and home adaptations, home help, meals on wheels, day centres, laundry, provision of a telephone, etc.).

Charitable assistance is also available in many forms outside the welfare system, e.g.:
- the loan of a wheelchair for travel on airlines or railways or for use in major shopping areas or theatres;
- advice on holidays for the disabled and other facilities through productions like *The Directory for the Disabled*;
- hire-cars adapted for disabled customers.

Industrial injury and diseases
The major benefits are:
1 *Sickness benefits*. These are SSP and sickness benefit, paid as for acute illness except that qualifying contributions for sickness benefit may be waived.
2 *Industrial injuries disablement benefit*. Paid for injuries arising during the course of work or for prescribed industrial diseases. Related to the degree of disablement and paid as a lump sum or pension or both (usually in addition to invalidity/unemployment benefit). Those people requiring daily care and assessed to be 100% disabled are entitled to a *constant care allowance* (similar to the attendance allowance payments for severe non-occupational disablement).
3 *Industrial death benefits*. A pension is paid to the spouse or children in two instalments: a short-term pension (first 26 weeks), then a permanent pension.
4 People who contracted their industrial disease or injury before 5 July 1948 may be able to claim:
    (a) various prescribed disease benefits (e.g. for pneumoconiosis or byssinosis);
    (b) a workmens' compensation supplement.

(The Industrial Injuries Act is outlined in Section 7.3, which also lists those industrial diseases that are notifiable by law.)

175
Chapter 5
Social
Medicine

Other welfare benefits

Some of the other principal welfare benefits are briefly described in Table 5.7. For information on the benefits available to war veterans, widows and pensioners, or for that matter a fuller discussion of *any* of the benefits described here, those interested are referred to the DSS pamphlet *Which Benefit?* — FB2.

Health benefits

In addition to the welfare benefits a range of health benefits are available to dependent groups such as:
- pregnant women and mothers in their first postnatal year;
- children under 16 years old;
- the unemployed;
- low-income groups (those on income support or family credit);
- the retired (men over 65 years old and women over 60).
  Benefits include:
- free NHS prescriptions, glasses and dental treatment; hearing aids on free loan (if prescribed by a consultant);
- free milk and vitamins (expectant and nursing mothers, children under school age from low-income families);
- hospital travelling expenses (means-tested).

Additional prescription charge exemptions

Certain other groups are exempt from NHS prescription charges by virtue of the chronic nature of their illness. These include:
1 Epileptics;
2 Those with continuing physical disability to the point where the patient cannot leave home without the help of another;
3 Patients with fistulae;
4 Those undergoing replacement/maintenance treatment, e.g. patients suffering from:
   (a) Addison's disease;
   (b) hypopituitarism;
   (c) myxoedema;
   (d) hypoparathyroidism;
   (e) myasthenia gravis;
   (f) diabetes mellitus;
5 War and service pensioners.

Exemptions are obtained either by age declaration or by Family Health Service authorities or DSS exemption certificates.

Prescription 'season tickets' are also available but are not free. They are prepayment certificates which can be purchased from the FHSA (application forms supplied by the DSS and post offices);

but they only save money if more than about 15 scripts are needed in 12 months (or five scripts in 4 months for the shorter 'season').

Help for the visually handicapped

About two people per 1000 are registered as blind and a further one per 1000 as partially sighted. These figures greatly under-estimate the true prevalence of visual handicap and it is thought that a further three people per 1000 have reading difficulties and four per 1000 severely limited distance vision.

Blind registration

For the purposes of *registration* the main factor is poor visual acuity (usually 3/60 or less for those registered blind and 6/60 or worse for the partially sighted), although allowance is also made for field loss. Registration requires a consultant's signature and is carried out through the Director of Social Services. Benefits of blind regis-tration include:

- an extra income tax allowance for those earning;
- additional supplementary benefit for those already qualifying for payments;
- entitlement to the severe disablement allowance for those of working age;
- a slightly reduced TV licence;
- parking concessions;
- concessionary travel fares;
- free postage on items specifically related to their incapacity;
- assistance through the Social Services with rehabilitation (mobility and orientation training), daily living skills (aids and training) and communication (e.g. learning braille).

Other services available include:

- large-print books (through public libraries and the National Library for the Blind), talking books (through public libraries and the British Talking Book Service for the Blind) and braille books (loaned by the National Library for the Blind);
- radios (on free extended loan from the British Wireless for the Blind Society);
- telephones (through the Blind Fund);
- advice from the Royal National Institute for the Blind.

Partially sighted

For the partially sighted most of the additional financial benefits are not available. However younger individuals may be entitled to education at special schools for the visually handicapped.

Help for the deaf

Deaf people may be entitled to some benefits through the Chronically Sick and Disabled Persons Act 1970. In particular it may be worthwhile registering with the local employment office and at the local Social Services department. The former depart- ment may assist through the DRO and any appropriate disable- ment resettlement schemes (see Section 5.6). The local authority Social Services department may help with personal problems and may be able to provide a range of special aids, including:

- louder doorbells, extra doorbells, visual doorbell systems or tone-modified doorbells;
- flashing-light alarm clocks and alarms that activate a vibrator pad placed underneath the pillow or mattress;
- sound-activated visual indicators (devices that flash in re- sponse to a predetermined sound, e.g. ringing phone, doorbell or crying baby);
- TV adaptors (e.g. headphones, induction loops and infrared transmissions);
- amplified telephones;
- travel concessions;
- holidays for old age pensioners.

These aids are available provided that there is a real need and the individual is formally registered with the department. In addi- tion anyone who has a hearing problem and could benefit from using a hearing aid is entitled to one through the NHS free of charge (through the ear, nose and throat consultant's outpatient clinic).

The Royal National Institute for the Deaf provides an informa- tion service, a wide range of reading material, a list of teachers of lip-reading, rehabilitative and longer-term residential care ser- vices, and training courses on behalf of the Department of Employment.

5.8 DEATH AND DYING

Attitudes to death
When life expectancy in the Middle Ages was 30 years or so, death, to coin a phrase, was a way of life. As life expectancy extended the taboo of the subject increased.

Doctors' attitudes
Doctors' attitudes are complicated by uncertainty (of true diag- nosis, of accurate prognosis, of whether the patient really wants to know). Questionnaires of the early 1960s and late 1970s suggest a complete reversal of doctors' attitudes from compounding the taboo to fighting it. In practice, however, and in part because of the uncertainty element, the strong tendency is still *not* to tell.

Patients' attitudes

Patients' attitudes are complex. Most patients harbour suspicions. Thus, Hinton (1980) interviewed patients in the 10 weeks prior to death and found that:

- 66% recognized death as a possibility;
- 8% were non-committal;
- 26% talked only of recovery.

In some studies two-thirds did not *really* want their suspicions confirmed and most wanted only messages that reinforced an optimistic view of their condition. These are of course generalities in the very individual experience of dying. Other interesting generalizations have been made about the so-called *awareness patterns* and *stages of dying* (Table 5.8).

Table 5.8 Patterns of dying.

The four awareness patterns	
1 Closed awareness	The patient does not recognize death, although everyone else does
2 Suspected awareness	The patient suspects that others know and tries to confirm it
3 Mutual pretence	All sides know but pretend the others do not
4 Open awareness	Everyone knows and openly admits it

Stages of dying (Kubler Ross 1970)	
1 Denial and isolation	Shocked and numbed: 'It can't be me'; 'It's a mistake'; intense isolation
2 Anger	'Why me?' Anger may be displaced or projected on to staff
3 Bargaining	A phase of good behaviour to try and postpone death
4 Reactive depression	Due to physical suffering or impending loss (of health, life, family, etc.)
5 Acceptance	

The place of death

Increasingly death has been removed from the community and hospitalized. However, much of the terminal illness is still spent usefully at home, e.g.:

- Ward (1974) found in 279 cancer deaths the mean stay in hospital was only 8.7 days.

Home care is still considered natural and preferable to the majority of patients, relatives and families, once they share the problem. Prior to this they often experience various worries in isolation:

1 The patient often prefers the home but worries that he will be a burden.

2 The relatives often prefer the home but worry they will be unable to cope.

3 The GP prefers the home but worries about both these things!

It *is* a balanced judgement since good-quality terminal care depends on:

1 Available resources (GP time, nursing time, aids and appliances, the ability to provide 24-h care).

2 The nature of the problem.

3 The attitudes of patient and carers.

Communications

During terminal illness patients, families and doctors tend to endure unpleasant feelings which they fail to share and which hinder effective communication.

The patient's feelings

Common reactions are:

1 *Anxiety*:

(a) for himself ('What is it like? Will there be pain and suffering? Will I lose control?');

(b) for his family ('Will they cope? Will they suffer and feel abandoned?');

(c) about his disease (ignorance and fear of the unknown).

This anxiety is totally understandable, but it may also become maladaptive and hence pathological.

2 *Depression*: a mourning reaction for loss of health, life, family, station, etc.

3 *Anger*:

(a) 'Why me? Can't the doctors do more?';

(b) frustration born of impotence;

(c) anger displaced on to the family or medical staff.

4 *Guilt*: at letting dependants down or being a burden.

5 *Denial*: 'There's been a mistake; I need a second opinion'.

6 *Dependence and regression*.

7 *Bewilderment* and the search for meaning.

8 *Withdrawal*.

9 *Paranoia*: patients who cannot cope with 'I'm dying' sometimes substitute 'They're killing me'.

10 *Isolation*, loneliness and loss of worth.

Family problems

1 All of the reactions felt by the patient may be experienced by the relatives in their own right or observed in their loved-one. Inevitably they cause distress, particularly the upsetting tendency of some patients to withdraw from their family.

2 Attempts from both sides to protect their loved-ones from stress actually exacerbate the situation: deceipt and tension disrupt family bonds.

3 Relatives particularly feel the sense of impotence and frustration.

4 A long terminal illness is exhausting.

5 Bereavement forces new roles on to the survivors.

6 Guilt feelings are very common:
   (a) guilt if illness occurs at a juncture when relationships were strained;
   (b) guilt in wanting a terminal illness to end;
   (c) guilt because of the human but selfish tendency to dwell most on one's own problems, etc.

7 Practical problems:
   (a) financial hardship;
   (b) time off work;
   (c) loss of the family driver, etc.

The doctor's problems

1 Should I tell?
   (a) does the patient really want to know?
   (b) do the relatives agree?
   (c) will they cope with the information?
   (d) if I hold back and don't tell, it will be hard to live the lie; and what will happen to my relationship with patient and family when the truth can no longer be hidden?

2 Do I really know?
   (a) uncertainty of diagnosis;
   (b) uncertainty of prognosis.

3 Can *I* cope? Terminal illness highlights to doctors:
   (a) their own failure and impotence;
   (b) their own mortality.

It also brings out their own defence mechanisms, e.g. *avoidance* by:
- the detached scientific approach;
- limiting contact to ritualistic conversational gambits;
- false cheeriness.

On top of these psychological problems there are the physical ones like:
- symptom control;
- 24-h availability;
- resource provision (aids, nursing time, access to a hospice, bereavement follow-up).

Management of death and the dying

The *objectives* of care are to:
- promote the patient's self-esteem (emphasize value and role);
- promote the patient's emotional comfort (relieve anxiety, depression and guilt);
- promote mutually supporting family relationships.

Needless to say these objectives are easier said than done and

require a deft touch, but certain management pointers are probably valid:

1 Listen to the patient:
   (a) this shows the patient he is valid (understood and not
   abandoned);
   (b) it allows him to ventilate unpleasant feelings (anger, frustration, guilt, shame, fear);
   (c) it enables the GP to gain a sense of what the patient knows
   and what he wants to know.
2 Encourage him to retain his role and responsibilities and to
participate in decision-making. This emphasizes he still has worth
and importance, undiminished by illness. Try to preserve his
dignity above all.
3 Work with the family:
   (a) encourage openness;
   (b) promote insight into the family's own feelings and those of
   their loved-one;
   (c) allow the family to vent their feelings;
   (d) encourage family care where this is possible;
   (e) prepare the family members for their new roles and
   responsibilities;
4 Control physical symptoms.
5 Remember practical problems; for example, if the patient is the
family breadwinner, financial hardship may require the social
worker's attention.

Bereavement
Normal grief
Normal grief reactions are said to encompass the phases of:
1 Shock; numbness; blunted emotion; incomprehension (this
lasts up to 2 weeks).
2 Physical distress; restlessness; withdrawal and grief. At this
stage the dead person is to all intents and purposes still with
them, to the point that the bereaved person may search for the
departed, set the table for him, talk to him, hear his footsteps
and even see him. There is a preoccupation with memories and
idealization and emotional reactions (depression, insomnia,
anorexia, guilt) are common.
3 Gradually a more realistic memory develops, depression lifts
and a process of disengagement occurs.
   Normal grief reactions last up to 6 months.

Abnormal grief
Abnormal grieving is said to apply when:
• grieving is prolonged (more than 6 months);
• the *intensity* of depression is extreme (patients who isolate

themselves from family and friends, take a lot of time off work, attempt suicide).

Post-bereavement mortality
Bereavement has a mortality which Parkes highlighted in his classical studies:
- morbidity and mortality are high in the first year and raised even after 2–3 years;
- widowers aged 55 years or more have an increased mortality of about 40% in the first 6 months and overall 20% of widowers die in the first year compared with 4% of matched controls;
- men are affected more than women and the risk for close relationships is greater than for distant ones.

Management of bereavement
The management of bereavement really begins with the preceding terminal illness:
- ensuring the family members are prepared and recognize their new enforced roles;
- making the terminal illness as painless as possible by promoting harmony, comfort and mutual support;
- encouraging family care: the family should be there at the end and see the body afterwards.

Afterwards the GP must be an available and sympathetic ear. A desire to vent feelings and to search for meaning are common sequelae, as are visits with emotional problems and minor ill-health. Close contact with the family also allows the pathological grief reaction to be recognized at an earlier stage. Referral to a self-help organization (e.g. The Compassionate Friends or Cruse) may be valuable.

Cot deaths

Cot deaths are a particular variant of the 'death and dying' theme which deserve special attention in their own right, and are a topical examination subject.

Cot death or sudden infant death syndrome (SIDS) has been defined as the sudden unexpected death of an infant or young child unexplained by post-mortem.

Epidemiology
1 There are about 1200 cases per year, i.e. approximately 2 per 1000 live births or one case for a GP every 2 years on average. It is therefore quite common, in fact the third commonest cause of death in the first 14 years of life in England and Wales after postnatal conditions and congenital abnormalities.
2 Relative risk is increased by:
(a) racial characteristics (e.g. it is more common in American Blacks; less common in Israelis);

(b) birth order (50% are second-born children, 25% first and 25% third or later);

(c) genetic similarity (the risk in twins is doubled and thought to be increased three to four times if a sibling has already died of it).

It also depends on:

(d) time of year (70% of SIDS occur between October and March);

(e) the child's age (nearly 80% occur between 1 and 6 months);

(f) the child's sex (by a slight margin: the male:female ratio is 1.4:1.0).

3 All social classes are affected but it is more common in the illegitimate and the poorly housed.

Aetiology

Aetiological theories are numerous and include:

- sleep apnoea;
- central nervous system immaturity;
- an abnormal larynx;
- minor viral infections;
- abnormal surfactant;
- febrile apnoea due to overheating;
- a fear-paralysis reflex;
- metabolic disorders;
- postulated toxins from PVC matresses.

'Near-miss' infants often show prolonged bradycardias, apnoea and autonomic dysfunction when subsequently studied.

Recent studies have focused on explaining the ethnic variations in incidence. In particular it has been suggested that lying babies supine rather than prone before sleep allows them to radiate more body heat in sleep (accounting for the low incidence of SIDS in Hong Kong where the practice is common). The exact cause of SIDS, however, eludes precise definition. Many believe it to be multifactorial and research, as ever, continues.

Supportive management in a case of SIDS

Questioned afterwards, 70% of people say initial GP support was good, but 30% say they found no real support and 10% claim that no contact was made at all.

Initial management includes:

1 Confirming death.

2 Offering sympathy and allowing venting of feelings.

3 Advising:

(a) the cause is unknown;

(b) the parents are *not* to blame;

(c) police enquiry and a post-mortem are painful but inevitable.

4 Making arrangements:

(a) the removal of the body;

(b) an anxiolytic?

(c) the care of the siblings;

(d) a follow-up visit.

Follow-up care includes:

1 Being available as a counsellor.

2 Monitoring the grief response.

3 Advising on post-mortem findings, on SIDS, on support groups, etc.

4 Referring the family to a paediatrician for counselling (do siblings need an apnoea monitor?).

5 Fostering a positive attitude to further pregnancies.

6 Attention to detail, e.g.:

(a) 5% receive immunization appointments for their dead child;

(b) remember the siblings: a high percentage undergo grief reactions, often manifesting as behavioural problems.

7 Referral to the Foundation for the Study of Infant Deaths.

6 Social Diseases

This chapter considers a number of conditions that are all produced by modern patterns of social behaviour. They are:
- smoking;
- alcohol abuse;
- obesity;
- drug abuse (including the misuse of tranquillizers);
- child abuse;
- acquired immune deficiency syndrome (AIDS).

These social diseases form an important proportion of the modern doctor's workload and are important exam topics.

6.1 SMOKING

The problem
Smoking is:
- responsible for 50 000–100 000 deaths per year with an average reduction in life expectancy of 10 years;
- the single greatest cause of premature death (e.g. 90% of lung cancer deaths and 75% of chronic bronchitis deaths in men under 65 years);
- the number one preventable cause of ill health (World Health Organization definition).

The overall cost to the NHS of smoking-related illness in 1984 was around £370 M.

The known medical health *risks* are summarized in Table 6.1. The *benefits* of stopping smoking are equally clearcut: all risks are significantly reduced and this effect is particularly rapid in the case of ischaemic heart disease.

Changing patterns
Recognition of the risk–benefit situation is slowly gaining ground and is reflected in the changing pattern of cigarette smoking.

1 More people are giving up (e.g. smoking among men aged 16 years or over fell from 52 to 35% between 1972 and 1986, and amongst women in the same age group from 41 to 31% (*Social Trends* 1989).

The effect is largely class-related, e.g.:
(a) in the 1960s smoking was equally common in all social classes; now it is three times less common in class 1 than class 5;
(b) 80% of doctors do not smoke (40% are ex-smokers).

Table 6.1 Medical health risks of cigarette smoking.

To the patient	To others
Lung cancer	*To the fetus*: growth retardation *in utero*
Cancers of oropharynx and bladder	*To the infant/young child*: recurrent upper respiratory tract infections
Bronchitis and emphysema	*To the child in later life*: a greater likelihood of smoking (because of parental example)
Ischaemic heart disease	
Peripheral arterial disease	
Aggravation of peptic ulceration	*To innocent bystanders*: risk from passive smoking

2   Health-conscious public attitudes and legislation have:
   (a) reduced the tar yields on all cigarettes;
   (b) increased the proportion of filtered cigarettes to more than 90%;
   (c) banned the overt advertising of tobacco on TV;
   (d) expanded the non-smoking facilities in public places.
3   In surveys:
   (a) at least 70% of smokers have tried to give up at least once;
   (b) 80% claim they 'would if told'.
In some countries (e.g. Norway) all tobacco advertising has been banned by law, a stance supported by overwhelming public opinion.
4   However, among older schoolchildren 31% of boys and 28% of girls are regular smokers by their final year.

Continuing obstacles
Political barriers
Political barriers are still considerable however:
1   Biting legislation is unlikely because of its unpopularity with a sizeable voting faction of the public.
2   Tobacco taxes raise a revenue of £5000 M in the UK and 50 000 people are employed in the tobacco industry.
3   Tobacco lobbies are very influential.
4   Tobacco companies spend more on promoting cigarettes than the anti-smoking lobby could ever raise to oppose them. Covert sponsorship advertising also still operates, circumventing TV restrictions.
5   While it is true that considerable savings could be made by the NHS if there were less smoking-induced disease, it is also likely that pension expenditure would have to rise if effective no-smoking policies were pursued.

Personal barriers
Personal barriers are no less important. As discussed in Section 3.1, before surrendering their cigarettes people carry out a personal cost−benefit appraisal. Amongst the sacrifices they count:

- the pleasurable pharmacological effects of cigarettes and their anxiolytic qualities;
- the social role they fulfil (relaxation rituals, social activities performed in groups, conversation fillers);
- the unpleasant withdrawal craving they face.

Appraisal of benefits depends on *knowledge* and *objectivity*. Some people are genuinely ignorant of the relative magnitude of risks in their life ('I'm just as likely to be knocked over'), and the health benefit of giving up ('It's too late now: the damage is done'). Others are not receptive to objective information: they belong to the fatalist school, the 'will of Allah' school or the 'someone else's problem' school.

What can the GP do?

Fowler (1982) proposed the following plan for GPs:

1 Record every patient's smoking habits in the notes.
2 Use every opportunity to advise them on how to stop and reasons why they should.
3 Supplement advice with a leaflet (e.g. the GUS or Give Up Smoking kit).
4 Follow up the patient's attempts.

Advice should cover certain basic ground:

- the health hazards of smoking;
- the benefits of giving up (and not just on lifespan but on quality of life, social acceptability and bank balance!);
- possible coping strategies (Table 6.2);
- formulating a plan, starting date and review interval.

Table 6.2 Some coping strategies for those giving up smoking.

1 Recruit a fellow and tell other people. Enlist family support
2 Avoid others who smoke
3 Record all cigarettes: where, why and whether enjoyed. Much smoking is habitual: cut out first the cigarettes smoked by rote and not really enjoyed
4 Look for alternative activities: something to nibble or chew; occupying the hands with something; relaxation exercises; deep breathing or yoga
5 Three commonly tried patterns of withdrawal are:
(a) the saturation method: smoking 2–3 times the usual amount for 2–3 days, until thoroughly sick of smoking
(b) the sudden withdrawal approach
(c) the gradual withdrawal approach: one cigarette less each day or taking the first cigarette 1 h later each day
6 Nicorette chewing gum

Does advice help?

Russell *et al.* (1979) found that advice given as part of a routine consultation (and supplemented with leaflet and warning of follow-up) persuaded about 5% of smokers to give up. This does not sound a great deal, but with more than 600 smokers per GP's average list this would represent 500 000 people per year if the effort were made nationwide.

Does Nicorette chewing gum help?
Controversially Nicorette is not available on NHS prescription, since the Advisory Committee on Borderline Substances advised that it is 'not a drug'. It is thought to act by relieving the withdrawal effects due to nicotine dependence. Early trials (e.g. Raw *et al.* 1980) were very impressive. Recent studies from specialist smoking clinics suggest 47–50% initial success rates. Nicorette:
● was better than placebo in five trials;
● produced blood levels of nicotine and fewer withdrawal effects.

Long-term abstinence seems to depend on the degree of support:
● with intensive specialist support it is 27%;
● with minimal GP support and some follow-up 21%;
● with minimal GP advice and no follow-up 10% (in some studies lower, say 4–9%).

It is difficult to translate the results obtained on the highly motivated clientele of specialist smoking clinics into everyday experience where motivation levels are often lower, and there are a lack of controlled trials in the ordinary general practice setting. Nevertheless, a case can be made for making Nicorette available on the FP 10 prescription, particularly since we are in the paradoxical position of being able to prescribe on the NHS for other forms of addiction (e.g. Heminevrin for the alcoholic, and methadone for the drug addict).

6.2 ALCOHOL ABUSE

Size of the problem
1 7.5% of consumer outlay goes towards buying alcohol (equivalent to 9 pints per adult each week, and over £10 000 M annually).
2 According to the Office of Population Censuses and Surveys:
   (a) 0.4% of the population are alcohol-dependent;
   (b) 2% have alcohol problems;
   (c) 8% are heavy drinkers.
3 Wilkins (1974) interviewed patients from general practice with at-risk characteristics, and found in a practice of 12 000:
   (a) 250 'abnormal drinkers' (2%);
   (b) 155 problem drinkers or addicts (1.3%).
4 Already alcohol is responsible for 5000–10 000 premature deaths per year, and all evidence indicates the problem is increasing, e.g.:

Table 6.3 Harmful effects of alcohol abuse:
(a) Physical.

System affected	Complication	Comment
Gastrointestinal	Carcinoma of the oesophagus	Increased threefold
	Carcinoma of the oropharynx	Increased fourfold
	Oesophageal varices	
	Peptic ulceration	
	Gastritis	
Hepatobiliary	Cirrhosis	Deaths from this increased 10-fold
	Alcoholic hepatitis	In 10–30% of cases
	Pancreatitis	25% of all causes
Neurological	Peripheral neuropathy	In 10% of cases
	Convulsions	In 10% of cases
	Korsakoff's psychosis	
	'Brain damage'	?in 40–50% on computerized tomography scanning
	Alcohol withdrawal reactions	
Cardiac	Alcoholic cardiomyopathy	
Respiratory	Pneumonia and tuberculosis	
Metabolic	Obesity	
	Vitamin deficiencies	Especially thiamine
Fetus	Fetal Alcohol Syndrome	

(b) Psychological and social.

Problem	Comment
Depression and suicide	Eightyfold increase in men; the overall risk is about 15%
Sexual problems	
Family and marital	High incidence of divorce and wife-battering
Employment problems	e.g. two and a half times as many working days lost
Accidents	Common, e.g. one-third of fatal driver accidents involve alcohol abuse
Crime	

(a) beer drinking has increased 45% since 1960 and the consumption of wine and spirits respectively by 290 and 135%;
(b) first admission rates with primary diagnosis of alcoholism rose from 2000 in 1952 to 10 167 in 1972;
(c) convictions for being drunk and disorderly have increased 28% in England and Wales and 91% in Scotland from 1960 to 1975.

5 Only the tip of the iceberg has been recognized: in some studies one-fifth of 'healthy' men attending screening programmes have abnormal LFTs, and probably one in 10 heavy drinkers is known in general practice.

The physical, psychological and social problems associated with alcohol abuse are summarized in Table 6.3. Several points are worth emphasizing:

1 Alcohol withdrawal is a serious and unpleasant condition, comprising tremor, nausea, insomnia, sweating, mood disturbance, hallucinations, hyperacusis, perceptual disturbances and convulsions.

2 Alcohol abuse probably causes brain damage long before gross deficits are seen: computerized tomography scans show sulcal widening/ventricular enlargement in 40–50% of apparently unimpaired male alcoholics.

3 Alcohol abuse affects more than one generation: children grow up in an environment affected by social, family and marital strife and are more likely to become or marry an alcoholic themselves; alcoholism in pregnancy may produce a baby suffering from the fetal alcohol syndrome, the risks of which are

(a) 17% neonatal mortality;

(b) mental subnormality and poor growth;

(c) craniofacial, limb and cardiovascular defects;

(d) premature delivery.

Identifying the problem drinker

GPs are well placed for spotting problem drinkers since two-thirds of their patients see them in a year, nearly 90% in 5 years, and the alcoholic probably sees his GP twice as often as other patients. Acres (1979) has highlighted several other advantages the GP has in this respect:

1 A long-standing and detailed knowledge of many of his patients and their families.

2 An opportunity to observe changes in behaviour, attitudes and attendance patterns.

3 A chance to visit and see the patient's home environment.

Barriers to recognition of the problem drinker

1 *Definitions.* There is no acceptable and universal definition of alcoholism, problem drinking or alcohol abuse, and no uniformity of opinion on 'safe' drinking levels:

(a) the working party of the Royal College of Psychiatrists (1979) recommended an upper limit of 56 units per week for both sexes;

(b) the Health Education Council (1983) recommended 21 units per week for men and 14 units per week for women;

(c) Anderson (1984) distributed a questionnaire to 70 people engaged in alcohol research, asking 'What is safe?': answers varied from less than 7 units per week to a maximum of 55 units per week.

If expert advice is so contradictory, is it so surprising GPs find difficulty in recommending limits to their patients?

2   *GPs' attitudes.* There are many problems:

(a) on average GPs themselves consume more than they should (standardized mortality ratio from cirrhosis 311) so they may not be best placed to advise;

(b) GPs often lack the experience of handling problem drinkers, and the sensitive counselling skills needed have been neglected in traditional medical school training;

(c) it is easier to avoid potential conflict and embarrassment in a consultation which is, in any case, too short to deal with the problem;

(d) alcoholism will be exacting to deal with; problems will be difficult and time-consuming; GPs are generally pessimistic about outcome; and alcoholics are help-rejecting complainers which leaves most GPs feeling helpless and frustrated;

(e) doctors are taught at medical school to distrust the drinking history they obtain: given a sensitive line of questioning and dubious returns it is simpler not to ask;

(f) the diagnosis is not straightforward: vague and protean patterns confuse the unwary, and making a connection between apparently unrelated events requires a methodical record system (when often there is none).

3   *Patients' attitudes.* Patients face many problems in common with their doctor:

(a) ignorance regarding safe drinking levels;

(b) a variety of vague effects that may not be linked with alcohol;

(c) psychological barriers (anxiety, guilt, shame, embarrassment) that result in denial;

(d) the perception of negative, censorious or uninterested attitudes in the family doctor;

(e) underestimation of true consumption: due to tolerance or cognitive impairment (if volunteers drink in simulated restaurant surroundings, the heaviest drinkers tend subsequently to underestimate their drinking by up to 12%).

4   *The unknown drinker.* Not all problem drinkers present to their doctors:

(a) teenagers may be better known to the police;

(b) professional people in competitive jobs may drink away from home;

(c) the elderly may drink in complete isolation.

The tools of detection

Unfortunately there is another barrier to detection: the absence of a cast-iron diagnostic test. The main tools of detection are:

1 *The honest question*: useful only if you get an honest answer back.

2 *Blood tests*: these are markers, but they are not particularly sensitive and have a high false-positive rate (Table 6.4).

Table 6.4 The value of gamma glutamyl transferase (γGT) and mean corpuscular volume (MCV) in assessing alcohol consumption (Chick *et al.* 1981).

	γGT ⩾ 50 iu/l	MCV ⩾ 98 fl	Both raised
True positives (men drinking more than 56 units/week)	50%	23–32%	62%
False positives (men drinking less than 56 units/week)	15%	5%	11.5–22.0%

3 *CAGE and MAST questionnaires*: these simple questionnaires are reproduced in Table 6.5. Their advantage is that they are quick, simple to administer and generally well received. Mayfield *et al.* (1974) have shown they have a useful discriminating power, greater in fact than the best laboratory tests. Thus:

  (a) the brief MAST questionnaire (scores ⩾6) has a sensitivity of 85% and a specificity of 86%;

  (b) the CAGE test (scores ⩾2) has a sensitivity of 93% and a specificity of 76% (Bernadt *et al.* 1982).

(It is likely, despite the value of these quick, convenient screening questionnaires, that they are little used in general practice; a small personal straw poll of local training practices indicated that very few trainers, principals and trainees knew, even in general terms, what problem the questionnaires addressed.)

4 *Postal questionnaires*. Potential shortcomings of this type of screening are:

  (a) the possibility of a poor response rate;

  (b) the administrative cost and effort;

  (c) the validity of the results: the main fear being that the people most in need of help are the least likely to respond honestly.

In practice, however, the postal questionnaire is surprisingly effective. Wallace and Haines (1985) distributed a postal questionnaire to 3000 patients in practices in North-West London asking:

  (a) whether people felt they had a drink problem;

  (b) for an estimate of drinking levels;

  (c) the questions of the CAGE screening test.

Table 6.5 The CAGE and MAST questionnaires:

(a) The CAGE questionnaire (Mayfield *et al.* 1974).

Have you ever felt you ought to **C**ut down on your drinking?
Have people **A**nnoyed you by criticizing your drinking?
Have you ever felt bad or **G**uilty about your drinking?
Have you ever had a drink first thing in the morning to steady your
    nerves or get rid of a hangover (**E**ye-opener)?

(b) The brief MAST questionnaire (Pokorny *et al.* 1972).

	Circle correct answer	
Do you feel you are a normal drinker?	Yes	No (2 pts)
Do relatives or friends think you are a normal drinker?	Yes	No (2 pts)
Have you ever attended a meeting of Alcoholics Anonymous?	Yes (5 pts)	No
Have you ever lost friends because of drinking?	Yes (2 pts)	No
Have you ever got into trouble at work because of drink?	Yes (2 pts)	No
Have you ever neglected your obligations, your family, or your work for 2 or more days in a row through drink?	Yes (2 pts)	No
Have you ever had delirium tremens (DTs), severe shaking, heard voices, or seen things that were not there after heavy drinking?	Yes (5 pts)	No
Have you ever gone to anyone for help about your drinking?	Yes (5 pts)	No
Have you ever been in hospital because of your drinking?	Yes (5 pts)	No
Have you ever been arrested for drunken driving?	Yes (2 pts)	No

Total score:

Positive responders were people who thought they had a drink problem, who gave at least two positive CAGE responses, or who admitted a consumption in excess of 42 units per week for men, or 21 units per week for women. Responders attended for further discussion and estimations of mean corpuscular volume, gamma glutamyl transferase and breath alcohol. They found that:

(a) the response rate was 72%;

(b) 7% of men and 3% of women expressed concern and thought they might have an alcohol problem;

(c) 10% of the practice were identified as positive responders: a substantial number of these were previously unknown;

(d) postal questionnaires were a viable alternative to other screening methods, with a high degree of sensitivity and specificity amongst respondents.

5 *The GP's checklist.* Many authors argue that early recognition of problem drinking depends on a low index of suspicion, and that

Table 6.6 Wilkins' suggested at-risk indicators for detecting alcoholism (after Wilkins 1974).

Categories	Subcategories	
Physical diseases	Pancreatitis, cirrhosis, peptic ulcer, gastritis, peripheral neuritis, tuberculosis, congestive cardiac failure (unknown origin), epilepsy (for the first time after age of 25 years), malnutrition/obesity, haematemesis/melaena	
Mental diseases	Anxiety, depression, attempted suicide, other psychiatric illnesses, sexual problems	
Symptoms of alcohol addiction	Morning shakes, blackouts/memory loss, delirium tremens, hallucinations, fugue states, morbid jealousy, withdrawal fits	
Blood tests	Mean corpuscular volume ≥ 98 fl, gamma glutamyl transferase ≥ 50 iu/l	
Occupations	Liver cirrhosis mortality (standardized mortality ratio, average = 100)	
	Publicans and innkeepers	1576
	Ships' officers	781
	Barmen, barmaids	633
	Fishermen	595
	Hotel proprietors	506
	Restaurateurs	385
	Medical practitioners	311
Work problems	Three or more jobs (over the last year), multiple short spells of absenteeism (over the last year), dubious sick note requests	
Accidents	e.g. road traffic accidents, accidents at work and at home	
Criminal offences	e.g. drunk and disorderly, drink–driving convictions	
Family and marital problems Marital status	Single males ≥ 40 years, married ≥ once, divorced or separated	
Family history of alcohol abuse		
Smelling of alcohol in the consultation		

GPs should be armed with a checklist of common alcohol presentations that prompt closer enquiry. Wilkins (1974) suggests an alcohol at-risk register based on a series of at-risk indicators (Table 6.6). Using his checklist, Wilkins noted in 1 year that 5% of his adult population consulted with one of the at-risk characteristics. Of these 546 patients, 28% were found to have alcohol-related problems or addiction, while the incidence in control patients was only 3%.

Several simple recommendations bear consideration for the GP who wishes to undertake screening:

1 It is feasible on an opportunistic basis to ask all patients about their drinking habits and to record them in the notes. The notes can then be tagged with the date of enquiry and the line of questioning repeated after an agreed interval. The aim should be 100% knowledge.

2 Self-administered questionnaires have a high response rate and yield about 10% of people expressing concern about their level of drinking. At present no tool of detection is much better than this, and the advantage to the GP is that patient self-administration makes no inroads into GP time, excepting of course the problems unearthed.

3 The CAGE and MAST questionnaires are quick, simple and fairly accurate screens, easily administered by nursing staff (e.g. in the context of a well-person clinic).

4 Practices could benefit from an at-risk checklist and register.

Is screening for alcoholism worthwhile?

In general, changing a patient's behaviour is one of the least rewarding areas of practice in terms of effort and returns. GPs are particularly pessimistic when it comes to the alcoholic, so is there any point to screening?

Available data tend to deal only with severely dependent individuals for whom the prognosis is clearly bad. However, detection at the earlier predependent, heavy drinking stage is more rewarding. Several studies suggest screening for problem drinking *can* be rewarding (Table 6.7). Furthermore a well known study by Edwards *et al.* (1977) comparing intensive conventional treatment (Alcoholics Anonymous referral, psychiatrists, social workers, drugs to cover withdrawal, etc.) with simple advice (and no significant follow-up) found no significant difference between the two groups at 12 months, suggesting that GPs do not require extensive time and facilities to help.

If we do not seek, we will not find. It is likely in the management of alcohol-related problems that the best dividends are realized when detection is early.

6.3 OBESITY

The problem

Obesity is measured in a variety of ways including:
- simple weight measurements;
- corrected weight (weight as a percentage of ideal weight for similar height, age, sex and build: 'ideal' according to insurance data);

Table 6.7 Studies of prognosis in alcohol abusers.

Study	Format	Results
Vaillant (1980)	456 Bostonian teenagers followed over 35 years	110 developed symptoms of abuse, but of these: • 48 later achieved abstinence for at least 1 year; • 22 returned to social drinking
Polich (1980)	758 men admitted to an American alcohol unit — a 4-year follow-up	14% had died. Of the survivors: • 28% were abstainers; • 18% were non-problem drinkers
Pollak (1978)	69 alcohol-dependent patients given several short therapeutic sessions. Independent assessment by relatives and a research worker	19% were sober at 2 years; 45% had 'improved'. Only three patients had sought help other than from the family doctor in that time
Costello (1975)	Analysed the results of 58 other studies involving 11 000 patients	After 1 year: • 1% were dead; • 25% had no current problem; • 53% were drinking continuously; • 21% were lost to follow-up

Table 6.8 Classification of body weight using the body mass index.

Weight:height ratio	Category
20	Underweight
20–24.9	Normal (grade 0)
25–29.9	Overweight/plump (grade I)
30–39.9	Moderate obesity (grade II)
40+	Severe obesity (grade III)

• skinfold thickness.

The preferred method for classifying body weight is the Quetelet index or body mass index. This is calculated by dividing weight (in kilograms) by the square of height (in metres; Table 6.8).

However it is measured, many people are overweight:

• at least 30% of adults are 10% or more overweight;
• 10% of children are overweight;
• on an average GP's list more than 300 individuals have a weight problem;

- at any one time 65% of British women and 30% of British men are trying to lose weight.

The risk to *mortality* has formerly been exaggerated; it increases only when men are more than 25% over ideal weight and women more than 30%. However, there is a considerable *morbidity* due to mechanical and metabolic effects (Table 6.9). *Psychological sequelae* are also common in this stigmatizing condition.

Table 6.9 Morbidity attributable to obesity.

Osteoarthritis — hips and knees; backache; flat feet	Abdominal surgery: postoperative difficulties with deep venous thromboses, pulmonary embolisms, chest infections, wound dehiscence, etc.
Impaired respiratory function; chronic bronchitis	
Reduced exercise capacity (fitness)	Childbirth: more chance of pre-eclamptic toxaemia, fetal loss, postpartum haemorrhage; reduced fertility
Varicose veins; varicose ulcers	Diabetes
Haemorrhoids	Gout
Gallstones	Coronary artery disease
Diverticulitis	Cirrhosis
Ventral hernias	Hypertension
Increased risk of carcinomas of colon, breast and uterine body	Psychological problems: teased, ridiculed, and treated by society as the model of unattractiveness

Aetiological theories

Many theories have been put forward including:

1 Psychological/behavioural models, e.g.:
   (a) emotional conflicts in childhood;
   (b) inability to distinguish the arousal of hunger from fear, anger, anxiety;
   (c) food received as a reward in childhood;
   (d) learning to eat by the clock and leave the plate clean;
   (e) eating when bored, lonely or miserable.
2 Social models, e.g.:
   (a) the 20th century diet — over-rich in refined carbohydrates and fats;
   (b) lack of exercise due to 20th century transport and labour-saving tools.
3 Developmental/biochemical models, e.g.:
   (a) a disturbance in the long-term weight control system of the hypothalamus;
   (b) an increase in the number of brown fat cells inherited;
   (c) the perpetuation of childhood obesity.

As usual when there are many theories to choose from, no one is entirely satisfactory.

Management

The pros and cons of whether a self-limiting minor disorder like obesity should occupy medical time are discussed elsewhere (see Section 4.3).

Assuming treatment is undertaken, the major options are: dietary advice and counselling; exercise; drug therapy; behavioural methods; group therapy and alternative medicine-type approaches.

1 *Dietary advice.* This consists largely of common sense measures, e.g.:

  (a) using artificial sweeteners;

  (b) choosing the low-calorie version where available (low-calorie drinks, low-fat cheese, skimmed milk, etc.);

  (c) increasing fruit and vegetable intake;

  (d) substituting white meat for red, wholemeal flour for white, and grilling for frying;

  (e) cutting out snacks, nibbles and notoriously high-fat foods.

2 *Exercise.* This has been under-rated as a method of weight reduction, since calculations based on their respective calorie equivalents suggest that considerable exercise produces only modest fat losses. However, we now know that after exercise the basal metabolic rate may be raised for several hours, so that true weight loss is probably greater.

3 *Drug treatment.* Appetite suppressants are now much out of favour because of their potential hazards, in particular the risk of addiction. In general, they should:

  (a) never be used in patients with known addiction/drug abuse tendencies;

  (b) only be used in the plateau phase when the rate of weight loss has slowed;

  (c) only then be used for a limited period to aid motivation, prescribing an exact number of tablets, and with regular (e.g. 2-weekly) review.

4 *Behavioural methods.* The main reason for failure to diet successfully is failed motivation. Various behaviour-modifying tips have been suggested to help maintain the all-important motivation element, e.g.:

  (a) eat only when hungry;

  (b) leave food on the plate;

  (c) use a smaller plate, knife and fork;

  (d) be last to start and last to finish;

  (e) eat only at the table and then leave it;

  (f) keep food out of sight;

  (g) keep a record;

  (h) have a reward system.

5 *Group therapy.* This also depends on the principle of stimulating motivation. Weight-watching groups use devices like:

(a) competitions, prizes, rewards or fines;

(b) pairing of individuals for mutual support;

(c) the example of successful group leaders.

They claim a better-than-average success rate.

6   *Starvation and very low calorie diets (VLCDs)*. Starvation has been used for many years under medical supervision in the treatment of massive obesity. It is no longer considered acceptable because:

(a) sudden unexpected deaths have occurred linked to K^+ depletion;

(b) weight loss in starvation is 50% fat and 50% lean (fat-free), whereas the excess weight comprises 75% fat and 25% lean: the inappropriate loss of lean in starvation lowers metabolic rate, making it harder to sustain weight loss. (Crash diets and self-imposed semi-starvation suffer the same drawback.)

VLCDs (diets supplying less than 600 kcal/day) have become popular of late. They are formulated to be nutritionally complete except for energy, and produce rapid weight loss with minimal loss of lean. However, concern has been expressed regarding their safety and efficacy. The Committee on Medical Aspects of Food Policy (COMA) report (1987) recommended that they were not a preferred option for weight loss, and were particularly unsuitable for people with a relatively small amount of weight to lose (body mass index <30), for children, the elderly and pregnant women.

Prognosis

The overall success rate is disappointing:

- on average about 1–12%;
- with *no* evidence that GPs are any more successful than anyone else (indeed weight-watching groups claim a 30% success rate).

6.4 DRUG ABUSE

The scale of the problem

Home Office notifications are rising, with a trend towards multiple drug abuse; for example, in 1960 there were 437 registered opiate users, but in 1978 the figure was 4122.

This is probably the tip of the iceberg:

- one-third of addicts attending Accident and Emergency departments are not officially registered;
- if solvent abuse (perhaps tried by one in five London schoolchildren) is included, the problem is huge.

The price of illicit heroin has increased 15- to 35-fold over 10 years.

Epidemiology and aetiology

1   *Sex*. Male to female ratio is 4:1.

2   *Age*. The peak is 20–35 years of age.

3 *Social class*. All social classes in the UK.
4 *Associations*. There is a higher chance of:
(a) family disharmony;
(b) alcoholism;
(c) peer group pressures and imitative behaviour;
(d) ready availability (witness the problem in the medical profession!).

These associated circumstances are thought to play a part in the *aetiology*. Reinforcement of drug-taking behaviour is then obtained from the stimulating or sedating properties of the drug.

Drugs of addiction can be subdivided according to their properties into stimulants, depressants and hallucinogens: *physical* dependence is a feature of the depressant group.

Detection
Recognition of drug abusers in general practice depends on a high index of suspicion and sensitive history-taking.

Physical clues
Nausea, malaise, sweating, stupor, constipation, pinpoint pupils, ataxia (the exact constellation depending on the drug abused); and other external signs, e.g. self-neglect, needle marks, facial/perioral rash (solvent abusers).

Psychological and social clues
Moodiness, irritability and personality change, inappropriate euphoria, confusion, hallucinosis and psychosis, furtiveness, drug-seeking behaviour, unexplained debts, criminal behaviour, parental concern ('something is wrong').

Legal obligations placed on the GP
See Section 7.2.

Management of drug abuse
The management of drug abuse requires expertise. Legal restraints on the prescribing of certain drugs and the inadvisability of blindly prescribing others pose some practical constraints on GP involvement. Nevertheless, the GP is, as always, able to offer support and counselling and referral as indicated. The ingredients of a treatment programme include:
1 The therapeutic contract (what is on the table and why; the duration and conditions).
2 The treatment of withdrawal symptoms (for depressant drugs).
3 Non-prescribing support (for stimulant drugs).
4 Long-term maintenance (under specialist supervision).
5 Specialist services — group and individual psychotherapy; social skills retraining and work rehabilitation; family/marital therapy; rehabilitation houses and therapeutic communities.

The prognosis depends on the drug abused but approximately 50% of opiate abusers develop long-term dependence and 2–3% die annually. (These figures may soon need to be revised upwards in view of the potent additional hazard of AIDS — in some localized areas of the UK, notably Edinburgh, infection rates of up to 80% have been found in intravenous drug abusers sharing contaminated syringes.) Solvent abuse is a quite separate situation.

Solvent abuse

Solvent abuse differs from 'hard drug' abuse in a number of important ways:
- it is very much a group activity;
- it involves a younger age group (14–16 years);
- it carries a much better prognosis (psychological dependence may occur but physical dependence is rare).

In general, misusers are more likely to come from a broken home, a large family or have an unemployed parent; and more likely to be involved in smoking, drinking, fighting, vandalism and regular truancy than non-users.

Agents abused included glues, modelling cements, petrol, cleaning solvents, paint cleaners and aerosols. The available concentration can be maximized by inhaling from a plastic bag or crisp packet (viscous products), or a handkerchief or plastic bottle (liquids). Mixtures usually contain acetone and toluene and produce a euphoria–drowsiness pattern that simulates drunkenness (but is achieved faster).

Rare toxic effects include:
- aplastic anaemia;
- polyneuropathy;
- cerebral and hepatorenal damage.

Large doses cause central nervous system depression with ataxia, nystagmus, dysarthria, drowsiness and coma. Perioral eczema and chronic upper respiratory tract infection may result from repeated contact with adhesives, and those inhaling petrol additionally risk lead poisoning. More important is the risk of fatal accident or serious injury while intoxicated. Occasional deaths have also occurred from arrhythmias and from asphyxiation after cold aerosol sprays have induced laryngeal spasm. A few solvent abusers progress later on to alcohol and other drugs.

Misuse of tranquillizers and hypnotics

Another familiar example of drug abuse is enacted daily in the surgery when tranquillizers and hypnotics are prescribed to dependent patients. The size of this problem is also daunting:
1 In one Oxfordshire study psychotropics comprised one-fifth

of all scripts: almost 10% of the men and 21% of the women (indeed, 33% of all women aged 45–59 years) received at least one psychotropic script in the year).

2   It has been estimated that 8.6% of adults in the UK had taken an anxiolytic for at least 1 month in the previous year.

3   In 1974 diazepam accounted for 4.3% of all NHS prescriptions.

Although physical dependence on bezodiazepines was first reported in 1961, the risk was considered low until an article in the *British Medical Journal* suggested otherwise in 1980. Since then the pressure to curtail prescribing has been building. In 1983 the legal profession began exploring the possibility of a patient compensation scheme and in 1987 the Council for Involuntary Tranquillizer Addiction was formed. Against this background, the number of prescriptions fell from 29.7 million in 1982 to 25.5 million in 1987.

Why do people take tranquillizers?

1   Foremost as a pharmaceutical crutch with anxiolytic and hypnotic properties at times of personal strain (stresses come in all forms — sexual, financial, marital, interpersonal).

2   However, a significant number commence taking tranquillizers to relieve a somatic symptom (not always related in their minds to stress), or under the strain of chronic ill health, or because of free-floating anxiety, anxiety-prone or inadequate personalities. In surveys people taking tranquillizers for the first time gave as the initial reason:

(a) a somatic symptom in 53% of cases;
(b) recognizable stress *alone* in 30% of cases;
(c) 'internal tensions' in 19% of cases.

The most common strains and conflicts mentioned by women centred around their roles as wife, mother and houseworker, while men tended to discuss problems in their work or work performance.

3   Ready availability and ready prescribing compound the problems. Prescriptions are offered for social reasons (see Section 2.2), in place of counselling, or because problems taken to a doctor tend to become 'medicalized'.

Are tranquillizers effective?

Initially tranquillizers are effective, but:

● Kales (1974) found their hypnotic effect can fall off or disappear over periods as short as 2 weeks;

● the Committee on the Review of Medicines (1980) pointed out that there is little convincing evidence that anxiolytics are still effective after 4 months' continuous treatment.

● Tyrer *et al.* (1988) found that when anxiolytics are used for more than 4 weeks they are less effective than antidepressants and psychological procedures.

Benzodiazepines are a very safe group of drugs, much safer than barbiturates. As a result the drawbacks of prescribing have been recognized late in the day.

1 *Withdrawal syndromes.* The overall incidence of the withdrawal syndrome is unclear: estimates vary from 30 to 100% depending on the population studied, the definition of abuse, duration of use, rate of withdrawal and length of follow-up (Pertusson *et al.* 1981; Tyrer *et al.* 1983). There is also evidence that withdrawal problems can occur after as little as 4–6 weeks' regular treatment. The syndrome appears within 3 days of stopping a short-acting drug and within 7 days of stopping a long-acting one. It usually lasts about 2 weeks but can go on for several months. It includes:

(a) anxiety;
(b) perceptual disturbances (including heightened sensitivity to all forms of sensory stimuli);
(c) a feeling of continuous movement;
(d) depersonalization and derealization;
(e) weight loss;
(f) electroencephalogram changes and epileptic seizures;
(g) psychotic behaviour (paranoid delusions, visual hallucinations).

2 *Psychological impairment.* Short-term usage impairs psychomotor function, and can produce anterograde amnesia. Chronic usage impairs performance in psychological tests, and abnormal computerized tomography scans have been found more commonly in chronic benzodiazepine users than in matched controls. Furthermore, it is likely that a significant number of accidents in the elderly are attributable to excessive sedation.

The implication is that it does matter that people take tranquillizers. Patients who have been taking a benzodiazepine for a long time should have their medication slowly withdrawn over 4–12 weeks, if at all possible (perhaps substituting a long-acting drug for a short-acting one in the first instance). People commenced on benzodiazepines for the first time should have treatment (preferably *intermittent* treatment) for periods less than 4–6 weeks. A firm decision on duration at the outset and a definite review date help to avoid the common pitfall of repeat prescribing by default.

In many cases the precipitating stress is still unresolved, which perpetuates drug-seeking behaviour. Non-drug-related approaches — counselling and relaxation — have more to offer, but demand from the doctor time and stamina which he may be ill equipped to provide.

6.5 CHILD ABUSE

Child abuse has received much publicity of late. It may truly be more common or may just be recognized more frequently.

Incidence

A GP sees one case every 2 years typically, but the true incidence is speculated to be much higher:

- perhaps 10–15% of all 'accidents' in children under 2 years old;
- perhaps 20% of all children are sexually abused.

Epidemiological features

1 *The home background*:

   (a) very young parents, often unmarried or with marital problems;

   (b) lower socioeconomic class (though not invariably);

   (c) financial problems and/or poor housing;

   (d) lack of support at home;

   (e) large family already;

   (f) parents who themselves had troubled childhoods and were battered;

   (g) step-parents.

2 *The circumstances of the pregnancy*:

   (a) termination requested but turned down;

   (b) poor antenatal attendance; difficult pregnancy;

   (c) a baby with physical handicap or prematurity;

   (d) a baby requiring Special Care Baby Unit care after birth.

   Nearly 90% of abused babies are the first or last in birth order. Mothers abuse more often than fathers. Meal times and bedtime are particular 'flashpoints'.

3 *The postnatal period*:

   (a) early maternal separation;

   (b) early signs of poor bonding;

   (c) lack of preparation at home; delay in choosing a name;

   (d) poor attendance at child health/immunization clinics;

   (e) unusual feeding practices (e.g. 'bottle-propping').

4 *Suspicious injuries*:

   (a) a history not consistent with the injury;

   (b) delayed reporting;

   (c) multiple injuries at different stages;

   (d) characteristic injuries (e.g. cigarette burns, fingertip bruises, strap marks, bite marks, black eyes, pull-injury with epiphyseal separation).

5 *The demeanour of the child*. 'Frozen awareness' is also said to be characteristic, and such children are unusually obedient in behaviour and often fail to thrive.

6 In childhood sexual abuse look for:

   (a) a clear statement from the child;

   (b) sexualized behaviour in the child at an inappropriately young age;

   (c) recent tears or bruising in the anogenital region.

   A report from the Cleveland enquiry concluded that anal

dilatation was a suspicious sign meriting investigation, but not in itself evidence of anal abuse.

Management of child abuse
Ethical problems abound, e.g.:
- breaches of confidentiality;
- when to involve the police;
- whether children should be taken into care for their own good, or left supervised at home for the parents' good;
- when does rigid discipline become cruelty or criminal abuse?

There is no simple answer but several general points of advice apply:

1 Have a low threshold of suspicion.
2 Get another opinion (colleague, health visitor, local police surgeon, paediatrician).
3 Try to confirm the diagnosis (e.g. skeletal survey showing multiple fractures of different ages).
4 Consider whether the child needs to be immediately removed to a place of safety. Hospital admission may avoid confrontation, otherwise a Place of Safety Order is obtained from a magistrate on application by the police, Social Services or NSPCC, and gives authority to remove a child to a place of safety (hospital, police station, community or foster home) for up to 28 days.
5 Consider calling a case conference (involving medical, social and perhaps psychiatric disciplines) and registering the child as 'at risk'.
6 Offer the family the support and care needed.

The most difficult decision on management is whether to attempt to reunite the child with his family, and work with them to repair the family unit, or whether the risk to the child is too great, when alternative arrangements (e.g. fostering) will need to be explored.

Prevention of child abuse
Prevention entails recognizing the needs of high-risk groups in advance of the event. They need to be seen often. The social worker may be able to improve home circumstances and provide the necessary support (e.g. childminders or playgroups). Unnecessary separation in the postnatal period must be avoided, and medical and Social Services follow-up is needed. The health visitor is a key figure in the prevention of child abuse, and will need to visit frequently in high-risk situations.

6.6 AIDS

The size of the problem
AIDS was first described following a handful of cases of pneumocystis pneumonia and Kaposi's sarcoma among homosexual men

and intravenous drug abusers in California and New York in 1981. From that tiny base the pool of infection swelled in the most dramatic fashion, and by the end of 1987:

- the World Health Organization (WHO) had been officially notified of 73 747 cases of AIDS from 129 countries;
- in the UK 1227 cases had been described, of whom 57% had died, representing one death in 30 among men aged 25–44.

These figures probably display only the tip of the iceberg: we know the pool of human immunodeficiency virus (HIV) sero-positive individuals is much greater — at least 5 000 000 worldwide (WHO) and 30 000–40 000 according to conservative estimates in the UK (DOH): and many of these (20–30% on current views) will also develop AIDS. The number of cases approximately doubles every year.

The *economic* consequences of the AIDS epidemic have also been highlighted, e.g.:

- in the UK the 3000 new cases in 1988 cost the Exchequer £88 M;
- the first 10 000 cases in the USA cost 1.6 million hospital days, 1.4 billion dollars in health costs and 4.8 billion dollars in lost economic activity.

Part of the problem with AIDS is the extent of our ignorance. While short-term extrapolations may be quite accurate, the long-term view is hazy and incomplete. For example:

- are we dealing with one or several epidemics?
- what are the limits of the incubation period? (The average of 8–9 years conceals a great deal of variation);
- does the infectivity of AIDS vary during that time?
- what is the ease of spread per sexual encounter? (Again there is a variability that suggests unknown biological factors are at work);
- what do we know of the frequency, intensity and types of sexual activity in populations?
- can sexual practices be modified by public education?

This last factor has a critical bearing on the validity of any mathematical projections. There is certainly encouraging evidence that homosexual behaviour has changed due to the AIDS situation, but it is not clear that the heterosexual population will follow suit until the virus becomes more prevalent and awareness levels are raised.

However, even taking the most optimistic viewpoint, it is likely that the death toll and the total burden of human suffering will be on an upward path for many years to come, and that we are facing the prospect of death and disease in fit adults, young women widowed, young children orphaned, parents attending their own childrens' funerals. Worst predictions include an economic crisis as a generation of workers is levelled, and perhaps radical changes in the future delivery of health care.

It is almost certain that a large part of the burden of care will fall on community-based services: 80% of the AIDS sufferer's time will be spent at home. GPs will in future find themselves more involved in aspects of care and prevention.

Clinical aspects

The presentation and clinical features of HIV infection are outlined in Table 6.10. It is important that GPs recognize the possibility of HIV infection in high-risk groups.

Table 6.10 Clinical features in HIV sero-positive individuals.

1 *Completely asymptomatic*

2 *Persistent generalized lymphadenopathy (PGL)*
Enlarged firm lymph nodes
Sometimes painful
No obvious cause
Present at least 3 months

3 *AIDS-related complex (ARC)*

Malaise	Mild diarrhoea
Pyrexia of unknown origin	Seborrhoeic dermatitis
Night sweats	Acne
Fatigue	Herpes simplex
Weight loss	Herpes zoster
Oral candida	
± PGL	
Immunosuppression	

4 *AIDS*

Encephalitis	Pyrexia of unknown origin
Meningitis	Wasting
Fits	PGL
Headaches	Opportunistic infections
Depression	Malignancies
Psychosis	Diarrhoea
Dementia	
Kaposi's sarcoma (25%)	
Pneumocystis pneumonia (60%)	

HIV testing

High-risk groups and those in need of the HIV test include the following individuals:

1 People with PGL, or features of AIDS-related complex (ARC) or AIDS (Table 6.10).

2 Men who have had sex with another man in the last 10 years.

3 Drug users who have injected drugs at any time in the last 10 years.

4 Haemophiliacs receiving unscreened blood products.

5 Prostitutes.

6 People who have lived in or visited areas of high prevalence (e.g. Africa, North America), and had sex with people living there.

7 Certain recipients of blood transfusions (blood has been screened in the UK since October 1985, but not always abroad).

8 People who may have been accidentally exposed (e.g. by needleprick injury).

9 Sexual partners of the above groups.

10 Children of infected mothers.

The Department of Health announced in 1988 an extensive programme of testing for HIV of unlinked anonymous samples. After all possible identifying tags were removed, the residue of blood collected for legitimate tests is to be randomly screened for HIV unless the patient has spontaneously objected. Data are being collected for community benefit, to monitor disease trends. The system is designed to ensure that everyone, including the donor, cannot identify positive cases.

The scientific, legal and ethical basis of this programme has been well reviewed (Gill *et al.* 1989).

Aspects of couselling and management

1 Prior to blood testing it is important that these people are appropriately and sensitively counselled. They should know the limitations of the test and have considered the implications of a positive test.

2 Post-test counselling is vital in view of the serious range of psychological reactions (shock, fear and anxiety, isolation, depression, guilt, frustration, obsessive disorders) that accompanies news of a positive result. About 10% of seropositive individuals will need to be referred to a psychiatrist or psychologist, and there is a real risk of suicide in patients left unattended around this time.

3 Follow-up must include common sense advice to patients and their partners (on safer sexual practices; the myths and truth about transmission and infectivity; and such diverse matters as how to cope with spillages of body fluid, and who to tell and what to say).

4 A number of support services exist to provide information and help (e.g. local special clinics and health education departments; AIDS help and advice lines; self-help groups). Doctors will need to develop close, effective working links with these bodies in future.

5 GPs will need eventually to deal with the complications of AIDS and will need to recognize those that are treatable and those that are not.

Aspects of prevention

1 As the epidemic spreads and anxiety levels rise, doctors will have to cope with the 'worried well' (people who remain well but have symptoms they attribute to AIDS), the 'worried ignorant',

Table 6.11 Advice on avoiding AIDS:
(a) The ladder of risk.

No risk
Solo masturbation
Massage away from genital area

Low risk
Mutual masturbation
Dry kissing
Body-to-body contact
Penis-to-body contact (except between thighs and buttocks)

Medium risk
Wet kissing
Fellatio
Urination
Coitus interfemoris
Anilingus
Fingering
Douches and enemas

High risk
Anal and vaginal sex
Fisting
Sharing sex toys and needles
Any sex act drawing blood

Risk *increases* with number of sexual partners
Risk *decreases* with use of a condom in intercourse
Risk *decreases* with the additional use of a water-based spermicide
(especially in anal sex)

(b) Using a condom.

7% failure rate (half due to incorrect use). Advice needs to be specific and full, e.g.

'Before
• Use before every act and put on before the penis touches the partner's vulva or rectum
• Wait until the penis is erect, then pinch the top of the condom with one hand; with the other put the sheath on the end of the penis and unroll it all the way down

After
• Withdraw the penis from the vagnia or rectum, holding the condom on the penis as you do so
• Take the condom off, taking care not to spill the semen, and dispose of it carefully
• Use a fresh condom next and every time'

Table 6.11 *Contd*

(c) Advice for the drug abuser.

Scale of increasing risk
Abstinence
Using drugs but not injecting them
Using sterile equipment only
Using but not sharing equipment
Using and sharing cleaned equipment
Using and sharing unclean equipment

Cleaning equipment
Aim: to flush the virus out
Method: rinse with hot water and washing-up liquid immediately; now
rinse in clean water

Table 6.12 Control of infection advice.

1 *Specimen-taking and handling*
● Adequate training first
● Wear gloves and disposable plastic apron
● Use minimum volume of blood
● Avoid spillages
● Dispose of sharps into a puncture-proof bin
● Do not resheathe needles
● Put specimen in robust leak-proof container in sealed bag and use
biohazard labelling
● Notify senior laboratory staff

2 *Hygiene/disinfection steps*
● Do not share between patients devices that can draw blood, e.g.
syringes and needles, electrolysis equipment, tattoo/acupuncture sharps
● Use disposable sterile equipment as much as possible
● Otherwise sterilize by heating (autoclave is better than boiling)
● Liquid disinfectants may do as second best, e.g. hypochlorite,
gluteraldehyde, alcohol

3 *Coping with spillages*
● Clean up immediately
● Use gloves and apron (as above)
● Use liberal amounts of household bleach diluted 1 : 10 (with hot water)
● Leave for 30 min
● Wipe up with disposable paper towels
● Carefully dispose of gloves, apron and towels
● Thoroughly wash and dry hands

4 *First aid for staff*
● Body fluid on skin, in eyes or in mouth — wash away as soon as
possible
● Penetrating wounds
  (a) encourage bleeding
  (b) wash with soap and water
  (c) notify employer

and the 'worried guilty'. They need to reassure and to educate, to engender appropriate degrees of concern and appropriate responses.

2 Most importantly they need now to give clear and explicit advice to the general public on the prevention of AIDS and safer

sexual practices (Table 6.11). Advice must be blunt and clear, but appropriate to the needs of the individual and the context of the consultation. GPs may be better placed than other health care personnel to fulfil this role.

3 Finally GPs (as good employers) will also need to educate their staff and to protect them from exposure to the virus through appropriate health care measures and protocols (Table 6.12).

Educating the carers

GPs clearly need to think out their advice and to ensure it is accurate and up to date. There is therefore a pressing need for further education and we appear to be starting from a distressingly weak base (Milne *et al.* 1988). Fortunately there is no shortage of information, and various initiatives have been proposed to help educate the carers:

1 Continuing education through the trade press, the journals and DOH circulars.

2 Seminars, symposia, lunch-time meetings and small-group debate, organized through the postgraduate centres of district hospital.

3 Distance learning courses (such as the Royal College CLIPP programme).

4 Information lines.

5 The appointment by district health authorities of a local liaison specialist to coordinate the effort.

6 Equipping GPs with all manner of public information material — display posters, leaflets, advisory material (and free condoms) to present to patients.

The Royal College of General Practitioners has committed itself to providing information, updates and original research for GPs, and to establishing close working links with other national organizations involved in the care of AIDS patients.

Attitudes must also improve. Surveys have suggested that seropositive patients fear a negative reaction from their GP, worry about confidentiality, and often conceal the diagnosis from him (King 1988). Steps must be taken to present a more sympathetic image to those in need.

7 Legal and Ethical Matters

7.1 THE 1983 MENTAL HEALTH ACT (ENGLAND AND WALES)

Definitions
Mental disorder (Section 1)
Included in the definition of mental disorder are:
- mental illness;
- arrested or incomplete development of mind;
- psychopathic disorder.

It *excludes* from the definition:
- promiscuity;
- sexual deviancy;
- dependence on alcohol or drugs.

Nearest relative (Section 26)
The nearest relative according to Section 26 of the Act is the first surviving person appearing in the following list:
1 Husband or wife (or co-habitee for more than 6 months);
2 Son or daughter (if aged over 18 years);
3 Father or mother;
4 Brother or sister (aged over 18 years);
5 Grandparent;
6 Grandchild (aged over 18 years);
7 Uncle or aunt (aged over 18 years);
8 Nephew or niece (aged over 18 years);
9 Non-relative living with the patient for 5 or more years.

'Approved' doctor and social worker
Doctor and social worker 'approved' under the terms of the Act as having special expertise and training in the area of mental health.

Principles
1 The *grounds* for admission under the various sections are similar, namely:
    (a) that the patient suffers from a mental disorder of a nature and severity which justify that particular section in the interests of the patient's own health and safety, and the safety of others;
    (b) that treatment has to be in hospital.
2 The applicant must be a social worker or nearest relative.
3 Usually two medical recommendations are needed (an approved doctor and a doctor with prior knowledge of the patient), except in the event of emergency, when one signature gives limited powers of detention.

4 Admission has a limited tenure and there are prescribed discharge powers and rights of appeal.

Details

For details of the main sections of the Act see Table 7.1. (Northern Ireland and Scotland have their own Mental Health Acts but the principles are similar to the English and Welsh Act.)

7.2 CONTROLLED DRUGS

Much legislation now exists regarding the use and misuse of controlled drugs, e.g.:

- Dangerous Drugs, Notification of Addicts Regulations 1968;
- Misuse of Drugs Act 1971;
- Misuse of Drugs Regulations (Notification of, and Supply to Addicts) 1973;
- Misuse of Drugs Regulations 1985.

Under the 1971 Misuse of Drugs Act three categories of controlled drugs were defined:

1 Class A: including opium, heroin, morphine, most opiates, pethidine, LSD and other hallucinogens, cocaine and methadone.
2 Class B: including cannabis, amphetamines and barbiturates.
3 Class C: including benzphetamine, chlorphentermine and diethylpropion.

These categories relate broadly to the degree of harm caused by misuse. The classification has limited significance for doctors and is used mainly in setting the penalties for unlawful possession and intent to supply.

Of greater importance to the medical profession are the 1985 Misuse of Drugs Regulations which define five groups of drugs (Schedules 1–5) and describe those regulations governing import, export, production, supply, possession, prescribing and record-keeping of controlled drugs.

1 Schedule 1: including drugs like cannabis and LSD which have no therapeutic use. Possession and supply are prohibited and availability is solely by Home Office licence for research purposes.
2 Schedule 2: including the opiates and major stimulants. GPs can possess these drugs for approved medical use but there are strict rules regarding safe-custody, record-keeping and the format of prescriptions (see below).
3 Schedule 3: including barbiturates, diethylpropion and pentazocine. The format of the prescription is regulated and invoices must be kept for 2 years.
4 Schedule 4: including benzodiazepines. Control requirements are minimal.
5 Schedule 5: controlled drugs combined with other drugs in

Table 7.1 The main sections of the 1983 Mental Health Act.

Section number and purpose	Application	Medical recommendations	Other conditions	Duration	Discharge powers
2: Compulsory admission for *assessment*	Nearest relative *or* approved social worker	Approved doctor *plus* doctor who knows the patient	1 Not more than 5 days between medical examinations 2 Application is valid for 14 days 3 The social worker normally interviews the nearest relative and/or informs him in writing	28 days. Not renewable	Responsible medical officer (RMO) *or* hospital manager *or* nearest relative. (The patient can also appeal to the Mental Health Review Tribunal)
3: Compulsory admission for *treatment*	As above	As above	As above	6 months (renewable for a further 6 months and then yearly)	As above. (If the patient does not appeal, the hospital managers *must* appeal on his behalf after 6 months)
4: Compulsory admission for *assessment in an emergency.* Compliance with Section 2 conditions would cause an undesirable delay	As above	*Either* approved doctor *or* doctor with prior knowledge of patient	1 The medical referee must have seen the patient in the last 24 h 2 Application valid for 24 h only	72 h. Not renewable	RMO *or* hospital managers. (Patient cannot appeal)

Other sections sometimes required

1 Section 5: the emergency detention of informal *inpatients* by the RMO or his nominated deputy for 72 h so that a Section 2 or 3 can be considered;
2 Section 7: reception into guardianship;
3 Section 115: right of entry of approved social worker into premises so he can remove a patient to a place of safety. (Section 135 is the same, with a police constable);
4 Section 136: removal of a patient from a public place by a constable to a place of safety (e.g. cell or hospital) for up to 72 h to allow medical examination.

amounts so small that they are not liable to produce dependence. Invoices must be kept for 2 years and manufacture is regulated by the Home Office.

The other points of relevance to the GP are as follows:

1   A doctor must notify the Chief Medical Officer at the Home Office, within 7 days, if he attends a person addicted to narcotic drugs. Addicts are entered on the Home Office's central register.

2   Doctors need a special licence (issued by the Home Secretary) to prescribe heroin, morphine or cocaine in the treatment of drug addiction [a special prescription form, FP 10 (MDA), has been introduced for this purpose].

3   Doctors must keep controlled drugs within a locked compartment, or if on their person, within a locked receptacle. (Note that a locked car boot is insufficient — it must be a locked case in a locked boot.)

4   Doctors must keep a register of the use they make of their controlled drug supply, and the police have the right to inspect this register.

5   It is an offence to issue an incomplete prescription for a controlled drug and the pharmacist will not dispense under these circumstances. The legal requirements are:

(a) scripts should be written in indelible ink;

(b) they should be signed and dated personally by the prescriber;

(c) the prescriber should write in his own hand: the name and address of the patient, the dose, the form of the preparation, the strength to be dispensed and the total quantity;

(d) all numbers must be in words and figures;

(e) the address of the prescriber must appear on the script.

6   Controlled drugs cannot be prescribed for patients leaving the country, and doctors cannot carry controlled drugs abroad unless endorsed by a licence from the Secretary of State.

Of course, careless or improper use of drugs must also lay the GP open to a charge of professional misconduct or incompetence. It is important to note in this respect that there is a black market for the resale of drugs obtained from GPs by deception, and also a black market for stolen blank scripts which can be forged to obtain drug supplies.

7.3 INDUSTRIAL INJURIES

Patients can claim for injuries 'arising out of and in the course of their employment' even if due to their own foolhardiness or carelessness. The Industrial Injuries Act lays down 47 'precribed' industrial diseases which are recognized for compensation purposes, and a schedule for prescribed degrees of disablement from trauma.

Compensation becomes payable through:

1 The State Industrial Injuries Scheme: this contributes *injury* and *disablement* benefits (on a 1–100% scale assessed by a medical board), and industrial *death benefits* (see Section 5.7);

2 An individual's private action against his employer (if he believes him negligent).

State claims can be made up to 5 years retrospectively.

In addition there are a group of diseases that are compulsorily *notifiable* by employers to the Health and Safety Executive when they occur in an industrial setting. Industrial diseases notifiable under the Reporting of Injuries, Diseases and Dangerous Occurrences Regulations (RIDDOR) 1985 include:

- poisoning by a number of industrial agents, e.g. arsenic, benzene, beryllium, cadmium, carbon disulphide, lead, manganese, mercury, phosphorus;
- chrome ulceration;
- skin cancers;
- folliculitis and acne (induced by tar, pitch and oils);
- occupational asthma;
- extrinsic allergic alveolitis;
- pneumoconiosis;
- byssinosis;
- compressed air sickness;
- vibration white finger;
- a number of occupational infections, e.g. leptospirosis, tuberculosis, hepatitis, anthrax, work with human pathogens;
- a number of occupational cancers (e.g. from ionizing radiation or asbestos).

Notes

1 The lists of *reportable* and *prescribed* diseases associated with occupation are similar but not identical. They are drawn up for separate and quite distinct purposes: the one to allow investigation and enforcement under the Health and Safety at Work Act 1974, the other to allow state compensation under the industrial injuries provisions of the Social Security Act 1975.

2 The obligation to report under the RIDDOR Regulations falls on the employer, not the doctor (except in respect of his *own* staff). However, if the employer is to do so, the doctor must make the diagnosis clear to him.

3 Other health and safety at work obligations imposed on GPs as employers (safety policies, accident books, insurance etc.) are described in Section 7.9.

7.4 THE CORONER

Notifiable deaths
Deaths that should be reported to a coroner include:

- all sudden or unexpected deaths;
- deaths where the doctor has not attended within the prior 14 days;
- deaths within 24 h of hospital admission (in most areas — some personal variation);
- accidents and injuries;
- industrial disease;
- medical mishaps (specifically including anaesthetics, operations and drugs, either therapeutic or addictive);
- deaths arising from ill treatment, starvation or neglect;
- poisoning;
- abortions;
- stillbirths (when there is doubt as to whether the child was born alive);
- service disability pensioners;
- prisoners.

Alcohol-associated deaths
Note that a new set of Coroners' Rules came into force on 1 July 1984, and this has made an important practical change to the regulations concerning the registration of alcohol-associated deaths: formerly *all* such deaths were notifiable, even if due to alcoholic cirrhosis in the chronic alcoholic; death due to chronic alcoholism is no longer notifiable *per se* as a coroner will no longer automatically hold an inquest. Of course the death is still notifiable if associated with one of the above listed conditions (e.g. the drunk who falls and fractures his skull qualifies for notification under the 'accidents and injuries' clause).

The Scottish system
In Scotland a slightly different system applies: deaths are reported to a procurator fiscal, in the same circumstances as for the coroner in England, with the addition of deaths of foster children and the newborn.

7.5 NOTIFIABLE DISEASES

Under the Public Health (Control of Disease) Act 1984 and Public Health (Infectious Diseases) Regulations 1988 the following infectious diseases in England and Wales must be notified to the local authority's Medical Officer for Environmental Health:

Anthrax	Food poisoning
Cholera	Lassa fever
Diphtheria	Leprosy
Dysentery (amoebic or bacillary)	Leptospirosis
Encephalitis	Malaria

Marburg disease
Measles
Meningitis
Mumps
Ophthalmia neonatorum
Paratyphoid fever A and B
Plague
Polio
Rabies
Relapsing fever
Rubella

Scarlet fever
Smallpox
Tetanus
Tuberculosis
Typhoid fever
Typhus fever
Viral haemorrhagic fever
Viral hepatitis
Whooping cough
Yellow fever

Note that in Scotland and Northern Ireland (where notifications are to the chief administrative medical officer) the list of notifiable conditions is amended.

1 In *Northern Ireland* it *includes*:
   (a) gastroenteritis (in those aged under 2 years);
   (b) infective hepatitis.

However, it *excludes*:
   (a) food poisoning;
   (b) leprosy;
   (c) malaria;
   (d) ophthalmia neonatorum;
   (e) tetanus.

2 In *Scotland* it *includes*:
   (a) continued fever;
   (b) erysipelas;
   (c) leptospiral jaundice;
   (d) membranous croup;
   (e) puerperal fever.

However, it *excludes*:
   (a) encephalitis;
   (b) tetanus;
   (c) tuberculosis.

A small fee is payable for each notification.

Acquired immune deficiency syndrome is not notifiable by statute. However doctors are urged to participate in a voluntary confidential reporting scheme.

7.6 THE ABORTION ACT

Under the Abortion Act 1967 and the Abortion Regulations 1991 termination of pregnancy is allowable if there is a risk:

1 To the woman's life (greater than if the pregnancy were to continue).

2 Of grave permanent injury to the woman's physical or mental health.

3   To her physical or mental health (greater than if the pregnancy were to continue).

4   To the physical or mental health of her existing children.

5   Risk of a handicapped child (rubella-damaged, Down's syndrome, etc.).

Clauses **3** and **4** can be employed only when the pregnancy does not exceed 24 weeks.

Two medical referees must sign the 'blue form' (form HSA 1).

Approximately 120 000 legal terminations are performed annually in the UK with an approximate mortality of 2.6 per 100 000.

The Abortion Act represents a middle ground between the extreme views of 'no abortion at all' and 'abortion on demand'. It does not place an absolute value on human life (human suffering coming higher in priority), but it places a *high* value — fetal destruction must be justified. Critics of the legislation point out that it is arbitrary and its application is inconsistent, e.g.:

● the 24-week time limit is based on notions of fetal viability which arguably occurs much sooner than this;

● under clause **5** Down's syndrome pregnancies are routinely terminated, but in a recent legal test case a life-saving operation was ordered on Down's syndrome baby Alexandra against the parents' wishes;

● clauses **3** and **4** are open to wide and subjective interpretation: practice varies widely throughout the country and from one doctor to another;

● the death rate from legal termination is lower than that for pregnancy, so it could be argued under clause **1** that *all* women should receive a termination on request.

(Exam candidates may be quizzed on their own attitudes to abortion. Obviously this is a question of convictions and belief rather than right and wrong answers, but you need to consider, from all sides, the practical implications of your views. If, for example, you regard termination as 'murder through a legal loophole', what do you do when faced by the patient requesting an abortion? Do you refer her to a colleague or a consultant? If you refuse to help her, are you within the terms of your service or within the ethical code of medical practice as a whole? And how do you stand with your colleagues? And what about postcoital contraception or the fitting of coils, or the prescription of RU 486?)

7.7 THE DATA PROTECTION ACT 1984

Users of computer-held data must register with the data protection registrar on a triennial basis. 'Users' obviously includes GPs installing a practice computer, but may also include those using computer bureau services from Family Health Service Authorities (FHSAs), District Health Authorities or accountants, for example. The key point is the *control* of personal data — automatically provided information which identifies individual patients.

Users need to comply with several principles. Data should be:

- obtained and processed lawfully;
- held for a specific lawful purpose;
- not otherwise used or disclosed;
- appropriate (and not excessive) for the purpose;
- dispensed with when no longer necessary;
- kept using appropriate security measures.

More taxing, perhaps, is the obligation for information to be accurate and up-to-date and — more significant for GPs — the principle of subject access. A 1987 amendment of the Act conceded that doctors could restrict access to personal health information when serious physical or mental harm might ensue. However, in view of the relentless march of computer systems into the surgery it is important to consider these problems and to get it right. Failure to register under the Act is a criminal offence.

7.8 ACCESS TO MEDICAL RECORDS

Access to Medical Reports Act (1988)
This Act allows patients to see medical reports prepared for prospective employers or insurers. Under the new rules doctors must allow those patients who wish to see the report 21 days to do so before it is dispatched. A copy of the report must be provided on request by the patient and a copy (to which the patient has access) kept for 6 months. Patients are allowed the opportunity to discuss the report with their doctors and to attach a codicil if they feel the report is inaccurate. The GP, however, is not obliged to alter his comments if there is still a difference of view. Ultimately the patient can refuse to allow the report to be sent, so if access is requested a further consent should normally be obtained prior to dispatch.

Access to Health Records Act (1990)
This Act allows patients aged 16 or over access to their medical notes (manual or computerized), but only notes written after 1 November 1990. It includes reports written by allied professionals (e.g. nurses, dentists, midwives). A copy must be provided, normally within 40 days of a written request, at nominal charge.

Doctors keen to avoid the pitfalls of these acts need to modify their working practices, for example to:

- ensure they receive (and keep) a written informed consent;
- date-stamp all requests for reports and correspondence;
- keep a dated record book and copies of all reports.

GPs can withhold information from the patient if they believe it is likely to risk serious physical or mental harm to the individual or others.

7.9 HEALTH AND SAFETY AT WORK LEGISLATION

The Health and Safety at Work Act 1974 applies to the GP employer and places on him the obligation 'as far as reasonably practicable' to ensure a safely maintained workplace. He must also display a statement of safety policy and notify certain categories of accident to the Health and Safety Executive. An accident book must be kept, insurance should be taken out against accidents to staff, and the inspectorate is entitled to enter and inspect premises to ensure they comply with the Act. (Interestingly, employees too have an obligation to comply with safety practices and it is an offence under the Act to put themselves or others at risk.)

The Control of Substances Hazardous to Health Regulations 1988 require employers to make a formal assessment of risk to employees arising in the workplace and adequately to control and monitor that risk. This might for example include the risk of dermatitis from biocides and sterilizing agents and the risk of staff contracting infection from patients and biological samples and waste.

There are clear implications for the counselling and training of staff, and policies are required for the cleaning of medical equipment and the safe disposal of drugs, contaminated needles, dressings and appliances. A written risk assessment is required.

7.10 MEDICAL CONFIDENTIALITY

Confidentiality has been a basic tenet of medical ethics for 2500 years and is embodied in the Hippocratic Oath, the International Code of Medical Ethics and the Declaration of Geneva (1947). There are several obvious *reasons* for confidentiality:

1 We set store by personal autonomy, the right of individuals to control their own lives and, in this case, to control disclosures about them.

2 Consultations have an assumed privacy built in to them. Indeed, although there are no legal precedents, there may be an

implied *legal contract* of confidentiality, and patients could theoretically obtain redress for breaches through the courts or through the General Medical Council Professional Conduct Committee.

3 Reciprocal respect and confidence are essential to obtain an honest history and meaningful doctor–patient relationship. This is to the mutual benefit of both parties and in some cases frankness may also serve the community best.

Exceptions

There are three general circumstances in which confidentiality may be breached:

1 *In the patient's own interests.* It is common practice to discuss some details of a patient's illness with his close relatives and friends outside his earshot when it is felt they should be told something the patient is not ready to receive (e.g. news of a terminal illness).

2 *When required by law.* Statutory disclosures include:

(a) poisonings under the Factories Act;

(b) terminations under the Abortion Act;

(c) drug addiction under the Misuse of Drugs Regulations;

(d) notifiable infections under the Health Service and Public Health Act;

(e) industrial injuries and diseases under the Reporting of Injuries, Diseases and Dangerous Occurrences Regulations;

(f) road traffic accidents under the Road Traffic Acts;

(g) births and deaths registration;

(h) coroner's cases.

Bodies with the power to order disclosures include:

(a) a court of law;

(b) an enquiry appointed by the Secretary of State;

(c) an NHS tribunal;

(d) the Health and Safety Executive.

3 *In the greater interest of the community at large.* This is a grey area, but includes the murderer who will not give himself up, the epileptic who risks serious accident by driving illegally when fit-prone, the child abuser, etc.

It is a source of concern among consumer groups that exceptions to the code of confidentiality are so numerous, in particular that much information on individuals is collected for administrative purposes, e.g.:

- the community health register and recall system collects birth information and distributes it to health visitors;
- many forms of hospital activity analysis are regularly performed;
- the Prescription Pricing Authority collects prescription details;

- the DOH and drug companies are informed about patients with suspected drug interactions;
- many authorities have access to child at-risk registers.

There is also pressure for confidential information to be available to police scrutiny. A Police and Criminal Evidence Bill to this effect failed, but consumers and doctors may be alarmed to hear that one NHS administrator, in a TV interview, admitted that as the Secretary of State's appointed custodian he would exercise his discretion and allow police access to confidential hospital files, without necessarily notifying the patient or his consultant.

The movement to computerize records, with its attendant security problems, has also caused concern and led to the Data Protection Act (see Section 7.7).

The rights of the underaged individual to medical advice in confidence (particularly when the advice relates to contraception) remains contentious.

7.11 MEDICAL RESEARCH

The discovery at the Nuremberg War Trials that Nazi doctors had perpetrated atrocities under the guise of medical research led to the declaration of a 10-point code identifying the main ethical principles on which true research should be founded. These principles were further refined in the Declaration of Helsinki (1964), which insists that:

1 Research must conform to generally accepted scientific principles and should be based on adequate laboratory and animal experiments.

2 The experimental protocol should be reviewed by an independent ethical committee.

3 Research should always be supervised by competent and qualified workers.

4 The importance of the objective is in proportion to the inherent risk to the subject.

5 The health of the patient is the prime and foremost consideration and should always prevail over the interests of science and society.

6 There is informed consent regarding aims, methods, risks and possible benefits.

7 There is no duress to participate and patients can abstain or withdraw at any time.

Despite these caveats medical research is littered with ethical problems.

1 Some authorities believe that 'informed consent' is an unobtainable ideal. It may be impossible to convey every facet of

knowledge and judgement to patients who vary in their interest in and capacity to comprehend complicated medical information. (In chemotherapy trials 40–50% of patients are unable to explain the purpose, nature and major complications of a procedure the day after they have been counselled, while informed consent for some cancer patients may result in an unpalatably blunt discussion of their prospects, or disclosures of uncertainty that may undermine their faith in medical care.)

2   Many patients cannot give informed consent, e.g.:
  (a) children;
  (b) the mentally handicapped;
  (c) the mentally ill;
  (d) embryos.

Problems then arise when their basic human right to self-determination is transferred to someone else.

3   Although medical research is undertaken to improve the lot of individuals and society it does not necessarily result in unmitigated good; for example, perinatal expertise may help to preserve damaged babies — is this truly in the best interests of patient or society?

4   Doctors experience ethical qualms in conducting controlled and scientific research when they have reason to believe beforehand that one trial treatment is superior to another. This problem arose in the Medical Research Council study undertaken in 1982 to establish whether vitamin supplements prevent spina bifida. Persuasive but inconclusive evidence had already suggested that this was so; under such circumstances randomization causes much soul-searching. However, is it ethical to prescribe *any* treatment without doing everything possible to assess its true worth?

5   Expensive medical research diverts funds from more easily treatable conditions; given limited resources someone must suffer in the short term in the expectation that more people will benefit in the longer term.

6   The most difficult dilemmas of all arise when research extends the realms of scientific possibility so far that they outstrip contemporary codes of morality. Embryo experimentation is a good example of this. Society has expressed great concern regarding the ethics of surrogacy, genetic engineering and experimentation on 'spare' embryos. There are many contentious issues, e.g.:
  (a) when does life start?
  (b) when does an embryo acquire rights?
  (c) what are those rights and who speaks for them?
  (d) how do we balance an embryo's rights against those of the prospective parents? And against the potential benefits that research brings to humanity?
  (e) is it acceptable for embryos to be implanted in a mother who bears no genetic relationship at all to them?

(f) is it acceptable for spare embryos to be frozen for future use, or killed, or used as tissue for research?

These ethical waters are so murky that the Warnock committee, appointed by the Government to consider them, was unable to reach a unanimous view, and had instead to publish two minority reports expressing differing views. It seems unlikely that the medical profession alone will resolve these issues. Society as a whole must shoulder the responsibility of deciding where to draw the line.

For interested readers the ethics of medical research and informed consent are discussed in more depth in *Doctors' Dilemmas: Medical Ethics and Contemporary Science* by Phillips and Dawson (see Further Reading).

7.12 GP CONTRACTS

GPs are independent contractors to the NHS, i.e. they contract with the FHSA to provide a particular service to patients accepted on to their list, but they do so on their own responsibility, and are largely free to run their business as they wish. This has certain *advantages*, e.g.:
- greater variety and flexibility;
- both doctor and patient have a choice;
- GPs can influence their working conditions to a greater extent than as salaried employees;
- GPs are taxed as self-employed (Schedule D rather than Schedule E).

The chief *disadvantage* is that GPs, as managers, must assume administrative and financial responsibilities as well as clinical ones.

Terms of Service
The FHSA still demands certain safeguards and standards from the GP, and these are layed down in its Terms of Service documents. The main points are summarized in Table 7.2. In return the FHSA contracts to remunerate GPs in accordance with its Statement of Fees and Allowances (see Table 1.6, p. 52).

Partnership agreements
According to the British Medical Association a sizeable percentage of practices have no formal written agreement. Partners are liable in law for one another's debts (especially tax liabilities), and practice disagreements are commonplace: on both scores a written contract is advisable.

The ingredients of a good partnership agreement include reference to:

Table 7.2 The GP's main terms of service with the FHSA.

Definition of a patient	Recorded by the FHSA as on the doctor's list (accepted and not cancelled, or within 7 days of application to cancel) Allocated to the GP by the Joint Allocation Committee Accepted as a temporary resident In the practice area and needing 'immediately necessary' treatment in an emergency
Number of patients	Not more than 3500 per partner (or up to 4500 for one partner in a group practice with an average ≤3500, temporary residents not included in this limit)
Terminating responsibility	By application to the FHSA: responsibility stops on the 8th day after application (unless the patient is being treated for something needing close supervision and reallocation is delayed) The same applies to accepted temporary residents For maternity patients *either* by the woman's consent *or* by representation to the FHSA who examines the grounds
Service to patients	GPs must render all necessary and appropriate medical services of the type usually provided by GPs This includes referral (if needed) but contraceptive and non-urgent maternity services are not obligatory The *standard* is that normally exercised by his GP colleagues (i.e. he is expected to make judgements to the standard of a reasonable GP, not a hospital specialist) This specifically includes: • advice regarding general health, diet and use of tobacco, alcohol, drugs and solvents • preventive physical examinations • offering immunization against measles, mumps, rubella, pertussis, polio, diphtheria and tetanus
Newly registered patients	Must offer within 28 days of registration a written invitation to attend a health assessment consultation of defined content (see Table 8.2, p. 235) Patients can refuse If undertaken, the findings must be recorded, an assessment made and discussed with the patient
Not seen in the last 3 years	Those aged 16–74 years who have not been seen by any doctor within the last 3 years must be invited to attend a health assessment consultation of defined content (see Table 8.2) Patients can refuse If undertaken, the findings must be recorded, an assessment made and discussed with the patient
Patients aged 75 and over	GPs must invite those aged 75 and over annually to participate in a health assessment of defined content (see Table 8.2) They must include the offer to make a domiciliary visit
Practice premises	Must be 'proper' and open to FHSA inspection at reasonable times (rent and rate reimbursements can be withheld if facilities are not up to standard) FHSA approval is needed regarding the place and time of any proposed changes to this

Table 7.2 *Contd*

227

*Chapter 7
Legal and
Ethical
Matters*

	Normally 'availability' is construed as: • over 42 weeks in any year • for not less than 26 h over 5 days in any such week • at times likely to be convenient to patients This includes time spent in clinics and home visiting, but not simply on call Those involved in training and approved health-related activities may be exempted from this rule to the extent of a day per week, while part-time pincipals may elect to be available to a lesser extent (either <26 h but not <19, or <19 h but not <13 h per week) with a suitable reduction in basic practice allowance Patients attending the premises at the agreed times must be seen except where an appointment system exists, the patient has no appointment and the GP feels his medical condition can wait
Practice area	Is defined with the FHSA; further changes require FHSA approval An accepted patient is entitled to treatment at the GP's surgery, his registered address or (as required) elsewhere in the practice area, but not outside it unless the address accepted at registration is outside the boundary
Absences and deputies	GPs must arrange adequate emergency cover and take reasonable steps to ensure continuity of treatment They must notify the FHSA of deputizing arrangements and obtain FHSA consent They must also notify the FHSA of cover arrangements if absent for more than a week A GP is generally responsible for all errors and omissions by his deputy (*except* where the deputy is already a principal on the FHSA list) He must also take reasonable steps to ensure his deputy is not disqualified by an FHSA or the General Medical Council (There are also conditions attached to the employment of assistants)
Records	Must be adequate and on FHSA-supplied stationery Are the property of the FHSA and must be forwarded on request, within 14 days of being told of the patient's death by the FHSA, or within a month of otherwise knowing
Certification	Certain statutory certificates (e.g. incapacity for work, registered stillbirth, pregnancy certification, etc.) are a contractual obligation, and no separate fee can be accepted
Fees	For most NHS work the GP cannot accept a fee from the patient: private medical reports, examinations and certificates, and immunizations not recognized for reimbursement by the FHSA are important exceptions
Employees	GPs must take reasonable care to ensure employees are qualified and competent and allow them refresher training opportunities

Table 7.2 *Contd*

Change of residence	Principals must notify the FHSA in writing within 28 days of moving hosue
Practice leaflet	Doctors on the medical list must compile a practice leaflet containing basic information specified by schedule (see Table 1.4, p. 44) This must be updated annually where appropriate, and made available to the FHSA and to the practice's patients
Annual reports	Doctors on the medical list must supply the FHSA with a confidential report containing basic information specified by schedule (see Table 1.3, p. 43), drawn up in the year ending 31 March and submitted by 30 June
Optional services	Separate medical lists are maintained for maternity, child health surveillance and minor surgery services Doctors must be suitably qualified and FHSA-approved Some activities are stipulated by schedule (e.g. minor surgery; see Section 1.7) while others are dictated on a local basis by FHSAs (e.g. child surveillance)
Local directory of principals	Doctors are obliged to provide sufficent information to enable FHSAs to compile and publish a local directory of family doctors, their qualifications, services and consulting arrangements (see Section 1.5)

1 The name of the parties.

2 The date their partnership commenced and the circumstances under which it can be dissolved.

3 The profit-sharing basis (ownership of premises and division of profits).

4 The division of expenses (including telephone, car, personal allowances and outside remunerations).

5 Basic working conditions like:
   (a) workload distribution;
   (b) holiday entitlement;
   (c) sick leave, study leave and maternity leave.

6 Practice policies, e.g.:
   (a) who signs the cheques;
   (b) who the practice solicitors/bankers/accountants are;
   (c) what private work and outside activity is allowable;
   (d) how far partners can place restrictions on acceptance of patients.

7 Voting rights of the partners in policy changes.

8 Provision for arbitration.

9 The condition on an outgoing partner that he will not set up practice within a close (defined) radius of the present one. (There has been difficulty in enforcing this last item, and in defining equality of workload, and practices often omit to make provision for arbitration.)

Commonly encountered problems include:

1   No written agreement to consult when there is disagreement.

2   A written contract different from the initial verbal offer.

3   Inequalities of workload or income contribution not reflected in partners' profit shares.

4   Unfairly restrictive clauses.

5   Disaffected ex-partners who set up practice down the road, taking their list with them.

Incoming partners can take advice from an independent solicitor and accountant, or seek guidance from the local medical council secretary, British Medical Association or other informed body. A correctly drafted agreement seeks to provide equity for all parties in all conceivable circumstances, and is in the interests of all partnerships with honourable intentions.

7.13 COMPLAINTS AGAINST GPs

In 1989 a total of 1361 complaints against GPs were investigated and 18% were upheld. The major cause of complaint was bad manners (35%), but the most frequent reason for successful complaint was failure to visit.

The stages involved in a complaint procedure are:

1   The FHSA receives an allegation from the patient, normally:
   (a) within 13 weeks (though certain circumstances are considered extenuating);
   (b) in writing (although oral complaints made in an FHSA office will be considered).

2   Attempts must first be made to achieve informal conciliation. (Typically a lay person contacts the parties.)

3   If this is unsuccessful the FHSA writes to the doctor inviting his account of what transpired.

4   This is submitted to the complainant to see whether the explanation now satisfies him.

5   If not, the chairperson of the Medical Services Committee (MSC) establishes whether there is a case to answer.

6   If there is, the correspondence goes before the entire committee (a chairperson and 4–6 other members, equally represented by medical and lay people) who decide the issue on the written accounts alone, or request a hearing.

7   The hearing differs from a court of law in that:
   (a) neither side can have a paid profesional advocate;
   (b) witnesses can be called, but are not compelled to attend;
   (c) no one is under oath;
   (d) members of the MSC can question anyone attending.

8   If the GP is thought to be in breach of his Terms of Service, the MSC may recommend:

(a) a caution;

(b) a fine;

(c) a restriction on the number of patients on the GP's list;

(d) referral to the General Medical Council or NHS tribunal (for possible removal from the medical list).

9 The FHSA may vary the penalty recommended; it sends copies of the verdict to the concerned parties and the DOH.

10 The GP has the right of appeal against the verdict, and can make representation to the Secretary of State.

7.14 PRODUCT LIABILITY

The Consumer Protection Act makes producers of defective products strictly liable for any harm caused, without need on the part of the injured party to prove carelessness or negligence in a law suit.

Normally in the event of mishap due to defective drugs and medical appliances the onus of liability falls on the manufacturer. However, if the manufacturer of personally administered emergency medicine cannot be identified the Consumer Production Act places liability on the immediate supplier, that is, the doctor himself.

The defence unions counsel that GPs should protect themselves through:

- proper container labelling;
- proper patient records;
- a separate personal record of the event, enabling the manufacturer or doctor's supplier to be identified (e.g. a log including data, patient's name, name of the drug, manufacturer's name, batch number and name of immediate supplier).

It is a hard but necessary fact of life that busy doctors need at antisocial times and in emergency situations to keep meticulous medicolegal records.

7.15 SHOULD DOCTORS ADVERTISE?

In 1989 the Monopolies and Mergers Commission decided that certain of the restrictions on advertising of medical services were anticompetitive and against the public interest. GPs have been allowed to advertise, subject to two broad caveats:

1 That advertising should not be of a form likely to bring the profession into disrepute.

2 That it should not abuse the trust of patients or exploit their lack of knowledge.

Thus, advertising should not disparage other doctors, or claim superiority over them, or include specific claims of cure. 'Cold calling' and undue pressure from over-frequent advertising are discouraged, and adverts are expected to conform to recognized standards — namely, that they are 'legal, decent and honest'.

Possible outlets for advertising include:

- the local media (newspapers, parish magazines, notice boards);
- yellow pages;
- mail shots.

Potential advantages

1 *To the consumer*: more information available when choosing a doctor.
2 *To doctors*: the opportunity to publicize their hard work and facilities and to be rewarded by higher capitation fees.
3 *To the tax-payer*: competition between doctors may raise standards of care and value for money.

Potential disadvantages

1 *To the patient*: choices made on the basis of this information may be shallow, as patients are not well placed to judge clinical competence. Efforts may be wasted providing gloss rather than substance. It has been suggested that the doctor–patient relationship is an impartial one, sometimes demanding the disclosure of unpalatable opinions, and that this is fundamentally incompatible with self-promotion and self-interest on the doctor's part.
2 *To the doctor*: the profession has misgivings that the code of good conduct will be difficult to police and ripe for exploitation.
3 *To the tax-payer*: the tax-payer ultimately funds advertising by doctors, as costs form part of the practice expenses pool.

A keen debate continues.

8 Schedules and Advice

The purpose of this chapter is twofold:

1 To present, mainly in tabular form, a lot of basic factual information that may be of help in the Multiple Choice Questionnaire (MCQ) and viva situation. The first part of the chapter tackles this and is very straightforward.

2 To cover some common clinical situations where GPs are required to give advice.

You can be sure that the examiners will be interested in establishing that you can give sensible and lucid advice to, say, the diabetic or epileptic, the foreign traveller, the driver and the asthmatic. Questions like this crop up in the viva (see Chapter 10). A good answer encompasses not just the traditionally taught physical aspects of the problem, but psychological and social ones, and examples are given to illustrate this point.

It is difficult to know where to begin and end, because effective communication is germane to every clinical contact and likely to appear under many guises in the examination. I would therefore encourage you to supplement the advice section liberally with your own examples.

It is, of course, a good principle to consider after every consultation how advice given could have been better phrased and delivered. It is probably also true that if you get into this habit, you will handle this aspect of the examination more competently.

8.1 SCHEDULES

Developmental milestones
Some milestones have well established predictive reliability (e.g. sitting unsupported — 90% at 8 months; using 2–3-word combinations — 90% at 24 months). Others have a wide range and may follow a particular pattern in families.

Developmental schedules
Developmental schedules widely used include:
- the Mary Sheridan developmental sequence (the 'average child at key ages' approach);
- the Denver screening test (the ages at which 25–90% of normals pass).

The key areas assessed are:
- vision;
- hearing;
- communication (comprehension and speech);

Table 8.1 Some common developmental milestones.

Age	Skills
2–4 weeks	Watches mother carefully when she speaks
4 weeks	Able to lift head from a surface
6 weeks	On ventral suspension, head held up on the same plane as body When pulled to sitting, marked but not complete headlag Can follow objects 1 m away over an angle of at least 90° Reacts to loud noises with a startle response Has the primitive reflexes (Moro, walking and grasp) Smiles (lack of a social smile by 12 weeks needs investigation) Gross symmetrical movements, but no fine ones
6–8 weeks	Vocalizes when talked to Eyes follow a moving person
12 weeks	When pulled to sitting, only slight headlag Will hold a rattle placed in the hand
12–16 weeks	Turns head to sounds on a level with the ear
5 months	No headlag Able to reach for an object and get it When prone, takes weight on forearms
5–6 months	Rolls over (supine to prone)
6 months	Sits supported When prone, takes weight on hands with arms extended Takes weight on legs if held up Begins to imitate Transfers a cube from one hand to the other Person preference developed
7 months	Feeds self with a biscuit Turns head to sounds below the level of the ear
8 months	Sits unsupported (75–90%) Picks up a raisin with a raking action (75–90%) (50–75% have hand transfer and finger-thumb grasp)
9 months	Crawls on abdomen
9–10 months	Plays 'peep-bo' Afraid of strangers
10 months	Creeps on hands and knees Pulls himself up to sitting Finger–thumb apposition and index-finger approach Waves bye-bye Plays patacake Assists dressing by offering an arm or foot
11 months	One word with meaning Walks holding on to furniture or with two hands held
12 months	2–3 words with meaning Walks when one hand is held
13 months	Walks unsupported (normal range 12–15 months)

Table 8.1 *Contd*

Age	Skills
15 months	Feeds himself from an ordinary cup Takes shoes off Builds a 2-cube tower
18 months	Manages a spoon Builds a 3–4-cube tower Points to three parts of the body Can climb stairs when one hand is held 10–12 words with meaning Jumps using both feet Asks for the potty
21–24 months	Joins 2–3 words to make a simple sentence
2 years	Runs without too many falls Can kick a ball or stoop and pick an object up while keeping his balance Builds a tower of 6–7 cubes Points to four parts of the body Puts on and takes off shoes and socks Speech is intelligible to friends and neighbours Tolerates children playing alongside him
2½–3 years	90% can scribble 15–20% of parents express concern regarding negative behaviour (temper tantrums, breath-holding spells and other outbursts and battles)
3 years	Plays with other children Can stand for a short period on one leg Can count up to three objects and state age and sex
4 years	Play is highly imaginative 90% can: • jump with feet together • pedal a tricycle • wash and dry their hands • copy a circle • give their first and last names
5 years	Can generally hop on one foot and count 10–12 objects

- social behaviour;
- neurological development (reflexes, gross motor movements, fine control and coordination).

Table 8.1 is a simplified description of some of the more memorable developmental milestones in the average child.

Well-person medical assessments

A series of new well-person assessments are required under GPs' Terms of Service. These contractual obligations are described in Section 1.5 and in Table 7.2, p. 226, and their clinical merit is considered in Section 3.3. Table 8.2 outlines the *content* of these scheduled examinations.

Table 8.2 Requirements of new medical assessments.

Newly registered patients and those not seen in the last 3 years
1   Consultation to establish relevant past medical and family history,
including:

Medical factors	Social factors	Lifestyle factors
Illnesses	Employment	Diet and exercise
Immunizations	Housing	Smoking
Allergies	Family circumstances	Alcohol and drug abuse
Hereditary factors		
Screening tests		
Current health		

2   Check of height, weight, blood pressure, urinalysis
3   Recording and discussing findings, giving appropriate advice

Over-75s
1   An annual invitation to consult, and offer of a domiciliary visit
2   Assessment, recording and discussion of matters relevant to health,
including:
  (a) sensory function
  (b) mobility
  (c) mental condition
  (d) physical condition (including continence)
  (e) social environment
  (f) use of medicines

Immunization

Types of vaccine
1   Toxoids, e.g. diphtheria, tetanus.
2   Inactivated vaccines, e.g. pertussis, cholera, typhoid, anthrax
and rabies.
3   Live vaccines — all viral (measles, rubella, polio, yellow fever)
except BCG.

Spacing and timing of vaccinations
At birth there is some passive immunity acquired when maternal
antibodies cross the placenta. At the same time the baby's own
immune system is immature, so babies are not vaccinated at birth.
(An exception is BCG vaccination given when a close household
member has tuberculosis.)

By 6 months passive immunity is lost and host immunity is
in the ascendance. Somewhere in between these two dates the
first triple and oral polio are given, representing a compromise
whereby maximum effect from vaccination is traded against the
increasing vulnerability to infection as passive immunity wanes.
Pertussis antibody (an immunoglobulin M antibody) is too large
to cross the placenta, so young unimmunized infants are particularly prone to this infection. Measles antibodies are slower to

be catabolized and the longer duration of immunity allows vaccination to be deferred.

Until quite recently it was advised that the optimum immune response for most vaccines required booster doses at approximately 6 weeks and then 6 months. However the schedule for primary immunization has been simplified (to start at 2 months with an interval of 1 month between each booster dose) because of theoretical and practical considerations — namely that:
- the old regimen was protracted, variable between authorities, and confusing, thus hindering uptake by highly mobile parents with young families;
- experience showed antibody responses to be perfectly adequate when the faster, simpler schedule was used.

In general, live vaccines have a prolonged duration of protection because they are more antigenic, and so booster doses are less important. (At first sight polio is an exception, since primary immunization follows the usual three-dose pattern: in fact three different strains of virus are employed, and so three spaced vaccinations are needed to ensure that antibody responses do not interfere with one another.)

It is from these principles that the familiar immunization schedules are constructed (Table 8.3).

Incomplete courses sometimes cause confusion. Generally speaking:

1 If only one dose is given, a further two doses with a month's gap between them will complete the course.

Table 8.3 A common immunization schedule.

Age	Vaccination	Route	Interval
2 months	DTP/Adv Plus polio	0.5 ml i.m./deep s.c. Oral (3 drops)	1 month and then . . .
3 months	As above (2nd dose)	As above	1 month and then . . .
4 months	As above (3rd dose)	As above	(Until school entry)
1–2 years	MMR or measles	0.5 ml i.m./deep s.c.	—
4–5 years	DT plus polio MMR*		(Until school leaving for tetanus and polio)
10–13 years	Rubella*	0.5 ml s.c.	—
10–13 years	BCG (if tuberculin negative)	0.1 ml i.d.	(3 weeks between rubella and BCG)
School leaving	Tetanus and polio (boosters)	0.5 ml i.m. and 3 drops orally, respectively	Tetanus — 5–10-yearly

*If not previously vaccinated.

2 If two doses have been given, the third will still be effective if given within 12 months of the second.

Contraindications to live viruses
1 Acute febrile illness;
2 Pregnancy;
3 Within 3 weeks of another live vaccine (except in emergency vaccination programmes);
4 Immunosuppression (e.g. immunodeficiency states, malignancy, cytotoxic treatment, steroids).

Points of importance individual to particular vaccines
1 *Diphtheria*. A safe vaccine. May cause transient local tenderness/redness. Not given over the age of 10 years unless Schick test positive and patient at risk.
2 *Tetanus*. Also causes occasional local reactions of a minor nature. Rarely a hypersensitivity response when injections are too frequent, hence a booster should not be given within 1 year of the previous injection.
3 *Pertussis*. Causes local reactions and mild fever/irritability. Encephalopathy and convulsions are very rare (about 1 in 300 000 vaccinations). Guidelines on the vaccine are prone to change.
    Absolute contraindications currently advised are:
    (a) severe local/general/neurological reaction last time;
    (b) history of cerebral irritation or damage in the neonatal period;
    (c) past history of fits/convulsions.
    Relative contraindications are:
    (a) parents or siblings with a history of idiopathic epilepsy;
    (b) children with neurological disease or developmental delay.
    Many children in whom there are relative contraindications can still be immunized, and referral to a specialist is usually warranted. It has been estimated that pertussis vaccination is contraindicated in 0.5–3.5% of children, and that a further 3.5% will receive an incomplete course due to problems arising from the first or second injection (Jelley & Nicoll 1984).
4 *Polio*. Contraindicated in cases of allergy to penicillin, streptomycin, neomycin and polymyxin. May cause diarrhoea and vomiting, and very rare cases of vaccine-related paralysis in contacts (a risk perhaps of one per million doses).
5 *Measles*. May produce a mild measles-like syndrome after about a week; rarely convulsions and an encephalopathy in about one in 87 000 cases (a 12- to 20-fold reduction over the natural complication rate of measles). Contraindicated when there is a severe anaphylactic allergy to egg protein and in tuberculosis (which it may reactivate); when there is a history of fits in the child, parents

or siblings, immunoglobulin should be given simultaneously in the other arm.

6 *Rubella*. May give a mild rubella-syndrome around day 9, arthralgia in women, and rarely thrombocytopenia. Contraindicated when there is allergy to polymyxin, neomycin and rabbits (Cendevax vaccine only). A risk of fetal damage in the first trimester, so pregnancy contraindicated and effective contraception advised for 3 months.

7 *Measles, mumps and rubella (MMR)*. As with measles the vaccine may cause malaise, fever, and/or a rash after about a week, lasting about 2–3 days. Parotid swelling occasionally occurs in the third week. This condition is not infectious. Contraindications are those for live vaccines; allergy to neomycin or kanamycin; or a history of anaphylaxis due to any cause (milder egg allergy is *not* a contraindication). If MMR is given to adult women, pregnancy should be avoided for 1 month. (The MMR vaccination programme is described below.)

8 *BCG*. Sometimes causes local reactions, including discharging skin ulcers and subcutaneous abscess formation. Contraindicated when there is local sepsis.

The MMR vaccination programme

In seeking to prevent rubella infection in pregnancy, two possible strategies could have been chosen. The first strategy, to eliminate childhood rubella altogether by infant vaccination, was adopted in the USA. The UK chose instead to protect in pregnancy, by immunizing 10–13-year-old girls and all women of child-bearing age found to be seronegative.

This approach was favoured at a time when the duration of immunity conferred by rubella vaccination in infancy was uncertain. However, it is now known that the modern vaccine's benefit will extend from infancy through the reproductive years; also that the UK policy failed to prevent nearly 400 cases per year, in part because of the reservoir of infection still circulating among the young offspring of seronegative mothers in their second pregnancy, and in part because it was difficult to achieve a 100% seroconversion rate in young women.

The argument has now swung in favour of the American programme under which a high uptake rate (80–90%) should virtually eliminate the infecting reservoir. Thus, infants will in future receive primary immunization against rubella.

The infection is most common in children aged 4–9 years, and to eliminate rubella speedily from this age group preschool children aged 4–5 years will be given the combined vaccine for the next few years (until the first cohort of infants reaches school age); schoolgirls will continue to receive monovalent rubella vaccine until the programme has caught up; and seronegative women will continue to be screened and vaccinated in the usual way.

The vaccine can be given to children of any age on request, and to non-immune adults, but since in 80–90% of cases disease is acquired before entry to secondary school, mass vaccination after the age of 11 would have little impact on incidence.

The mumps component of the vaccine has been included because of the considerable morbidity caused by mumps, e.g.:

• over 1000 hospital admissions per year;
• the commonest cause of meningitis and encephalitis in children under 15;
• permanent sensorineural hearing loss on occasion. Experience in the USA indicates that the mumps vaccine is successful and popular, and combining it with the measles vaccine has improved the uptake of the less popular measles component.

Preliminary studies indicate that the MMR vaccine is effective with a high seroconversion rate (90–100%). The overall benefit and progress of the MMR campaign will be closely monitored.

Vaccination for foreign travel

Recommendations
Recommendations change from time to time, so it is important to keep abreast of the latest ones, which are published regularly in the medical press. The current Red Book vaccination recommendations (accepted for reimbursement) are listed in Table 8.4.

Reimbursement
Reimbursement comes from two sources:
1 *The Family Health Service Authority (FHSA)*: claimed on form FP 73 for vaccinations given in accordance with the Red Book recommendations (as above).

Table 8.4 Red Book vaccination recommendations.

Area	Vaccinations
Northern Europe, Southern Europe (excluding Turkey), North America, Australia, New Zealand and Japan	No specific needs Update standard domestic vaccinations, e.g. tetanus For special high-risk groups ('living rough') polio, typhoid, tetanus or human immunoglobulin
Turkey	Polio
Central and South America, Central Africa	Polio, typhoid, yellow fever (mandatory)
Middle East, North Africa	Polio, typhoid, cholera
South Africa, India, South-East Asia and China	Polio, typhoid

2   *The patient* for:

(a) vaccines and the service (if outside the FHSA guidelines);

(b) private prescriptions related to foreign travel (prescriptions issued solely for the purpose of foreign travel, as distinct from normal maintenance prescribing, should be *private* prescriptions);

(c) summary certificates and international cholera card.

Vaccination schedules

Vaccination schedules depend on the countries being visited, the degree of risk of contracting the disease and the amount of time left before travel. Full and abridged schedules appear in Table 8.5. (Abridged schedules are a compromise, affording reasonable protection when time is short.)

Points of importance relating to specific vaccines
See Table 8.6.

Table 8.5 Full and rapid vaccination schedules for foreign travel.

Time	Vaccination
Full schedule	
First visit	Typhoid 0.5 ml deep s.c./i.m. *plus*
	Cholera 0.5 ml i.m.
	Tetanus 0.5 ml deep s.c./i.m.
	Polio 3 drops p.o.
3 weeks (if visiting a yellow fever area)	Yellow fever 0.5 ml s.c. (from specialist centre)
4–6 weeks (must be 6 if yellow fever given)	Typhoid 0.1 ml i.d. (booster)
	Cholera 0.1 ml i.d. (booster)
	(Polio 3 drops p.o. — if part of a primary immunization course)
7–9 weeks (and 2–4 days before travel)	Human normal immunoglobulin 0.5 ml deep i.m.
(6–8 months later)	(Further tetanus and polio boosters if part of a primary immunization course)
Rapid schedule	
Day 1	Typhoid, cholera, tetanus and polio (as above)
Day 5	Yellow fever (as above — if applicable)
Day 13	Cholera booster (and polio booster if part of a primary immunization course)
Day 28	Typhoid booster (and tetanus/polio if part of a primary immunization programme)

(In a true emergency, even the last visit can be omitted, since one typhoid injection gives reasonable immunity)

Table 8.6 Details relating to specific vaccines used in foreign travel.

Vaccine	Dose/route	Spacing	Side-effects	Contraindications	Efficacy
Polio	3 drops p.o.	5- to 10-yearly	Rarely paralysis in recipients or contacts	Those for any live vaccine	Excellent
Tetanus	0.5 ml deep s.c. or i.m.	5- to 10-yearly	Rare hypersensitivity reactions with too frequent boosters Transient local pain	A tetanus injection within the last year	Excellent
Typhoid	0.5 ml i.m., then 0.1 ml i.d. (first course) 0.1 ml i.d. (for boosters)	If 3 years or more since last one (*Not* after age 35 years)	Local redness and swelling; malaise, nausea, fever, headache — 36 h Rare neurological complications	Not under the age of 12 months	70–90% effective for 3–7 years
Cholera	0.5 ml i.m., then (after 4 weeks) 0.1 ml i.d.	6-monthly (Certificate valid from 6 days to 6 months)	Local pain, redness, swelling (i.d. injections give less reaction)	—	40–80%, declining after 3 months
Yellow fever	0.5 ml s.c., in special regional centre	10-yearly (Certificate valid from 10 days to 10 years)	Rare — sometimes redness/swelling; myalgia and headache (5–10 days) Rare encephalitis in the under-1-year-olds	Not under the age of 12 months; those for any live virus; egg hypersensitivity	Very good

Incubation and infectivity periods of communicable diseases

For details see Table 8.7.

8.2 ADVICE

Medical advice to travellers

Medical contraindications to flight

Physiological problems produced by air flights include:

1 Reduced atmospheric pressure: aircraft cabins are not pressurized to sea level, and cabin pressure drops with ascent until about 7000 feet, hence gas trapped in body cavities *expands*.

2 Hypoxia: reduced atmospheric pressure means a reduced partial pressure of oxygen (P_{O_2}). At 6000 feet oxyhaemoglobin is reduced by 3–4% — a small amount if you are healthy, but not if you are an unhealthy hypoxia-sensitive individual.

3 An upset in the normal circadian rhythms (jet lag).

Other problems can arise from the risk of spreading contagious disease in a confined space, and the impossibility of providing anything other than the most basic medical care during travel.

Most of the contraindications can be remembered by applying these principles in a common sense way. The following is a simple *aide-mémoire*.

This problem . . .	*. . . may exacerbate these conditions*
Expansion of gas trapped in body cavities	Asthmatic attack
	Recent middle ear disease, middle ear surgery, and sinusitis with catarrh
	Unresolved pneumothorax
	Recent chest surgery (within 3 weeks)
	Recent abdominal surgery (within 10 days)
	Diving (within 12 h for aqualung divers, and 24 h if diving depth is more than 100 feet)
Hypoxia	Recent myocardial infarction (within 3–6 weeks)
	Uncontrolled cardiac failure
	Severe anaemia (e.g. haemoglobin less than 7 g/dl)
	Severe respiratory disease
	Recent cerebrovascular accident (within 3–6 weeks)
	Sickle cell disease

Table 8.7 Incubation and infectivity periods of communicable diseases.
(a) Incubation periods.

Disease	Range: max. (days)	Usual (if different)
Short incubation (<7 days)		
Bacillary dysentery	1–7	2–4
Gonorrhoea	1–12	2–6
Influenza	18 h to 3 days	18–36 h
Anthrax	1–7	1–3
Cholera	Hours to 6 days	2–3 h
Diphtheria	2–5	1–7
Scarlet fever	1–3	—
Intermediate incubation (7–21 days)		
Chickenpox	10–21	14–17
Measles	7–14	9–11
Mumps	12–21	18
Whooping cough	7–10	7
Tetanus	1–14	4–13
Rubella	14–21	18
Amoebiasis	14–28	21
Malaria	10–14	—
Polio	3–21	7–14
Typhoid	7–21	10
Long incubation (>21 days)		
Infectious mononucleosis	4–6 weeks	––
Hepatitis A	2–6 weeks	4 weeks
Hepatitis B	6 weeks to 12 months	12 weeks

(b) Infectivity periods.

Disease	Infectivity period
Scarlet fever	10–21 days after rash onset (but only 1 day if penicillin given)
Chickenpox	5 days before rash until 6 days after the last crop
Measles	From onset of prodromal illness to 4 days after the rash onset
Mumps	3 days before salivary swelling to 7 days after
Whooping cough	7 days after exposure to 3 weeks after onset of symptoms (but only 7 days if antibiotics given)
Rubella	7 days before onset of rash to 4 days after

(c) Interval between disease onset and rash.

Disease	Interval in days
Scarlet fever	1–2
Chickenpox	0–2
Measles	3–5
Rubella	0–2
Typhoid	7–14

Spread of infection in a confined space	Contagious diseases in their infectivity period
Remoteness from medical care	Recent gastrointestinal haemorrhage
	Pregnancy (after 35 weeks for long flights and after 36 weeks for domestic ones)
	Acute mental illness (unless the patient is escorted and sedation is to hand)

Motion sickness

1 *Who?* One-third of the populus, especially children (peak age 10 years).

2 *What?* Various symptoms, including: pallor; cold sweats; nausea and vomiting; malaise; yawning; headaches; drowsiness.

3 *Why?* Probably multifactorial, but a mismatch between motion information from the eyes and vestibular apparatus/proprioceptors is the main stimulus.

4 *Advice?*

    (a) sit children up high, so they can see out;

    (b) provide good ventilation;

    (c) provide activities (e.g. games), but *no* reading;

    (d) limit alcohol intake;

    (e) if severe, lie down with eyes closed;

    (f) choose the most stable part of the vehicle to sit (car — front seat; boat — the middle; plane — between the wings).

5 *Drugs?*

    (a) take preparations 1–2 h *prior* to travel (otherwise absorption may be impaired).

    (b) either an anticholinergic or antihistamine. Anticholinergics are very effective, but associated with more side-effects. The antihistamines offer a choice in the duration of action (e.g. cyclizine — short-acting; promethazine — once-daily preparation). Tailor the time course of the drug to the duration of travel.

Jet lag

1 *What?* An upset in the circadian rhythms (e.g. sleep cycle; hunger pattern; bowel and urinary habits). Occurs if the time difference is greater than 5 h. *Less* marked when the day *lengthens* (i.e. going westwards).

2 *Advice?*

    (a) avoid unnecessary stress (e.g. arrive in good time);

    (b) avoid smoking, food and alcohol;

    (c) maintain a good fluid intake (non-diuretic beverages);

(d) sleep on the plane if you can;

(e) allow an easy first 24 h to adjust after arrival. Remember that performance may be impaired for a week after travel (businessmen beware!).

Food hygiene

1   *The problem.* Food-borne and water-borne infections, e.g.:

(a) contaminated drinking water may transmit *Escherichia coli*, *Shigella*, cholera, typhoid, hepatitis A, amoebic dysentery or giardiasis;

(b) poultry are notorious sources of *Campylobacter* and *Salmonella*;

(c) shellfish may transmit typhoid;

(d) unpasteurized milk is a possible source of tuberculosis, brucellosis and Q fever.

2   *Advice?*

(a) boil drinking water or chlorinate it (remember — *all* water);

(b) avoid unpasteurized milk;

(c) do not buy food or icecream from street vendors;

(d) avoid salads and unpeeled fruit and vegetables;

(e) eat only food that has been recently cooked (and is hot and steaming);

(f) be wary of seafood, especially shellfish.

Other precautions for travellers

Table 8.8 summarizes some of the more common hazards and strategies for reducing the risk.

Malaria

1   *General advice.* The standard insect bite avoidance advice (Table 8.8) is appropriate. Also:

(a) start tablets 1 week before departure and continue for at least 4 (possibly 6) weeks after return;

(b) if you omit any doses, you are taking a risk;

(c) drugs are prophylactic, not curative; furthermore protection is not 100%, so report fevers within 2 months of return.

2   *Drugs.* The appropriate choice is not straightforward. Recommendations change frequently, so get up-to-date information from an expert source. Two currently favoured preparations are compared in Table 8.9.

In *falciparum*-endemic areas both chloroquine and Fansidar should be taken (the chloroquine because of its better protection against *vivax*).

Other drugs include:

• *Maloprim* (contains dapsone, which is sulphonamide-related and so is also contraindicated in sulphonamide hypersensitivity);

Table 8.8 Common holiday hazards and how to avoid them.

Problem	Advice
Sunburn	Limit the exposure in very hot climates to 15 min at first, doubled each day thereafter (longer if sunscreens are used, less if fair-skinned and sun-sensitive) Avoid the midday sun Reapply sunscreens after bathing
Prickly heat (a pinhead itchy rash due to keratin plugs blocking sweat ducts which extravasate sweat into the tissues). Mainly in areas of non-evaporation (chest, back, axillae and groins)	Maintain a high fluid and salt intake Reduce sweating, e.g.: • wear loose cotton clothes • swim and shower often • keep in the shade and limit exertion • use the room-fan, if one is provided Dust with talc or apply calamine. Antihistamines for the itching
Insect-borne infections (many problems from local reactions through to rickettsial infections and leishmaniasis!)	Wear long-sleeved shirt and long trousers after dark Do not walk barefoot Use any mosquito net provided Apply insect repellant to *all* exposed skin
Sexually transmitted diseases	Barrier contraception and postcoital douching or micturition offer some partial protection. The high prevalence of acquired immune deficiency syndrome in parts of Central and East Africa and North America makes casual sex very risky: it should be avoided
Accidents	Common sense precautions (e.g. do not drink to excess; do not approach stray animals; drive with extra care) Take important spares (contact lenses, dentures, Ventolin inhaler, diaphragm, etc.) Arrange adequate medical insurance. Leaflet T1 (DSS) lists countries with reciprocal health care arrangements
Travel vaccinations	Covered separately in Table 8.5, but remember: • consult the latest guidelines • allow adequate time to complete the course

• *proguanil and pyrimethamine* (which cause occasional folate antagonism).

Traveller's diarrhoea

1 *Where?* Worldwide, but most commonly in Africa and Asia.

2 *What?* 70% of cases are due to enterotoxic *E. coli* strains; other culprits include *Campylobacter*, rotavirus, *Salmonella*, *Shigella*, *Amoeba* and *Giardia*.

Symptoms, which usually only last a few days, include:

Table 8.9 Two common antimalarial preparations.

Preparation	Form	Availability	Contraindications	Efficacy	Side-effects
Chloroquine	300 mg base/ week	No script needed	—	Very good versus *vivax*, but not *falciparum*	Chronic use can produce corneal and retinal changes
Fansidar (pyrimethamine and sulfadoxine)	1/week	Prescription only	Sulphonamide hypersensitivity First few weeks of life Third trimester (neonatal jaundice)	Best for *falciparum*	Typical sulphonamide side-effects

(a) nausea and vomiting;
(b) colic;
(c) watery diarrhoea.
3 *Drugs?*
(a) *prophylactic antibiotics* (e.g. Streptotriad and doxycycline) have been shown to be beneficial but consideration of possible side-effects and drug resistance suggests they are best reserved for the elderly, infirm and high-risk cases.
(b) *in treatment* Lomotil or Imodium will reduce stool frequency and abdominal pain, and Septrin/trimethoprim reduces symptoms considerably if taken early. The mainstay of treatment, however, is fluid replacement. Electrolyte mixtures (e.g. Dioralyte) are very useful.
(c) *medical advice* may be needed in severe cases (prostration, severe vomiting, fever and blood per rectum) and for the very young.

Medical advice on fitness to drive

Medical fitness to drive is a favourite examination topic. Some of the more important aspects are summarized in Table 8.10, which is adapted from the definitive and detailed account *Medical Aspects of Fitness to Drive* published by the Medical Commission on Accident Prevention.
    Note that according to the law:
1 It is the duty of the *applicant* (not his doctor) to declare:
(a) prescribed (relevant) disabilities, e.g. epilepsy and subnormality;
(b) intermittent or progressive disabilities which may become relevant (prospective disabilities).
2 Licence-holders are also obliged to notify the Drivers and Vehicle Licensing Centre (DVLC) as soon as they develop relevant

Table 8.10 Medical advice on fitness to drive.

Disease or symptoms	Advice to the holder of an ordinary driver's licence	Advice to the holder of an HGV or PSV licence
Cardiovascular system		
Myocardial infarction	Avoid driving within 2 months Notify the DVLC	Very exacting restrictions — disbarred: • if his ECG is abnormal (typical Q waves, ST and T wave changes, left bundle branch and complete heart block) • if it is his 2nd myocardial infarction (*or* first *with* peripheral vascular disease) • if a coronary angiogram shows significant occlusions or his treadmill test significant ST depression • or if any of the host of complications listed below applies
Angina	Avoid driving if angina is easily provoked by it	There should be no anginal pains at all (and no significant ST changes on treadmill testing)
Complete heart block	Driving is *forbidden*. Notify the DVLC. After pacemaker implantation driving is allowed (from 1 month) as long as the pacemaker function is checked regularly	Driving is permanently forbidden, even with a pacemaker *in situ*
Transient faintness, impaired concentration, syncopal tendency, postural hypotension	Avoid driving until the problem is resolved	Depends on the cause but generally driving is not allowed if there is any vasovagal/syncopal tendency or any arrhythmias (except occasional ectopics disappearing with exercise)
Other problems	Heart surgery, aortic aneurysms, hypertension, peripheral vascular disease, valvular lesions and arrhythmias — no special restrictions (unless they provoke the problems covered above)	Many conditions cause a ban on driving: • any significant cardiomegaly (CTR ≥ 0.5) • any features of aortic aneurysm • blood pressure $\geq 200/110$ mmHg • complicated congenital heart disease • current anticoagulant treatment • almost all paroxysmal arrhythmias • many exclusions after heart surgery

Table 8.10 *Contd*

Disease or symptoms	Advice to the holder of an ordinary driver's licence	Advice to the holder of an HGV or PSV licence
Endocrine/metabolic system		
Diabetes	Notify the DVLC. A limited licence (1, 2 or 3 years) will normally be issued, depending on quality of control, complications and follow-up. Insulin-dependent diabetics in particular should show: • a reasonable understanding • reasonable control of their blood sugar • no frequent, sudden or unexplained hypoglycaemic attacks	Following the WHO Expert Committee report (1980) and the EC Driving Licence Directive: *Existing drivers* need to report to the licensing authority only if: • their control worsens • they switch to insulin *but* they need individual review; *New entrants* must not be insulin-dependent
	For all driving diabetics Driving should be avoided (or carbohydrate taken) at times when hypoglycaemic risk is greatest. Drive by the clock and stop for regular meals. Carry sugar lumps or glucose tablets and at the first hint of hypoglycaemia pull over, switch off, take the ignition key out and vacate the driving seat (*then* take the sugar)	
Neurological system		
Epilepsy	Notify the DVLC. Under the Road Traffic Act a limited duration licence (1, 2 or 3 years) is granted, providing: • the patient has been fit-free during the previous 2 years, *or* • has only had attacks while asleep for the last 3 years, *and* • is not likely to be a source of danger to the public	Road Traffic Act regulations bar people from holding a vocational licence if they have had an epileptic attack since attaining the age of 5 years. (When there is doubt that the event was a true fit, the Honorary Medical Advisory Panel will arbitrate)
1 If a further daytime fit occurs after a licence is granted	Another 2 fit-free years must elapse	
2 During treatment changes	Epileptics are advised not to drive for 6 months	
3 The patient with a single fit (diagnosis in doubt)	Driving should be suspended pending investigation. If clinical or EEG evidence of a primary cerebral cause emerges this is regarded as epilepsy. If no cause is found, the DVLC must still be notified (and will probably ban driving for 1 year)	
4 After severe head injuries or craniotomy	Due to the high frequency of fits in the next 12 months it is advised not to drive for this period	
Migraine	Do not drive from the onset of the warning period	(No additional restrictions)

Table 8.10 *Contd*

Disease or symptoms	Advice to the holder of an ordinary driver's licence	Advice to the holder of an HGV or PSV licence
Sudden disabling giddiness/syncope (e.g. due to Menière's disease, vertebrobasilar insufficiency)	Notify the DVLC who will normally ban driving for 12 months	These patients are debarred from holding a vocational licence
Vertigo and TIAs	Notify the DVLC who normally insist on 3 symptom-free months	
Muscle weakness, post-CVA, sensory defects, multiple sclerosis, Parkinson's disease	Individual assessment of competence and disability	Persistent or recurrent deficits and most disorders of a progressive disabling nature result in a driving ban
Vision	All drivers must pass the standard number plate test: 3½" figures at 25 yards in daylight: this is a visual acuity of about 6/10 (glasses are allowed) Significant disabilities (e.g. poor visual acuity, diplopia, impaired night vision) will normally debar. Special assessment and review are needed for prospective disabilities (e.g. field defects, cataracts, glaucoma, macular degeneration, diabetic retinopathy)	Uncorrected visual acuity must be at least 6/60 in each eye, and corrected must be 6/9 or better in one eye, and 6/12 in the other. Applicants with any field defect, or diplopia, or a single eye will be banned. Patients may be allowed to drive within 2 months of cataract surgery if their vision fulfils the required standards
Psychiatric aspects Psychosis	Should not drive until the illness is controlled and compliance with treatment is satisfactory	Suspension of a licence for at least 5 years following cessation of treatment (and 10 years for hypomania/mania)
Neurosis	Should avoid driving in the early stages of acute illness	Caution is advised
Mental handicap	Depends on the severity of the handicap	An absolute ban
Alcoholism	The law on drinking and driving is clear: the legal blood alcohol limit is 80 mg/100 ml. In many road accidents alcohol plays a part, so do not drink and drive!	The same recommendations apply as for acute psychosis
Personality disorders	Together with drinkers account for more accidents than the other categories combined. Unlikely to accept advice	

Psychotropic drugs (covered separately under the heading 'Drugs')

Table 8.10 *Contd*

Disease or symptoms	Advice to the holder of an ordinary driver's licence	Advice to the holder of an HGV or PSV licence
Locomotor system	Largely a matter of common sense and individual assessment. Even amputees can drive safely in adapted vehicles. Prospective disabilities must be notified to the DVLC	The same is true, but assessment is likely to be more stringent
Drugs CNS depressants (e.g. hypnotics, sedatives, neuroleptics, many antidepressants, antihistamines, anticholinergics, narcotic analgesia)	Impair motor skills and reaction time. Patients should exercise special care, especially when starting drugs for the first time. Sedation is potentiated by alcohol	In general, driving is excluded because of the medical condition for which the drug was taken. Also in general, taking CNS-active drugs, insulin and most hypotensive drugs is felt to be incompatible with vocational driving
Stimulants and appetite suppressants	Avoid driving: they promote risk-taking behaviour	
Anaesthetics	Patients should not drive for 24–48 h after anaesthesia for minor outpatient surgery	
Antihypertensives	May cause hypotension, sedation and fatigue. Exercise care at the outset of treatment	
Age	Drivers over 70 years have to renew their licence and make a health declaration every 3 years, but their insurance companies may demand annual medicals. Common diseases rendering the elderly unfit to drive include: TIAs, vertigo, syncope, arrhythmias, severe angina, Parkinson's disease and senile dementia. (Elderly drivers are advised to avoid peak traffic periods, overlong journeys and a lot of night-time driving)	*HGV licence holders* must apply for a renewal at 60 years, and then every 3 years. They must supply a medical certificate *PSV drivers' licences* are reviewed at 46 years, 5-yearly to 65 years, then annually. Again a medical report is needed

HGV, Heavy goods vehicle; PSV, public service vehicle; DVLC, Drivers and Vehicle Licensing Centre; CTR, cardiothoracic ratio; WHO, World Health Organization; EC, Economic Community; EEG, electroencephalogram; TIAs, transient ischaemic attacks; CVA, cerebrovascular accident; CNS, central nervous system.

or prospective disabilities, and if a previously notified disability becomes worse.

3   Temporary disabilities (e.g. fractures) are excluded, if they are expected to last less than 3 months.

Failure of the licence-holder to notify the DVLC places the doctor in an awkward position, as he may regard the physical safety of other road users to be at risk. This is one of the acknowledged circumstances under which breach of confidentiality may be justified (see Section 7.10).

The Transport Act 1981 states that drivers and front-seat passengers must wear a seatbelt; children must sit in the back and wear seatbelts if fitted. Exemptions are allowed:
- for drivers who have to get in and out frequently (e.g. from a milk float);
- while carrying out manoeuvres (e.g. reversing);
- for holders of medical exemption certificates. Since wearing a seatbelt reduces fatalities and injuries by 50%, very few conditions genuinely justify an exemption and very few exemptions have been approved. The following are *not* generally accepted:
- pregnancy;
- colostomies (seatbelts are adjustable);
- recent abdominal surgery (if a scar prevents the wearing of a seatbelt the person should not be driving).

Advising the person with epilepsy

Epilepsy is a very common problem. It is estimated that one in 20 people have a non-febrile seizure at some stage; 80% of those having more than one fit become seizure-free, leaving one in 200 with chronic epilepsy. In a practice list of 2500 this means 125 patients with a non-febrile seizure and 12 with epilepsy.

The psychological and social impact of the diagnosis may pose more problems than simple stabilization to a fit-free state. Advice will be required on drugs and compliance, the likely restrictions on activity and employment, the genetic implications, and to the carers in the first-aid situation. Epileptics will need intensive education and emotional support. Some of these points are now considered.

Driving

Epileptics cannot legally drive until entirely fit-free for 2 years (or experiencing fits only while asleep for 3 years). People who have fits after age 5 years are ineligible to hold a vocational licence. After a single fit it is recommended not to drive while under investigation, and for a year after if the cause is unknown. Epileptics should not drive while treatment is being altered (see Table 8.10).

Certain occupations exclude epileptic patients, for example, air traffic controllers; surgeons, high-speed machinery operators; the armed forces and police; those debarred by driving restrictions.

Activities

Most young epileptics risk being cocooned in a restrictive environment by overprotective relatives. Activities should be as free as possible with the exception of a few common sense guidelines:

- do not swim alone;
- do not climb trees/ropes, or take up mountaineering;
- do not bathe babies whilst alone, etc.

Bicycle riding is generally felt to be an acceptable risk, and little restriction is advised in games and school activities.

Genetic advice

If one parent is epileptic, the chance of producing an affected child is about 3% although there are some variations: the risk is higher if the epilepsy is idiopathic or generalized, and lower if focal or structural. However it is still less than 5%, and therefore no reason to advise against child-bearing. The incidence of congenital malformation is increased from about 2.7–7.5% (though abnormalities are often mild).

Epileptics should continue taking their drugs in pregnancy. Although there is a small teratogenic potential, the risk to pregnancy is greater from uncontrolled epilepsy.

First-aid advice

Simple guidelines are required to help carers cope with a frightening situation, e.g.:

- restrain the patient and prevent him from hurting himself;
- try to prevent him biting his tongue, by putting something in his mouth: this may not be possible in the tonic phase so do not force the issue (you may break a tooth!);
- if possible, try and move the patient into the recovery position;
- if in doubt, and particularly if the fit is prolonged, phone for medical assistance.

Emotional support and education

The patient should be treated as normally as possible. Remember that he (and especially his family) may be experiencing a variety of emotions, e.g.:

- anger and rejection;
- anxiety;
- a sort of bereavement reaction (following loss of health, job, etc.);
- shame or embarrassment.

Offer easy access and a sympathetic ear. Educate at every opportunity: referral to the British Epilepsy Association and books like *Epilepsy — the Facts* may help.

Follow-up
Well organized GPs are armed with a checklist of areas to cover (perhaps a flow sheet or cooperation card) and this may include such aspects as:
- drugs and compliance;
- side-effects;
- blood levels of drugs;
- control;
- social and psychological problems.

Febrile convulsions
Febrile convulsions are very common. It has been estimated that 30 per 1000 children under 7 years have a seizure associated with a fever. (About 5 per 1000 have recurrent non-febrile seizures.) Febrile convulsions are very alarming for parents, who naturally suspect the unpalatable diagnosis of epilepsy or worse.

Characteristics of febrile convulsions include:
- association with fever;
- rarity after age 6 years;
- a strong genetic element (25% in siblings and 50% in identical twins).

The association seems to be with the *rise* in temperature rather than its absolute height.

First-aid measures designed to lower temperature include taking clothes off, sponging with tepid water, fanning and administering antipyretic drugs. Fits can be controlled with Valium 0.2–0.3 mg/kg i.v. or rectally. Many authorities would admit to hospital on the first occasion to rule out meningitis.

Parents' major concerns will be with the likelihood of recurrence and of the child being a long-term epileptic. The following information may be given:

1 About 30–40% have a recurrence.

2 Prophylactic medicines are generally disappointing; they may have significant side-effects and do not reduce the risk of subsequent epilepsy. Attempted prophylaxis during a febrile episode is worth trying but often too late.

3 There is an increased risk of epilepsy in adulthood (increased about fourfold compared with the general population) but the risk is still only about 2 or 3 in 100. The risk is higher (perhaps 10%) if seizures:

    (a) are focal;
    (b) are prolonged (more than 15 min);
    (c) run in the family;

(d) start before age 1 year;
(e) are associated with developmental or neurological abnormalities.

Advising the person with diabetes
In the complicated and common metabolic disorder of diabetes much ground needs to be covered by way of education and information. There are several important areas.

General information
1 Explanation of the disorder (the underlying principles of the disorder and its management).
2 The dangers if neglected (hypoglycaemia, hyperglycaemia, long-term complications).
3 The range of treatment (diet, drugs, insulin).
4 The need to learn self-monitoring and to make it a way of life.
5 The relevance of follow-up to health.
6 If insulin is prescribed, specific help with needles, syringes, self-injection, dose adjustments, etc.
7 Important 'dos and don'ts', e.g. *Do*:
   (a) always carry a readily absorbable glucose store (e.g. sugar lumps);
   (b) carry a medic-alert bracelet in case of collapse;
   (c) seek medical advice when ill with persistently raised urine or blood tests (more than 1% sugar in the urine or fingerprick blood tests 13 or more mmol/l);
   (d) develop a regular routine;
   (e) take extra sugar if extra exertion is planned;
   (f) contact your doctor in the event of persistent vomiting;
   (g) contact your doctor at the earliest opportunity if pregnancy is suspected (or better still see him before conception to plan management);
   (h) have your feet and your eyesight checked regularly.
   Do not:
   (a) reduce insulin when unwell and taking a reduced diet: it generally needs increasing, so increase the frequency of self-monitoring and seek advice;
   (b) miss meals;
   (c) drive if you feel a hypoglycaemic episode coming on;
   (d) walk barefoot;
   (e) smoke.

Pregnancy
1 Diabetes is associated with an increased perinatal mortality (PNM) due to an increase in the incidence of:
   (a) congenital abnormalities;
   (b) long difficult labours (because of big babies);

(c) unexplained intrauterine death in late pregnancy;
(d) respiratory distress syndrome;
(e) neonatal hypoglycaemia;
(f) hydramnios;
(g) pre-eclampsia;
(h) urinary tract infections.

Some of these problems can be ameliorated by stringent control of the blood sugar. However in gestational diabetes (which is symptomless) the PNM is about 5%, and in full-blown diabetes, even with excellent control, it is around 10%, rising significantly in the poorly controlled diabetic and the diabetic with vascular complications.

2   Preconceptual counselling and planning are important:

(a) because of her decreased life expectancy and because of the relationship between PNM and complications, the diabetic woman should be encouraged to start her family earlier rather than later in life;

(b) her diabetic control should be perfected prior to conception (as there is evidence that the incidence of congenital abnormalities can be reduced);

(c) she should be warned of the likely sequence of events (shared care with consultant unit delivery; the need for insulin, and frequent fetal and blood sugar monitoring throughout pregnancy; induction of labour around 38 weeks, etc.).

3   The chance of a child developing diabetes is about 0.5%; the chance of a woman with gestational diabetes developing the full-blown condition is about 20% at 5 years.

Driving

See Table 8.10. Basically, *ordinary licence holders* need to notify the DVLC and are given a restricted licence, but may be barred if:

- they do not understand their condition and act sensibly;
- they are poorly controlled;
- they default on follow-up;
- they have major complications.

New regulations apply to *vocational drivers*: fresh applicants may be turned down if they are insulin-dependent, as may existing holders if their condition worsens.

Psychological and social problems

In addition to the practical problems of diabetes there are common psychological and social problems (many of which can be overcome with preparation and education). These may include:

- fear of diabetes;
- fear of coping with all the complicated facets of management;
- mourning for lost health, shortened lifespan, increased risk of complications in later life, restricted freedom, etc.;

- fear of needles and self-injection;
- bewilderment (diabetes *does* take a long time for patients to understand);
- resentment ('Why me?');
- the stigma and embarrassment of being different from every-one else;
- overprotective instincts shown by parents, relatives and friends;
- the inconvenience of regular attendance for medical follow-up;
- vocational problems;
- interference with normal social activities and rituals (e.g. eating what your guests eat; eating when your host eats).

Follow-up
Doctors need to be well organized because they have much ground to cover at follow-up. Flow sheets may help. Points to consider include:
- quality of control (symptom episodes, self-monitoring results, urinalysis, blood sugar, glycosylated haemoglobin);
- physical examination (fundoscopy, visual acuity, foot pulses, foot care, weight, etc.);
- discussing problems and reinforcing understanding.

Prescription exemption
Diabetics are exempt from prescription charges and can obtain a prescription charge exemption certificate.

Sources of information
1 Many District Health Authorities provide diabetic district nurses to help with problems, especially relating to the use of insulin.
2 Education leaflets of various kinds are available from the British Diabetic Association.
3 Some drug companies produce flow charts and cooperation cards to assist doctors and diabetics in the task of systematic follow-up; the Royal College of General Practitioners also offers a comprehensive information folder.

Advice for women with frequency and dysuria
To counsel individuals with the symptoms of frequency and dysuria, the GP must have an overview of the problem.

The size of the problem
1 500 consultations per GP per year;
2 One survey of 3000 women aged 20–60 years indicated that 50% had experience of dysuria.

The causes

Two-thirds of patients do not have a significant bacteriuria but a urethral syndrome (?traumatic urethritis, ?infective organisms that are hard to culture). Among the bacterial causes, *Escherichia coli* is the most common (80–90%); others include *Staphylococcus*, *Proteus* and *Klebsiella*, and the frequency of chlamydial infection is increasing. Occasionally a chemical cystitis develops due to allergy (e.g. to rubber, foams, jellies, soaps and vaginal deodorants).

Mechanical factors come into play, since women are more often affected than men, sexually active individuals more than the celibate, and highly parous women more than those of lower parity. A short urethra, sexual intercourse and the pelvic changes that follow childbirth are implicated in the aetiology.

Natural history

The natural history depends on the sex and age of the patient, and for women on their gestational state. Four different situations can be defined:

1 *The usual situation* (frequency dysuria in a sexually active, non-pregnant adult woman). About 5% of women have asymptomatic bacteriuria, and in any 1-year period about 30% of these go on to suffer an attack of cystitis. Less than 2% then get acute pyelonephritis, and although cystitis is very common, chronic renal failure from pyelonephritis is very rare (20 per million per year). Long-term studies in sexually active young women, in the absence of an abnormal urinary tract or pregnancy, show that both asymptomatic bacteriuria and cystitis are benign, common and self-limiting.

2 *In pregnancy*. Perhaps 5% have asymptomatic bacteriuria and this tends *not* to resolve spontaneously. Some 30–40% of pregnant women with this condition go on to develop a pyelonephritis (with increased risk of abortions, small-for-dates babies and premature deliveries), but the risk is substantially reduced (say by 80–90%) if antibiotics are given.

3 *In children*. Some 25% of children with urinary tract infections (UTIs) have grossly scarred kidneys and about 30% show vesicoureteric reflux on investigation. Chronic renal failure due to pyelonephritis is clearly related to UTIs and reflux in the first 5 years of life, so UTIs in children, as in pregnant women, cannot be dismissed as benign.

4 *In adult males*. Because of the low incidence of UTIs in this group, the strong possibility is either that the man has a sexually transmitted disease (e.g. non-specific urethritis) or a structural abnormality of his renal tract.

Advice

The advice to the groups listed above is clearly different. Groups **2–4** need to see their doctor, have their urine cultured and receive treatment and/or investigation whereas, in the common situation outlined for group **1**, self-help has much to offer. Suitable advice for the sexually active, non-pregnant young woman with symptoms of dysuria and frequency might therefore be as follows:

1 *In an attack*:

(a) drink copious fluids to flush the bladder, dilute the infection and prevent stasis;

(b) alter the pH of the urine to discourage bacterial growth (using, for example, lemon barley, mixture of potassium citrate or 2 teaspoons of sodium bicarbonate 2-hourly);

(c) otherwise, consult the GP regarding antibiotic treatment, and take a urine specimen along.

The clear advantage of the first two approaches is that they do not require a medical appointment and possible delay, and offer over-the-counter remedies available without prescription from the chemist. Self-help also benefits the woman without easy access to medical care (e.g. the foreign holidaymaker).

2 *In prophylaxis — in women prone to recurrent attacks*:

(a) urinate after intercourse;

(b) ensure adequate lubrication in intercourse;

and in particularly difficult recurrent cases:

(c) pay close attention to perineal hygiene (use a separate perineal flannel, regularly boiled; wash the perineum twice a day; wipe from the front to the back);

(d) wash the genitalia before sex, urinate beforehand, drink copious amounts and urinate again afterwards;

(e) avoid tight clothes and nylons;

(f) double micturition;

(g) consult a doctor regarding a prophylactic antimicrobial.

(Not all these measures have been strictly validated, but the latter approach is certainly effective in stubborn cases.)

3 *In general*:

(a) this is a common, benign, nuisance condition — very unpleasant, but not dangerous;

(b) self-help tips may alleviate or palliate, or prevent attacks.

Advice to women with a vaginal discharge

For advice to be appropriate, the diagnosis must be clarified. Is the discharge physiological, pathological or blood-stained?

1 *Physiological discharges* are:

(a) clear;

(b) odourless or non-offensive;

(c) non-irritant;

(d) associated with the Pill, the midcycle preovulatory cascade, pregnancy, the coil or sexual excitement.

2 *Pathological discharges* are:

(a) purulent;

(b) odiferous and offensive;

(c) irritating;

(d) a significant and abrupt change from normal;

(e) associated with the Pill, recent antibiotics, recent delivery or abortion, or possible contact with venereal infection.

3 *Blood-stained discharges* may be due to all manner of problems from retained tampons and atrophic vaginitis, through to salpingitis, endometritis and cancer of the cervix or uterus.

4 *Thrush* is likely if the discharge is white and scanty with intense itching, and predisposing factors are present (the Pill, broad-spectrum antibiotics, possibly tight-fitting clothing and nylons). Women who have had the characteristic symptoms on several occasions usually know their own diagnosis.

Advice

1 If the discharge has physiological characteristics and the predisposing factors are plain, patients can be reassured.

2 If the discharge is pathological, and especially if bloody, they should see their doctor, who will examine, investigate and treat as appropriate.

3 Patients with *recurrent thrush* can be advised on self-help. Possible measures include:

(a) regular or cyclical prophylactic antifungal pessaries (e.g. at midcycle);

(b) simultaneous treatment of any bowel reservoir of organisms with oral antifungals, in stubborn cases;

(c) simultaneous treatment of the male partner, even if asymptomatic (again to clear any possible reservoir of infection);

(d) exclusion of diabetes via the doctor;

(e) avoidance of precipitants (e.g. broad-spectrum antibiotics; the Pill as a method of contraception; tight-fitting clothes and nylons);

(f) natural yoghurt orally or intravaginally (apparently the bacteria in natural yoghurt produce favourable pH changes discouraging the growth of pathogens).

9 Allied Services

The primary health care team is only one cog (albeit a central one) in the complex and interactive machinery of the country's medical services. Many other bodies provide support for primary care and for patients directly or indirectly, through administration, fiscal planning, resource provision and other activities. Table 9.1 attempts to list some of the principal agencies whose main characteristics will now be described.

Department of Health
The NHS is run basically on a three-tier management system. The DOH is the first tier. The Secretary of State for Health has responsibility to Parliament to effect national policies for the NHS through the NHS Management Executive and its Policy Board. Its principal role is planning, budgeting and health service management at a national level. Its sister department, the DSS, administers the large, complex and important Welfare Benefits System.

Regional Health Authorities (RHAs)
RHAs represent the second tier. Their location and size are set so that each region has at least one university medical school within it and encompasses several District Health Authorities (DHAs) and their associated county councils.

Composition
- a chairperson appointed by the Secretary of State;
- five non-executive members (one from the FHSA), appointed by Region;
- five executive members (including the Regional General Manager, chief finance officer and other directors or senior managers).

There is no longer trades-union representation at this level.

Function
Their main role is the purchasing of health care services at a regional level. Except in the case of certain 'super-specialties' patient services are indirect. RHAs also support teaching and research, assume responsibility for new construction work, and appoint consultants and certain DHA members.

District Health Authorities (DHAs)
The third tier of the NHS, DHAs provide or purchase patient services at the district level.

Table 9.1 Principal agencies involved in health care.

Indirect patient services
1 Department of Health
2 Regional Health Authorities

Direct patient services
1 Family Health Service Authorities
2 NHS trusts
3 Primary care teams
4 District Health Authority services
5 County Council and County District Council services
6 Voluntary services
7 Others — including private medicine, industrial and occupational health services and alternative medicine

---

Composition
Normally 11 members, namely:
● a chairperson appointed by the Secretary of State;
● five non-executive members;
● five executive members (comprising a finance officer, chief administrative medical and nursing officers and two other senior district managers).

Functions
The main role of the DHAs is the purchase and provision of inpatient, day-patient and outpatient hospital services for the common specialties within the district. A number of community services are also purchased provided which are supportive both to consultants and GPs. These may include:
● key health care personnel (district nurses, midwives, community psychiatric nurses, stoma specialists, health visitors, diabetic nurses, community physicians, etc.);
● open-access services for primary care (e.g. physiotherapy, occupational therapy, direct-access investigative facilities);
● cervical cytology services;
● child health clinics;
● child and family psychiatry;
● chiropody and dental care;
● clinical psychology services;
● family planning clinics;
● health education services;
● medical referee services;
● psychosexual counselling;
● school health services.
The DHA has been provided with a budget out of which hospital, primary care and other community services are jointly funded. These services in a sense compete for a common purse.

The aim is to allow a more direct comparison of different approaches (community-based versus hospital-based) to the solution of common health problems.

NHS trusts
The recent NHS Act has allowed hospitals and community care units to assume a 'trust' status. Trusts are managerially independent of district control, but as health care providers, enter into service contracts with RHAs and DHAs.

Family Health Service Authorities (FHSAs)
In 1974 each Area Health Authority (as then) was obliged by statute to establish a Family Practitioner Committee (FPC, as then). From 1982 the FPCs related to one or more DHAs and from April 1985 they became independent employing authorities responsible directly to the Secretary of State. Recently their powers have been extended and their name changed to that of Family Health Service Authority.

Composition
There are 10 members constituted as follows:
- an FHSA general manager appointed by the Secretary of State;
- five non-executive members appointed by the RHA;
- one GP, one dentist, one pharmacist and one nurse.

Functions
Traditionally:
- to enter into service contracts with medical, dental and ophthalmic practitioners and pharmacists;
- to supervise their payment;
- to ensure practice premises and services meet basic minimum standards;
- to deal with disputes and ensure contractual obligations are fulfilled.

However, FHSAs have a newly extended range of powers, notably:
- to administer a budget from which expenditure on GP staff and surgeries and the needs of primary care are met, according to assessed need and priority;
- to maintain a register of local practitioners;
- to compile lists of doctors eligible to offer maternity, paediatric surveillance and minor surgery services;
- to vet and license health promotion clinics;
- to vet indicative prescribing budgets;
- to vet and assist fund-holding by participating practices;
- to coordinate audit in primary care through Medical Audit Advisory Groups (MAAGs).

The FHSA is served by four professional committees who advise on matters concerning their own field of experience:

1 The Local Medical Committee (LMC).
2 The Local Dental Committee (LDC).
3 The Local Pharmaceutical Committee (LPC).
4 The Local Ophthalmic Committee (LOC).

Formerly FPCs had their expenditure reimbursed by the DOH and, in distinction to other branches of the health service, administered an open-ended budget. The new-look FHSAs are effectively cash-limited and primary care expenditure is subject to tighter fiscal control.

Local authorities

Local authority responsibilities include the promotion of social care and a healthy environmental background for daily living. Provision includes:

• social services (meals on wheels, social workers, home helps, childminding and fostering services, etc.);
• special educational facilities for the handicapped;
• environmental health services;
• rented housing for general needs, sheltered housing for the elderly, and residential homes for children in care.

Voluntary associations

There are numerous voluntary associations. The best known include the Red Cross and St John Ambulance Brigade, the Samaritans, Alcoholics Anonymous and the MacMillan Nursing Service. However voluntary associations have been formed to provide support and advice for families and individuals with a wide range of problems. Table 9.2 illustrates the breadth of support available.

Referral to a voluntary association is a valid, often valuable adjunct to other treatment, and in the MRCGP examination it is well worth rounding off the answer to a management question with a reference to this.

Health Education Services

At a *national* level the principal responsible agency (other than the DOH) is now the *Health Education Authority (HEA)*. This replaced the old Health Education Council (HEC) from April 1987, forming in its own right a new authority of 'region' status accountable to the Secretary of State.

Functions
• to organize and institute health education campaigns (in concert with health authorities);
• to promote training schemes for health education workers;

Table 9.2 Some well known voluntary associations.

Problem	Voluntary body
Alcoholism	Alcoholics Anonymous Al-Anon (self-help group for relatives and friends) Alateen (for teenagers with alcoholic relatives)
Alzheimer's disease	Alzheimer's Disease Society
Asthma	Asthma Research Council
Back pain	Back-pain Association
Blindness	Royal National Institute for the Blind
Bereavement	Compassionate Friends (bereaved parents) CRUSE (for the widowed and their children)
Cancer	Cancer relief (MacMillan Cancer Relief Foundation) Marie Curie Memorial Foundation
Child cruelty	NSPCC
Coeliac disease	Coeliac Society of the UK
Colostomies	Colostomy Welfare Group
Deafness	Royal National Institute for the Deaf
Diabetes	British Diabetic Association
Down's syndrome	Down's Childrens' Association
Drug Abuse	Turning Point Drug Line
Dyslexia	British Dyslexia Association
Elderly	Age Concern Help the Aged
Epilepsy	British Epilepsy Association
Gambling	Gamblers Anonymous
Haemophilia	Haemophilia Society
Ileostomies	Ileostomy Association of Great Britain and Ireland
Leukaemia	Leukaemia Society
Marriage guidance	Relate
Mental illness	Depressives Anonymous National Association for Mental Health (MIND) Samaritans
Migraine	British Migraine Association
Multiple sclerosis	MS Society of Great Britain and N. Ireland
One-parent families	Association of One Parent Families (Gingerbread)
Parkinson's disease	Parkinson's Disease Society of the UK
Rape	Rape Crisis Centre
Smoking	ASH
Spastics	Spastics' Society
Tinnitus	British Tinnitus Association

- to offer a consultative service with special expertise in all relevant matters;
- to promote related research.

At a *local level* health education has become the responsibility of DHAs. They employ full-time health education and health promotion officers, but health education is offered in addition by health visitors, social workers and community physicians. Many of the functions of the HEA at a national level are reflected by the DHA at a local level but with special emphasis on local needs.

Medical Audit Advisory Groups (MAAGs)
Established in April 1991 by FHSAs acting in cooperation with their LMCs.

Role
A local body charged with the task of directing, coordinating and monitoring medical audit activities within all general practices and in hospital services in their area.

Each MAAG is accountable to its FHSA, which is in turn accountable to its RHA. The aim is to demonstrate professional commitment to securing the highest quality of service within available resources through programmes of audit.

Composition
Although the precise size and composition are locally determined and flexible, a MAAG would normally comprise no more than a dozen members, including:
- representatives from the LMC and local Royal College of General Practitioners faculty;
- GP principals with special experience of audit (e.g. regional or associate GP advisers; academic staff of the local medical school's department of general practice);
- a public health physician;
- FHSA representatives.

Prescription Pricing Authority (PPA)
Within the NHS the PPA has the status of a special health authority.

Its functions include:
1 Feedback to prescribers:
   (a) annual PD2s;
   (b) detailed PD8s on request;
   (c) quarterly PACT reports;
   (d) monthly reports to assist the Indicative Prescribing Scheme.
2 Information for the DOH on high prescribers and prescribing patterns and costs.

3 Pricing arrangements which enable pharmacists and dispensing doctors to be paid.
4 Assistance in research, post-marketing surveillance and even police investigations!

Composition
The PPA is a large organization with 2000 employees and one of the largest computer systems within the NHS — it processes a million prescriptions a day. Its board has a chairperson, chief executive and representatives from the DOH, FHSAs, Community Health Councils (CHCs), as well as pharmacists and GPs.

The General Medical Council (GMC)
Prior to 1858 the regulation of medical practice in the UK was chaotic: 19 separate licensing bodies conferred various professional titles after tests of competence whose standards varied widely, and more than one-third of UK practitioners were not qualified. The Medical Act of 1858 laid down minimum standards of medical education and established a new regulatory body called the General Council of Medical Education and Registration of the UK. In later years this body became known as the GMC, but did not receive its first major overhaul until more than a century had passed. These changes (in composition, size, structure and function) came with the Medical Act 1978 and left the GMC in its present form.

Composition
The GMC has approximately 95 members:
- more than half are elected by the profession;
- about one-third are chosen by universities and other bodies empowered to grant registrable qualifications;
- a few others are nominated by Her Majesty on the advice of her Privy Council.

The Council is served by various professional and disciplinary committees including:
- the Preliminary Proceedings Committee (PPC);
- the Professional Conduct Committee (PCC);
- the Health Committee.

Functions
The GMC is the watchdog for professional standards.
1 It maintains a medical register.
2 It provides guidelines on expected standards of care.
3 It judges on cases of professional misconduct and disciplinary matters, and decides in such cases on fitness to remain registered.
4 It is empowered to vet overseas doctors for linguistic competence prior to registration.

The Royal College of General Practitioners

The College of General Practitioners was founded in 1952 and obtained 'Royal' status in 1967. In 1992 it had a membership of about 17 000 doctors.

Function

Its main function since inception has been to serve as a think-tank for the setting of standards and the improvement of general practice. The Royal College of General Practitioners seeks to achieve this broad aim through its main activities, important among which are:

- the setting of a postgraduate examination as a benchmark of expected standards;
- the organization and conduction of general practice research;
- the publication of an academic journal based on original research and frequent special reports;
- the provision of reference and advisory material to aid good practice;
- the stimulation of debate through policy statements and its national and local educational meetings;
- to exert its influence on the structure of vocational training.

The Royal College represents the academic voice of general practice. Although it does not speak for the whole of the medical profession, and critics level against the membership the charge of elitism, it has contributed significantly to the state of improved esteem and morale that exists now within general practice. It has proved a successful breeding ground for fresh and innovative thinking (see Section 4.10), and is likely to remain at the forefront when it comes to future developments within the profession.

10 The MRCGP Examination

10.1 THE SYLLABUS

The 1972 publication *The Future General Practitioner — Learning and teaching* provided an outline of educational objectives for vocational training programmes. According to the *Royal College of General Practitioners* these educational aims have been adopted for assessment purposes as the basis of the examination.

Of course the interpretation of this syllabus is a subjective exercise, but it is important to note that pure clinical material (symptoms, signs, investigations, treatment) forms only perhaps one-fifth of the syllabus. The examiners also wish candidates to show a grasp of:

- *business methods:* the GP as policymaker and manager; as the organizer of practice services; as a self-employed business person;
- *the handling of people:* communication; attitudes; appreciation of human behaviour; teamwork;
- *the global view:* ethics; the law; consumer rights; resources; epidemiology;
- *a critical approach:* dogma or fact? What are the alternatives? What do my colleagues do?

This book has tried directly to address these areas. Broadly speaking, practice matters are discussed in Chapters 1 and 3, communication in Chapter 2, the wider issues in Chapters 5, 6, 7 and 9, and matters of debate are examined throughout, but with specific emphasis in Chapter 4.

In general, pure clinical material (symptoms, signs, investigations, treatment) has been passed over because experience suggests that candidates with several years of experience and exams behind them have least difficulty with this part of the syllabus. It is also true to say [with the exception of the highly factual Multiple Choice Questionnaire (MCQ)] that greater emphasis is placed on the non-clinical areas of general practice than on classical medical school teaching in the examination itself.

In deciding how to allocate his revision time, the candidate would do well to remember this. Revising the whole broad canvas of clinical medicine is a disheartening business and may not be rewarded much outside the MCQ. Given a reasonable competence in the MCQ (this can be tested using mock papers) the candidate would do better devoting the majority of his time to the sorts of issues and areas that this book covers.

Table 10.1 The MRCGP syllabus (from Walker *et al.* 1983, with permission).

A 1 *Clinical practice — health and disease*
The candidate will be required to demonstrate a knowledge of the diagnosis, management and, where appropriate, the prevention of diseases of importance in general practice:
(a) the range of the normal
(b) the patterns of illness
(c) the natural history of diseases
(d) prevention
(e) early diagnosis
(f) diagnostic methods and techniques
(g) management and treatment

2 *Clinical practice — human development*
The candidate will be expected to possess a knowledge of human development and be able to demonstrate the value of this knowledge in the diagnosis and management of patients in general practice
(a) genetics
(b) fetal development
(c) physical development in childhood, maturity and ageing
(d) intellectual development in childhood, maturity and ageing
(e) emotional development in childhood maturity and ageing
(f) the range of the normal

3 *Clinical practice — human behaviour*
The candidate must demonstrate an understanding of human behaviour particularly as it affects the presentation and management of disease
(a) behaviour presenting to a GP
(b) behaviour in interpersonal relationships
(c) behaviour of the family
(d) behaviour in the doctor–patient relationship

4 *Medicine and society*
The candidate must be familiar with the common sociological and epidemiological concepts and their relevance to medical care and demonstrate a knowledge of the organization of medical and related services in the UK and abroad
(a) sociological aspects of health and illness
(b) the uses of epidemiology
(c) the organization of medical care in the UK — comparisons with other countries
(d) the relationship of medical services to other institutions of society
(e) ethics
(f) historical perspectives of general practice

5 *The practice*
The candidate must demonstrate a knowledge of practice organization and administration and be able critically to discuss recent developments in the evolution of general practice
(a) practice management
(b) the team
(c) financial matters
(d) premises and equipment
(e) medical records
(f) medicolegal matters
(g) research

Table 10.1 *Contd*

271

Chapter 10
The MRCGP
Examination

B The examination is designed to assess in a variety of ways the skills of the candidate in:
(a) interpersonal communication
(b) history-taking and information gathering
(c) selecting examinations using investigations and procedures
(d) recording information
(e) interpreting information
(f) problem definition and hypothesis formation
(g) early diagnosis
(h) defining the range of intervention
(i) selecting therapy
(j) providing continuing care
(k) interventive and preventive medicine in relation to: the patient, the family, and the community
(l) the organization of his practice and himself
(m) teamwork, delegation, and in relating to other colleagues
(n) business methods
(o) communications

C The candidate will be expected to demonstrate appropriate attitudes to his patients, his colleagues and to the role of the GP. He must demonstrate his ability to develop and extend his knowledge and skills through continuing education.

10.2 THE CARDIOPULMONARY RESUSCITATION CERTIFICATE

In order to sit the MRCGP exam candidates must demonstrate proficiency in basic cardiopulmonary resuscitation (CPR). In practical terms, a certificate of competence has to accompany their entry form. The Royal College provides a list of regional centres at which testing can occur. Training is available too (though candidates would have to bear the costs of this). As an alternative to the certificate, the printed report from an electronic testing machine may be accepted. Certificates remain valid for 3 years.

The CPR certificate is reproduced in Table 10.2. It carefully details the requirements, so candidates should read it with some care. An excellent general account on cardiopulmonary resuscitation, representing the recommendations of the Resuscitation Council (UK), is to be found in the *British Medical Journal* (see Further Reading).

It is worth noting that the College proposes to introduce some random testing of CPR skills when candidates attend for the vivas. (This is probably to validate the scheme of pre-exam assessment, but you should remain on your guard for some sort of question.)

It is also worth considering how CPR skills need to be adapted because of the unique position GPs are in providing immediate care in the surgery and the home rather than a hospital.

Table 10.2 The cardiopulmonary resuscitation certificate (reproduced by permission of the Royal College of General Practitioners).

EXAMINATION FOR MEMBERSHIP
CARDIOPULMONARY RESUSCITATION PERFORMANCE TEST

Candidate's name: ....   Date: ....

Activity	Ideal performance	Acceptable variation	Pass	Fail
1 Determine responsiveness Call for help	Shake by shoulders Call for help immediately	None Call within first 60 seconds		
2 Open airway Determine breathlessness	Head tilt with chin support Look, listen and feel for breathing for at least 3 seconds	Head tilt with neck lifted None		
3 Initial ventilations	2 slow ventilations Vol per ventilation 0.8–1.2 litres Inspiratory time per ventilation 1–1.5 seconds	1–5 slow ventilations		
4 Determine pulselessness	Palpate carotid artery for at least 5 seconds	For at least 3 seconds		
5 Cycles of chest compressions and ventilations	15 chest compressions of 1.5"–2" each on the lower part of the sternum avoiding pressing the xiphisternum and the ribs. Compression rate 80 per minute. Followed by 2 slow ventilations	70% correct ventilations 70% correct compressions Compression rate 50–110 per minute Average compression: ventilation ratio over assessment period 10–20:2–3		

6 Reassessment of pulselessness

Palpate carotid artery for at least 5 seconds after 4 cycles of compressions and ventilations

Reassessment after 3–5 cycles

7 Timing of activities

Steps 1 to 5 (to end of first 4 cycles of compressions and ventilations) to be performed in 90 seconds

Performed with 80–120 seconds

Vol per ventilation 0.8–1.2 litres. Inspiratory time per ventilation 1–1.5 seconds. At least 4 cycles of compressions and ventilations must be performed

A ratio of 4–6:1 is acceptable if at least 10 cycles are performed

Examiner: Signature ....

Name ....

Address ....

....

Result: Pass .... Fail ....

Candidates must obtain a pass in each activity

Candidates who fail the test may be re-tested after instruction

ATTACH MANIKIN PERFORMANCE RECORD IF AVAILABLE   THIS CERTIFICATE REMAINS VALID FOR THREE YEARS

- what resuscitation facilities should be available in surgeries?
- what equipment and drugs should GPs carry around with them?

It is conceivable that a question or two on this theme might arise in the viva.

10.3 THE FORMAT

The examination is in two parts. Part 1 consists of three written papers which are completed on the same day. These are:

1 The Multiple Choice Questionnaire (MCQ);
2 The Modified Essay Question (MEQ);
3 The Critical Reading Question Paper (CRQ).

Part 2 consists of two consecutive oral examinations conducted on a later date. The content of these vivas is based on:

1 The practice Log Diary (first viva).
2 Any matter pertinent to medicine and general practice, but often based on management problems the examiners have personally experienced (second viva).

All five parts of the examination have approximately equal weighting. The overall pass mark is probably an average over 50%. It is not generally necessary to pass all parts of the exam to achieve an overall pass, although a dangerously incompetent viva performance could jeopardize the final outcome!

Each section will now be considered in detail.

10.4 THE MCQ

Time allowed
2 hours.

Format
Sixty five-part answers (hence 300 answers altogether). Each question is of the true/false variety. A stem statement is followed by the five completion statements; each complete statement can be answered 'True' or 'False' or 'Don't know'; answers are transferred to a computer card by colouring in the appropriate lozenges with a pencil; marking can then be performed automatically by computer-scanning of the answer sheet.

Marking scheme
Correct answer scores 1 mark.
Incorrect scores *minus* 1 mark.
Don't know scores no marks.

Pass mark
The pass mark is not known for certain, but many people have problems with MCQs, and it is probably less than 50% (it is not necessary to pass on the MCQ to pass overall, although *very* low scorers who have lost too much ground to make up in the vivas may be spared that ordeal).

Content
Clearly the proportion of the 60 questions devoted to different areas of knowledge is relevant to the time spent revising those areas. Approximate guidelines are provided by the Royal College of General Practitioners as follows:

general medicine	10 (questions)
therapeutics	6
obstetrics and gynaecology	6
psychiatry	6
paediatrics	5
dermatology	4
practice organization	4
eyes	3
surgical diagnosis	3
physical medicine/trauma	3
ear, nose and throat	2
care of the elderly	2
epidemiology/statistics	2
infectious diseases	2
social and legal aspects	2

Past papers
Past papers are not available, but many practice papers are (including: *The MRCGP Examination*, MTP; *The MRCGP Study Book*, Update; *MCQ Tutor for the MRCGP Examination*, Heinemann; *The Multiple Choice Question in Medicine*, Pitman; regular MCQs in *Pulse* and *Doctor* magazines). Never let a practice paper pass by without trying it!

Points of technique
1   Read the question carefully. This is mundane advice but many mistakes are made by answering what it was *thought* the examiner asked, not what was asked.
2   Read the stem and *the item in question,* and consider them in isolation: they have nothing to do with the stem and any other completion. Always go back and read the stem as well as the completion so it makes *a complete sentence,* otherwise by item 5 you may have forgotten the exact intonation and sense of the stem statement.

3   The exact wording is important; indeed, a paper published on the linguistic significance of questions in MCQ exams (Slade & Dewey 1983) suggests that by attention to this alone a candidate with little knowledge of the subject can pass. I will leave the reader to make up his own mind on this, but the importance of wording cannot be overemphasized. To take a typical example, 'always' and 'never' are in most cases wrong, because in medicine there are usually exceptions. Expressions like 'is associated with' cause more problems because able candidates can often construct a tenuous link between even the most distantly related events. In Table 10.3 guidelines are given on the interpretation of some common question wordings.

4   The most important thing is to trust the examiner and accept questions at face value: the obvious meaning of the statement is the intended one. Slightly more difficult is the situation in which you know both the commonly accepted answer, and the exceptions and qualifications to it. Consider in this case what the examiner intended you to answer: in most cases the straightforward answer is the intended solution, and the questioner did not spot the ambiguity (or anticipate your sophistication!).

5   Answers can be subdivided into:

(a) those you are *confident* you know;

(b) those you have *no clue about at all*;

(c) those you have a *feeling* are true or false for some reason, but cannot swear to;

(d) those you feel you can *rationalize* the answer to, without knowing;

(e) those you find *ambiguous*.

These should be tackled differently.

(a) The answers you are confident about are probably right assuming you read the question carefully. They may not *all* be right, but the vast majority should be, so answer them.

(b) When you have no clue at all, the question is best left as 'Don't know'. Guessing should be avoided for very good reasons: when there is no penalty for wrong answers, with average luck you could score 50% but with a negative marking scheme for incorrect answers average luck scores 0%; worse than this, the penalties for incorrect guessing quickly eat into the gains made on answers you do know, as illustrated in Table 10.4.

(c and d) Those questions you have a feeling about or feel you can rationalize are, by contrast, not usually guesses. They usually relate to something you know or have heard sometime, but cannot freshly recall. There is a school of thought that says these guesses will be more often right than wrong and that you should not give up too easily, but can you rely on this? The approach I adopted in preparation for the MCQ was to practise

Table 10.3 Interpretation of the wording in exam MCQs.

Wording	Interpretation
Always	Invariably and without a single exception (usually the answer to this is false)
Never	Not in one single person nor on one single occasion (again usually false)
The majority	At least 50% and strictly speaking *more* than 50%
A characteristic feature	A feature that occurs with sufficient frequency as to be of some diagnostic significance. Absence of the feature might make you doubt the diagnosis (NB: Not a feature that *characterizes* the disease: this means occurring in that condition and no other, i.e. a *specific* or *pathognomonic* feature)
A typical feature	A feature you would expect to be present (this is more or less the same as a characteristic feature, but perhaps not so diagnostically absolute)
Usually	In the majority of cases
A recognized feature	One that has been reported and that is a fact the candidate might reasonably be expected to have heard of (NB: Not necessarily a *common* or *characteristic* feature, but one mentioned often in textbook accounts)
Is associated with	Well recognized (not necessarily common, though) This implies information which has been repeated so often as to gain an accolade of accepted truth or could be demonstrated by reference to an authoritative paper on the subject
In 25% of cases	When figures are quoted they are usually 'true' or very wide of the mark. (Thus, some studies may say 24% of cases, some 26%, some 27%, and so on. When examiners quote a figure there must be some leeway in what they regard as true to account, so if you think the answer is 30% of cases, the answer is probably true; if you think 50% it is probably false)

Table 10.4 The penalties of wrong guessing in the MCQ.

Number of True/False answers attempted (out of 300)	Percentage score if:			
	All correct	10 wrong	25 wrong	35 wrong
150	50	43	33	27
175	58	52	42	35
200	67	60	50	43
225	75	68	58	52
250	83	77	67	60

with as many mock papers as I could find, carefully noting my performance at questions in this category. I found, after allowance for negative marking, that my score was much better than zero (the score for blind guesses) and concluded in my own case that it paid to answer this sort of question. I would recommend trying this for yourself, to assess in advance of the exam your aptitude for this sort of question.

(e) Ambiguous questions are answered as described in **4** above or left alone.

6 How many questions should you answer? Experts on exam technique often advise you not to waste time trying to tot up your score, but to concentrate on answering each and every question objectively and to the best of your ability. There are two clear drawbacks to the totting-up approach:

(a) you do not know the pass mark with certainty;

(b) you cannot count your own score with certainty, since even the 'dead-certs' will probably contain some wrong answers.

These objections are clearly valid: they emphasize the element of chance in counting up your score and electing to answer no more questions than you consider necessary to pass. However, the other side of the coin is that trying to work out answers you do not know (and may not need to answer) also contains an element of risk. And it may be possible using intelligent guesswork to allow a margin of error. It is reasonable, for example, to assume you need to score 50% (any less would be a risk in its own right), and to assume that 10% of the answers you are 'certain' about are actually wrong, marking yourself down 20% (you could perhaps get a better idea of this figure, as I chose to do, by noting your performance in a wide variety of MCQs). The decision is clearly a personal one, best assessed by practice under exam conditions, but note carefully the words in a recent Royal College occasional paper on the MRCGP: 'it has been repeatedly shown that most candidates improve their scores if they are forced to commit themselves on all the items previously marked as "don't know"'.

10.5 THE MEQ

Time allowed
2 hours.

Format
A loose-leaf book with questions fairly evenly spread over the pages. After each question blank spaces are left for the answers. There are about 10–12 questions. As a rough guide you are warned when approximately halfway through the paper.

Each page is independently marked. The questions carry equal
marks.

The examiners have a marking grid in front of them specifying
the points you are expected to make. This is fairly rigid: if you do
not make those particular points, they cannot allocate the mark.
However, there is also a discretionary allocation (perhaps 10–
30% of the total) given to candidates who present their answer
cogently, and create the impression of overall perspective and
grasp of the subject matter.

Pass mark
The pass mark is not known for certain, but probably around 50%.

Past papers
Past papers are reprinted in the *British Journal of General Practice*
some time after the examination, so past questions can be obtained
by careful scrutiny of back issues. The College also provides a set
of past papers on request, at a modest price. Mock questions with
sample answers are offered by some of the books named under
Further Reading.

Content
According to the *Journal* the MEQ has been used to test the skills
of: information gathering, hypothesis formation and testing,
evaluation of data, definition of problems in physical, psychological and social terms, decision-making, recording and com-
municating, management planning, mobilization of available
resources, follow-up and anticipation of future problems. In more
practical terms, it is a problem-solving exercise.

Note that although some of the questions have a clinical bias,
the paper also places great emphasis on sensitivity to psychological and social aspects of the problem, ethical dilemmas and the
wider considerations and implications of decision-making. Clinical
expertise is only one of the attributes being examined, and the
questions reflect this; for example, candidates are often quizzed on
the advantages and disadvantages of particular courses of action
and generally 'put on the spot' in awkward practical situations:
- the liberated rebel demanding natural childbirth in a swimming
pool or caravan;
- the patient who demands tranquillizers (and insists your colleague has always prescribed 'without this bother');
- contraceptive conundrums;
- ethical conundrums;
- non-compliers and problem families;
- liaison (and potential conflicts) with colleagues;
- 'unreasonable' patient requests, etc.

- controversial and 'hot' topics (e.g. alcohol, acquired immune deficiency syndrome, alternative medicine).

In recent years the content has been slightly modified. Instead of working through the trials and tribulations of a single family, evolving over an extended time period, the format has tended towards that of a 'typical surgery' or single working day, in which a succession of problems is presented.

Recent MEQ papers have included supplementary material on which questions can be based (e.g. a problem summary card or a protocol for a well-person clinic).

Points of technique

As already emphasized, examiners are looking for broad answers, and a global grasp of the problem. If you just deal with the physical aspects, and the marking schedule includes psychological and social aspects, implications for the primary health care team, the law, society and the NHS, you have missed the boat! No marks are deducted for being over-inclusive, only for omissions, so the implications are several:

1 You must think and write from all aspects: see it from the doctor's point of view, from the patient's, from that of the primary health care team, society and any other viewpoint you can think of. *If it might be relevant write it down.*

2 This is easier to do if you memorize a checklist of areas to consider. You can then scribble down in rough the main headings of your *aide-mémoire*. These might be for example:

    (a) physical, psychological, social;

    (b) options, implications, choice;

    (c) doctor's angle, patient's view, profession's view, other view (e.g. society, solicitor, defence union);

    (d) pros and cons (to all relevant parties);

    (e) any relevant studies?

Regarding management it is easy to construct a similar *aide-mémoire*, e.g.:

    (a) clarify the problem (in physical, psychological and social terms);

    (b) investigate if necessary;

    (c) treat:

- counsel and advise;
- prescribe (drug and/or appliance);
- carry out a procedure (e.g. intrauterine device fitting, vaccination, injection of tennis elbow, minor surgery, etc.);

    (d) refer:

- within the primary health care team (e.g. health visitor, midwife, practice nurse, district nurse);
- to hospital services (e.g. inpatient, outpatient, day hospital, consultant, domicillary visit, physiotherapy);
- to the social services (e.g. social worker, social services, day

centre, part 3 accommodation, meals on wheels, home help, orange badge, welfare benefits department);
- to the community services (e.g. dentist, optician, chiropodist);
- to other agencies (self-help, voluntary, local authorities, etc.);

(e) follow up;

(f) preventive action desirable? health education possible?;

(g) liaison needed (e.g. with colleagues, school, community physician, solicitor, etc.)?

By practising a few MEQs you can identify questions with a common theme; for example, if a patient asks you to do something that could be construed as controversial, your options are: agree, disagree, refer, bargain/counsel/educate — and each has predictable implications. Advance planning allows you to offer polished and comprehensive answers.

3 As usual read the questions very carefully.

4 Write in note form: it takes less time, allows you to write more, and is easier for the examiner to mark.

5 Be prepared to repeat yourself from one answer to the next: the answers are marked independently, so the same point, if relevant, may score points in more than one question. If you omit to repeat yourself, you may miss out.

6 Be honest and say what you would really do, not simply give the textbook answer. We do not X-ray all children who are chesty for a week because general practice requires a modified and pragmatic approach, and your answer should reflect this (although it is reasonable to consider and reject alternatives as long as you justify it). Similarly differential diagnoses must list common things first and rarities in passing.

7 You are advised not to read through the MEQ booklet before you start, or alter your answers on the basis of questions asked later on. The argument is that it may distort your natural judgement and lead you to stray from the common sense surgery approach stressed in (6) above. Like all sound advice, this should be tempered with common sense. If you discover as you go along that you have gone down a stupid blind alley, and omitted to mention the glaringly obvious conclusion on page 9, you would be well advised to 'adjust' your answer!

8 There is less time than you think for this exam: practise as many mock papers as you can find, and time yourself. You have about 10–12 min per question, as a very rough guide.

10.6 THE CRQ

Time allowed
2 hours (plus 15 min to read the written material presented).

Format
Three questions. No choice. Essay or expanded note form.

Marking scheme
Like the MEQ, examiners follow fairly rigid marking guidelines which itemize the points expected to be made. There is also likely to be a discretionary allowance for a logical and well ordered approach, showing grasp of the subject.

Pass mark
The pass mark is about 50%.

Past papers
As for MEQs, i.e. available from the Royal College of General Practitioners, and published periodically in the *Journal*. (The CRQ is a relatively new addition to the examination and there is a shortage of past material. Some additional examples are provided in the Royal College's occasional paper 46: Examination for Membership of the Royal College of General Practitioners: Development, Current State and Future Trends.)

Content
Questions cover the areas of health and disease, medicine and society, and practice management:
1   *Question 1* presents candidates with a published paper from an established general medical journal. Candidates are tested on their ability to:
    (a) identify the main issues;
    (b) discuss aspects of study design;
    (c) discuss the implications and practical application of findings in general practice.
2   *Question 2* examines candidates' familiarity with published literature in areas of current interest in general practice.
3   *Question 3* presents candidates with some written material commonly encountered in general practice (letters; practice protocol, report or audit; advertising material). A critical appraisal is sought.

Points of technique
1   Read the questions very carefully.
2   Have a *plan* to answer each question. Allot 40 min total time: say 5 min making a skeleton outline, 30 min writing and 5 min reading over the final answer.
3   It helps to break the reply up into logical subdivisions: paragraphs, subparagraphs, underlined headings and the obligatory introduction and conclusion. This promotes a logical approach and makes it much easier for the examiner to follow your line of thought.

4 Write concisely. If you make a valid point you can only score the mark once, while flowery elaboration can waste a lot of time. In the same vein, stick to the point: you will fail to impress and cannot score if you wander off at a tangent.

5 Answer *all* the questions. This is really an aspect of time management: the questions carry equal marks, so allow equal time to answer them. It is a cardinal error to write excessively on one question to the exclusion of another. Practise your timing under exam conditions. You have about 40 min per question, less if you wish to read over your answers at the end.

6 In *question 1* the examiner is really asking you to write an abstract to the paper concerned, and then to comment on it. The first part of this exercise is easy if you follow the format commonly used by recognized journals when presenting their abstracts. Sir Austin Bradford-Hill first suggested that the key ingredients should be:

(a) introduction: why did the author start?
(b) methods: what did the author do?
(c) results: what did the author find?
(d) discussion: what does it mean?

In a similar vein, if you look at recent papers in the *British Medical Journal* you will see that abstracts contain the following structured points:

- objectives;
- design;
- setting;
- subjects;
- interpretation;
- end-points;
- measurement and main results;
- conclusions.

An *aide-mémoire* of this sort will ensure that all the main points are considered.

The candidate is asked to place the findings in context, and three useful supplementary questions will help:

1 What is the message?
2 Do I believe it?
3 If true, how does it affect what I do at present?

Remember in considering the implications for general practice to examine it from the relevant angles (doctor, patient, community; legal, ethical and practical; options, implications, choices; pros and cons).

This is an area the candidate can easily practise beforehand — simply choose a paper from a mainstream journal, read it (excluding the abstract), attempt to write your own abstract, and then compare it with the published one.

There remains the problem that some candidates will feel

unfamiliar with points of study methodology and statistical analysis. Chapter 11 provides a simple overview of this subject, and has been written for such candidates.

7   *Question 2* probably relates to a 'hot topic' of current interest to GPs. The emphasis is on British general practice and British journals.

A careful study of recent major editorials and reviews in the *Lancet, British Medical Journal* and *British Journal of General Practice* is likely to yield a useful list of possibles. Look for topics with some factual background, which are both important and controversial in general practice. Some examples are provided in Chapter 4. Candidates can start (but not finish) here.

The examiners have stated that some marks will be awarded for pure factual knowledge (reference-quoting etc.), but that the majority are awarded to those showing they have read and *understood* the relevant literature. So, concentrate on the *concepts*. (If you can cite the evidence too you will earn the 'icing on the cake'.)

8   *Question 3* requires critical assessment of common written material from general practice. Likely issues can be anticipated, e.g.:

This material . . .	*. . . may well raise these issues*
Letters between colleagues	Confidentiality
	Communication
	Interprofessional relationships
	Hidden agendas
Practice protocol or audit	Defining objectives and standards
	Defining valid methods
	Colleagues' attitudes to peer review
Advertising or promotional material	Worthwhile question asked
	Valid study method and analysis
	Context established
	Credibility
	Practical importance

[Material on audit (Section 1.3), evaluating health promotion (Sections 3.1 and 3.3) and rational prescribing (Section 2.2) may be of practical assistance in preparing for this exam question.]

10.7 THE FIRST VIVA

The vivas are held about a month after the written papers and approximately 16 out of 20 candidates get through to this stage.

Time allowed
Just under 30 minutes.

An oral examination conducted by two examiners (and possibly a third, or a video camera, invigilating not your performance but that of the examiners).

The first viva is structured around the practice Log Diary which candidates must complete and submit in advance of the examination. This asks basic questions about the workload, services, equipment, staffing, organization, health promotion and audit arrangements of their own practice, and also for a list of 50 patients the candidate has recently seen and treated in practice (comprising 25 surgery patients, 15 home visits and 10 out-of-hours emergency consultations). Candidates are allowed to take along to the viva their own crib or *aide-mémoire* regarding these patients, and are not expected to carry in their heads specific details like laboratory findings and social history.

Marking scheme
The first viva represents about 20% of the total marks. Because of the nature of the viva it is difficult to have a rigid marking scheme. However examiners have some general guidelines. In particular they seek in their marking to assess whether candidates:
• are competent, safe and reasonably well read;
• in their decision-making consider reasonable alternatives, the implications, and present a coherent argument;
• in their attitudes tolerate alternative attitudes;
• are aware of their own limitations.

Content
The first viva is structured around the candidate's Log Diary and therefore on what he has written. However, this only forms the starting point for discussion. Examiners are likely to digress and extend the realm of discussion towards principles, rather than getting bogged down in the details of a particular case. Thus, if your Log Diary records a high list size, an unusually high number of home visits or home deliveries, a practice nurse, diabetic clinic, ECG machine or hospital assistantship, be prepared to discuss the pros and cons and practical implications of these things. Similarly a Log Diary case of acute otitis media may be used as a springboard to discuss the pros and cons of antibiotic prescribing, the management of glue ear, and the limitations and frustrations of being a school medical officer (as happened in my own viva!).

Points of technique
1 Usual points of viva technique (dress conservatively, be courteous, do not argue, be punctual, sit up, do not mumble) are particularly valid in this exam, since GPs are innately conservative, and often entertain quite stereotyped views of the fitting dress, deportment and manner of prospective College members.

2   Do not raise a topic unless you are prepared to talk about it. The converse is to bait the examiner into asking you a question that you have thoroughly prepared. The Log Diary viva gives reasonable scope for this, as you can include or omit from your submission as you see fit.

3   Quote-dropping is useful in small amounts. Examiners read the same journals as you, so scrutinize the main ones in the lead-up to the exams. 'Hot topics' are likely to be in the forefront of their minds and may well surface in some form.

4   Do not express your view too early in proceedings. You may be left defending only one side of the argument! In this exam you score best by teasing out the reasonable alternatives, so introduce the pros and cons first, talk about them at some length, support them with evidence if you can, and then give your qualified view.

5   As always, thorough preparation pays dividends: although you cannot anticipate every question, with wide preparation you should be able to say *something* about most topics. It then becomes an exercise in organizing packets of knowledge into a sensible argument. Practise your viva technique regularly with a colleague.

6   Make sure for the Log Diary patients that you have your own common sense limited prescribing policy which you can justify and cost.

7   Ensure the list of patients for the Log Diary is balanced and representative (but interspersed with one or two interesting cases). The notebook you take into the exam should be concise and comprehensive; you should be able to locate the relevant entry without a lot of fumbling and searching and not appear to read excessively from it.

10.8 THE SECOND VIVA (PROBLEM-SOLVING ORAL)

Time allowed
Just under 30 minutes.

Format
After the first viva a bell rings and the examiners hand you a piece of paper to take on to the next viva, which is conducted immediately afterwards with a new pair of examiners. This paper informs the second pair of the ground already covered, so there is no accidental duplication of questioning.

Marking scheme
As for viva one. This part of the exam represents about 20% of the total marks available.

The second viva is loosely based on the experiences of the examiners who are practising GPs. Cases may be clinical or may be widened to include any issue that impinges on general practice. There is free rein: examples from my own viva (including the legal requirements for prescribing to addicts, the problem of a partner propositioned by means of a love letter, the counselling of a patient demanding inappropriate emergency referral, and the role of the family in schizophrenic illness) illustrate this point very well! In general the presentation follows the lines of the problem-solving MEQ.

Sometimes use is made of role-play (although candidates should not be failed as a result of this alone) and sometimes the candidate is presented with a record or tracing or a piece of equipment.

Points of technique
The general points made concerning the first viva apply equally here. However, in this viva, more than the Log Diary one, the battleground is chosen by the examiner. It is still possible with care to lead the questioning into the relative calm of prepared backwaters. Remember as always the emphasis is not so much on facts but options, alternatives and implications: your chances of success will be enhanced if you keep this firmly in mind every time you speak.

11 Epidemiology and statistics

In 1990 the College introduced into the MRCGP examination a new section called 'Critical Reading' — in part designed to determine candidates' ability to understand and critically evaluate written material relevant to general practice.

A reading list has been proposed by the College, with heavy emphasis on statistics and epidemiology. Furthermore, one section of the new paper requires candidates to write an abstract from a published paper, summarizing the principal findings and commenting intelligently on the methods used to collect and analyse the data.

Medical statistics is perhaps an area of the syllabus from which most doctors ordinarily shy away (exam considerations apart), but it is of increasing importance for those wishing to:
- read original papers critically (understanding their methods and limitations);
- plan appropriate research and audit studies;
- validate and report findings in a scientific manner.

Suggestions for tackling the Critical Reading Paper as a whole are made in Chapter 10, alongside other pointers on exam conduct. This chapter offers a simple overview of statistics and epidemiology for the uninitiated.

11.1 BASIC DEFINITIONS IN EPIDEMIOLOGY

1 *Epidemiology* is the study of the distribution and determinants of disease and other indices of health in human populations.
2 *A population* is a circumscribed group of individuals sharing one or more defined characteristic in common. Several groups may exist, e.g.:

These groups . . .	. . . are	. . . for example
The target population	All people everywhere who share the characteristic(s) defined	Men aged 40–50 years with diastolic blood pressures >100 mmHg
The study population	A fraction of the target population selected for study	All such men in region X
A study sample	The fraction of the study population sampled when the numbers are large	All such men in practice Y from region X

Epidemiology seeks to infer from the *particular* (study sample or population) to the *general* (target population). Whether it can do so depends critically on whether the study population is *typical* of the target population.

3 *A measuring instrument* means (speaking epidemiologically) any technique used to collect data.

(a) examples might equally include:
- blood samples;
- X-rays;
- spirometric graphs;
- questionnaires;
- agreed sets of diagnostic criteria;

(b) good measuring instruments must be:
- valid, i.e. provide a true assessment of what they purport to measure;
- repeatable, i.e. provide the same result when remeasured under the same conditions;

(c) validity is measured in terms of *sensitivity* and *specificity*, as compared with the gold-standard of all measuring instruments (see Table 3.2);

(d) repeatability may be less than perfect because of:
- within-observer variation (e.g. although the blood pressure is the same, I read it differently after coffee than I did before it);
- between-observer variation (e.g. I tend to make the same blood pressure higher than you do);
- within-subject variation (his blood pressure changes anyway).

(e) Measuring instruments should be chosen, refined or tested by pilot study to ensure that they are as valid and repeatable as possible. (The best existing ones, e.g. the Medical Research Council Respiratory Questionnaire, have been developed in this way and should be used where appropriate and possible.)

11.2 STUDY DESIGNS

Longitudinal versus cross-sectional

1 A study in which events evolve and are enumerated over a period of time is said to be *longitudinal* — case control and cohort studies are of this type.

2 A study which takes a snap-shot picture of the state at a particular point in time is said to be *cross-sectional*, and is also known as a survey.

3 Some examples should make the difference clear:

Longitudinal study
In a study from general practice patients with backache were randomized between receiving an education leaflet or not. Over

the next year the numbers presenting with backache were counted for the two groups.

Cross-section study
In another study doctors from practice X examined a randomly chosen selection of patient records to establish the proportion of patients currently being treated for backache.

Cohort versus case control
1 The cohort study (also called a prospective study) is a longitudinal study which follows forwards over a fixed period of time two groups of people who have different exposures to an agent of interest (e.g. Pill-takers and non-Pill-takers), but are otherwise matched. The incidence of disease is compared in the two groups.
2 In practice two basic approaches are possible:
(a) we could start today and count events occurring over the next 10 years (a so-called *truly* prospective design);
(b) we could finish today and look at disease in Pill and non-Pill-takers over the *last* 10 years (a so-called *historically* prospective design).
3 The case control study (or retrospective study) compares people who have a specific disease (cases) with those who do not (controls) to establish whether their past exposure to possible disease risk factors (e.g. Pill-taking) differed.

The essential difference between cohort and case control studies is illustrated in Figure 11.1. Note particularly that groups in a cohort study are compared with respect to *disease*, while those in a case control study are compared with respect to *exposure*.

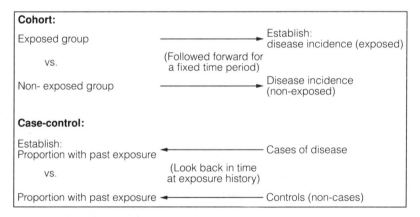

Fig. 11.1 Cohort and case control study designs.

Randomization, placebos and blind trials
1 If the purpose of a study is to compare two groups receiving different treatments (e.g. chemotherapy versus placebo), patients

would ideally be randomized between the groups. This design would be called a randomized controlled trial.

2 If the patient does not know which treatment he is receiving but the doctor does, this is called single-blind randomization.

3 If neither the patient nor the doctor knows which treatment is being given, this is called double-blind randomization.

The purpose of randomization is to iron out any chance differences that exist between the groups. The double-blind design removes one source of bias — that due to patient and doctor expectation.

Error and bias

These terms have distinct and separate meanings. *Bias* is a form of systematic error, leading to consistent over- or under-recording of the true situation. *Random error*, because of its chance nature, leads to neither.

This is a more important distinction than it seems. Random error leads to a less precise estimate of the study parameter, but the degree of imprecision can be statistically estimated, and the effect can be offset by making the study larger. The effect of bias is harder to estimate and its magnitude cannot be reduced simply by including more subjects. A study beset with random error may be salvaged; a biased study may not, unless the bias is recognized and removed.

Designing questionnaires

Designing a good questionnaire is an art — bad questions beget bad answers. There are a few cardinal rules:
- keep questions short, clear and concise;
- use language which is unambiguous but intelligible to its readership;
- ensure that possible answers are restricted in choice and can be objectively interpreted (e.g. yes/no, or a number);
- do not seek too much information from one question (it often confuses).

It is important too to get a good response rate (inevitably when studies are incomplete there is suspicion that the participants differed from the non-responders in important ways — 'they had an axe to grind'). Response rates can be improved by making the survey more acceptable to the target group:
- by prior publicity;
- by convenient timing;
- by polite and full explanation of the use that will be made of the information;
- by assurance of confidentiality.

11.3 MEASURING RATES

1 *Incidence* — the rate of occurrence of new cases. (Note that you need to exclude old cases at the outset of the study as they must not be counted.)

2 *Prevalence* — the proportion of the population at risk affected at a given time (point prevalence = at a given point in time; period prevalence = within a stated period).

3 *Age standardization* — Age is such an important determinant of ill health that it would be very misleading to compare two study populations with different age structures. Suppose, for example, we suspected that the medical standards exercised in preventing cerebrovascular accidents differed in Bournemouth and Milton Keynes. We could attempt to test this hypothesis by comparing the incidence of cerebrovascular accidents in each population, but the comparison would be meaningless unless some account was taken of the age groups found in each community. Age standardization is a technique that allows the comparison to be made (the details need not concern us). It is from this technique that the standardized mortality ratio (SMR) is derived.

4 *Expressing results* — In comparing the incidence rates of disease in exposed (Ie) and non-exposed (In) populations we are asking, what is the risk in the one population compared with the other? This comparison can be expressed in several ways, e.g.:

(a) the absolute difference between the rates (Ie − In);

(b) the proportionate difference in rates [(Ie − In)/Ie];

(c) the ratio of the rates (Ie/In).

The latter is usually chosen. It is called the *relative risk*.

The SMR is an important example. It is also a product of convenience: because of the expense and difficulty of following groups through a cohort study convention allows the control group to exist only on paper, a reference population whose mortality experience can be *looked up* in tables of national statistics. After age standardization the rates are compared:

$$\text{SMR} = \frac{\text{Observed deaths in study population}}{\text{Expected deaths in study population}} \times 100$$

Expected is understood in the sense of 'the number of deaths that would occur in the study population if it experienced the same age-specific mortality as the reference population'.

A mortality experience equivalent to that of the reference population gives an SMR of 100. If >100, the mortality experience was greater, and so on.

Because the starting point in the design of a case control study is quite different, we cannot calculate relative risk in quite the same way. The *odds ratio* is an approximation to relative risk suitable in interpreting the findings of case control studies.

$$= \frac{\text{Odds of developing disease in the exposed}}{\text{Odds of developing the disease in the unexposed}} \times 100$$

Its interpretation is broadly similar to that of the SMR.

11.4 BASIC PRINCIPLES OF MEDICAL STATISTICS

Definitions

1 Statisticians divide their field into:

(a) *descriptive statistics* — the summarizing, enumerating and presenting of data in meaningful forms;

(b) *inferential statistics* — the use of data from study groups to draw inferences concerning target populations.

2 Statistical data can be:

(a) *quantitative* — data to which an exact number can be ascribed (blood pressure, episodes of backache);

(b) *qualitative* — data to which a quality can be ascribed but not an exact number (sex, blood group).

Quantitative data may be:

• *discrete* — assuming only certain discrete values (e.g. number of children);

• *continuous* — assuming any value along a continuum (e.g. serum cholesterol).

It is subject to the normal rules of arithmetic.

Qualitative data may be grouped into categories that have an order (ordinal data, e.g. clinical severity grading scales for breathlessness), but cannot be treated in a simple arithmetic way.

3 Data can be summarized in tabular or graphical form by means of contingency tables, bar charts or frequency histograms.

4 It is conventional in describing statistical data to measure central tendency and distribution or dispersion of the data points.

(a) Measures of central tendency include:

• the *mean* — the average value;

• the *mode* — the most commonly occurring value;

• the *median* — the middle observation when all the values are ranked in ascending or descending order.

The mean is the most widely used of these measures, because it can be mathematically manipulated. In a normal distribution all three have the same value.

(b) The most important measure of dispersion around the mean is called the *standard deviation* (SD).

(The square of the deviation from the mean is taken for each data point. The results are summed and averaged. The square root of this value is the SD.)

The SD has convenient properties where values are normally distributed (as in many biological systems):

- 66% of values lie within the range of X ± 1 SD;
- 95% of values lie within the range of X ± 2 SD;
- 99% of values lie within the range of X ± 3 SD.

Correlation and regression

If we wished to assess the association between two quantitative variables (say height and blood pressure) we might start by plotting height against the blood pressure for each of the individuals studied. The variables height and blood pressure would be X and Y coordinates on the graph and each subject would be represented by a single point. An immediate visual inspection of this graph (which is called a *scatter diagram*) might give the impression that a linear association existed. Correlation is the mathematical verification of this impression.

A *correlation coefficient* is a measure of the strength of linearity between two quantitative variables. It has a value on a scale of −1 to +1:

- +1 indicates a perfect direct association;
- −1 indicates a precise inverse association;
- 0 (and values close to it) indicate no association.

The process is a descriptive one.

Regression, by contrast, is a predictive process. The line of best fit in the scatter diagram is found mathematically, and used to *predict* the value of one variable given the value of another.

Notes

1 The processes are complementary. Regression can always find a line of best fit — even if the fit is very poor and in all probability no linear relationship exists. A high correlation coefficient tells us that there probably *is* a line there, so the regression result is credible.

2 Strictly speaking this is *linear* regression. Non-linear regression is also possible, but here the association is assumed to be non-linear and calculations are based on formulae describing the form of relationship between the variables.

Sampling statistics: standard error of the mean

If we take a study sample and ascertain its mean and standard deviation we have an approximation of the true population mean and standard deviation. If we took another sample and repeated the exercise we would probably end up with a slightly different estimate.

According to the theory of sampling statistics, if we take an infinite number of samples our estimates of the population mean would show a normal distribution around the true mean. The standard deviation of this sampling distribution could in turn be described and is called the *standard error of the mean*.

This standard deviation of the sampling means gives us an idea of the dispersion of our estimates around the true value, and a better statement of the range in which the true value is likely to lie.

Significance tests

1 Tests of statistical significance, though varied, are based on a common line of reasoning. The so-called *null hypothesis* contends that no true differences exist between population groups in a study and that any apparent difference is due to the effects of chance alone. This results, for example, in their sample means lying at different points on a single normal distribution of sample means.

2 The probability (P) of getting values as far apart as those observed, while still belonging to the same family of sampling means, can be deduced.

3 If the probability appears extremely small we would contend that the null hypothesis is unlikely and that the two populations are indeed different; if the probability does not appear small enough we would contend that the null hypothesis could still be true and the differences observed could be due to chance alone. The value of P at which we make this distinction is chosen arbitrarily, and is called the *significance level* of the test. Usually:

$P < 0.05$ leads to rejection of the null hypothesis and a *significant difference*, and
$P < 0.01$ is regarded as *highly significant*.

Notes
1 Even if $P > 0.05$, the difference could still be genuine, but such a study would have failed to prove it so.
2 A statistically significant difference may not be a *clinically* significant one: while it is likely to be a genuine difference, the magnitude of effect may be small and the consequences clinically unimportant.

Type I and type II errors

Significance testing only indicates the balance of probabilities. A conclusion based on it can still be wrong:
1 A *type I error* occurs if the test leads us to conclude that there is a difference when one does not actually exist. The risk of this occurring depends on the significance level we choose for the test: the lower it is, the more convinced we require to be, the lower the risk of a false positive.

2 However, if we are too strict we may miss a genuine difference between compared groups. Because we insisted on a value of $P < 0.0001$ when we could only demonstrate $P < 0.01$, we draw a false-negative conclusion. This is a *type II error*.

3 Type II errors can be reduced by increasing the size of the study. They are not normally quoted, but they are used beforehand by statisticians in this way to establish the minimum size worthy of study.

Confidence intervals

Many published articles now report their findings using *confidence intervals* rather than tests of statistical significance.

1 A confidence interval is a range of values within which it can be stated, with a certain degree of confidence, that the population statistic lies.

2 A 95% degree of confidence is often chosen, though this is arbitrary and could be higher or lower.

3 The confidence interval is preferred because it contains useful additional information: the likely upper and lower limits of the range in which the statistic is to be sought.

4 The value of this can be illustrated by reference to a fictitious study of relative risk: suppose that a study suggests the relative risk of a cerebrovascular accident in Bournemouth compared with Basingstoke is 1.5:

(a) if the 95% confidence intervals are 1.0–2.0 this is consistent with a twofold increase in risk (relative risk = 2) but also with no increase in risk at all (relative risk = 1)!

(b) if the 95% intervals are 1.3–2.0 we can at least say that an increased risk exists (assuming we have designed and conducted the study properly and compared age-adjusted figures).

(Table 3.7, p. 114 provides examples of confidence intervals used in this way to cast doubt on the conclusions of major mammography screening trials.)

11.5 THE ROLE OF THE STATISTICIAN

If the reader is confused by my explanations, I hope it will at least be clear that it is worth consulting a statistician or epidemiologist from the outset in a planned study worth its salt. This would help in:

- selecting appropriate controls (often the most difficult exercise);
- choosing the right numbers;
- eliminating sources of bias;
- applying the statistical tests appropriate to the circumstances in question.

This chapter has been difficult to write and, if unfamiliar, the concepts make for difficult reading. If you feel at sea but out of your depth, do not lose heart! The objective is to pass the MRCGP and in this context more information has been provided than is strictly necessary. If you find the material straightforward it may earn you an extra mark or two; it may even have stimulated your interest(!); if not there are other more important fish to fry!

12 Facts and Figures

This chapter lists some of the major statistics relating to the clinical and administrative content of general practice and the provision of health care under the NHS. It is not essential to memorize all the figures, but it may well be useful to quote one or two statistics in support of, or to provide perspective for your arguments. (Most of these figures are derived from the meticulous records that John Fry has kept over many years in general practice.)

Levels of care

1 75% of ill health is dealt with by 'self-care', made up roughly as follows:
- 25% upper respiratory infections;
- 20% aches and pains;
- 20% emotional upsets;
- 10% gastrointestinal upsets;
- 5% rashes.

2 20% dealt with by GPs.

3 10% by hospitals.

Vital statistics of workload

List sizes

The trend is towards smaller list sizes. The averages have been, respectively:
- 1969   2495;
- 1981   2200;
- 1989   1917;

There is a spectrum across the country; for example, average list size in Scotland ≪ 2000 per GP, in the Trent area ≫ 2500 per GP.

Consultation rates

1 Average consultations per patient each year: approximately 3.5 (men 3.2; women 4.0).

2 Average home visits per patient each year: approximately 0.3–0.5.

3 Average surgery consultation time: approximately 5–6 min.

4 Average time per home visit: approximately 15 min.

5 60–70% of the practice consults over a 1-year period, and 80–90% over 5 years.

6 The *range* is large between different practices. For doctors with a list of 2500 patients the range is from 5000 to 17 500 consultations

per year, i.e. assuming 230 working days per year, from 22 to 76 per day taking from 5 to 12 h per day.

Practice size
The trend is towards bigger practices with fewer 'single-handers', e.g.:

	1969	1988
1 doctor	22%	12%
2 doctors	25%	15%
3 doctors	26%	20%
4 doctors	15%	18%
5 doctors	7%	15%
⩾6 doctors	5%	20%

Areas are categorized according to the average list size within them:

Category	Mean list size
Restricted	0–1700
Intermediate	1701–2100
Open	2101–2500
Designated type 1	2501–2999
Designated type 2	3000+

In 1983 there were 1570 areas, of which about 250 were open and only 6 designated.

Provision of staff and premises for primary care
In Britain there are approximately:
30 000 GPs (81 000 doctors);
9000 surgeries (25% of which are Health Centres);
3200 dispensing GPs;
20 000 district nurses;
3500 practice-employed nurses;
9000 health visitors;
45 000 secretarial staff;
2000 trainees per year (25% of practices undertake training);
50% of GPs making use of deputizing arrangements.

Clinical content of general practice
Each year, in an average list of 2500 patients, the following clinical events would typically be seen.

Births and deaths
32 births: 30 in hospital and 2 at home.
25 deaths made up of:

1 infant death
8 coronaries
5 cancers
4 strokes
1 accidents
6 others

25% of deaths at home, 65% in hospital, 10% in other places, e.g. nursing homes, public places.

Minor illness
600 upper respiratory tract infections
325 emotional upsets
200 gastrointestinal upsets
100 cases of tonsillitis
 75 cases of otitis media
 50 urinary tract infections
 50 acute backs

Major illness
100 cases of acute bronchitis
 20 pneumonias
 10 coronaries
  5 strokes
  1 suicide per 4 years

Chronic illness (prevalence figures)

450 chronic mental illness	20 peptic ulcers
100 chronic rheumatism	10 epilepsy
100 hypertension	20 diabetes
50 coronary artery disease	10 thyroid disease
35 chronic bronchitis	2 multiple sclerosis
30 asthma	>1 chronic renal failure

Overall:
65% of disease is minor/self-limiting
15% of disease is major/life-threatening
20% of disease is chronic with permanent disability

Social pathology
200 patients receiving welfare benefit
 70 physically handicapped patients
 40 unemployed patients
 30 mentally handicapped patients
 30 single-parent families
 25 deaf patients
 10 blind patients
 10 alcoholics
  5 schizophrenics

New cancers
1 lung every 6 months
1 breast every 12 months
1 colorectal every 18 months
1 skin every 18 months
1 stomach every 18 months to 2 years
1 prostate every 2 years
1 cervix every 5 years
1 leukaemia every 5 years
1 ovary every 6 years
1 larynx every 6 years
1 uterus every 7 years
1 brain every 10 years
1 lymphoma every 15 years
1 thyroid every 20 years

Congenital disorders
1 cardiac disorder every 5 years
1 pyloric stenosis every 7 years
1 spina bifida every 7 years
1 mongolism every 10 years
1 cleft palate every 20 years
1 congenital hip dislocation every 20 years
1 phenylketonuria every 200 years

Non-illness events
Contraception	100 per year
Immunization	100 per year
Smears	50 per year
Postnatals	30 per year

The special demands of the young and old
Children (under 15 years) are 15–20% of the population, but 25% of GP consultations; 90% of the under-5s are seen each year.
The elderly. 15% of the population are over 65 years (9% 65–74 years, 6% over 75 years), but 40% of GP consultations are for this age group. As the proportion of very elderly in the population rises, the workload will rise.

Obstetric and gynaecological trends
1 Delivery in hospital is increasing and home confinements are far less common; for example, in 1962 65% of deliveries were in hospital, whereas in 1979 the figure was 95%.
2 The average family size is 2.3 children.
3 About 180 000 terminations occurred in 1989, and 60% of these were in non-NHS hospitals.

4 Since 1950 the perinatal mortality rate has fallen from 35 to 18 per 1000.

5 The maternal mortality rate is about 11 per 100 000 (with a regional variation of 6–17 per 100 000).

6 10% of couples are involuntarily infertile, the mean number of cycles to conception is 6, and 80% of couples achieve a pregnancy in 12 months.

7 In contraceptive methods are used to the following degrees:
- Pill   25%;
- Sheath   16%;
- Withdrawal   4%;
- Intrauterine device   6%;
- Diaphragm   1%.

8 66% of single women and 53% of married women are said to show a preference for the Family Planning Clinic over their own GP.

Practice administration

1 88% of practices now have appointment systems.

2 Approximately 50% have an ECG machine.

3 Nearly 70% have attached nurses, and nearly 90% have attached health visitors. A majority now employ treatment room nurses of their own.

4 Facilities are said to bear some crude relationship to the social class of the practice population (with a tendency to find increased use of deputizing, lower doctor qualifications and less equipment where the socioeconomic class is lower).

Referral rates and the use of hospital facilities

1 One in three people visit hospital outpatient departments each year, comprising:
- 1 in 6 referred by their GP;
- 1 in 5 self-referred to casualty.

2 Each elective outpatient department referral generates 4.2 follow-up visits (8.5 for psychiatry).

3 Referral rates vary greatly between doctors: one study (Last 1967) suggests that two-thirds of doctors refer 10–35 per 1000 each month, but this varies from 5 to 115 per 1000 each month.

4 The provision of hospital beds is 9 per 1000 populus.

5 One in nine of the population is admitted to hospital (i.e. 11%) over a 1-year period.

6 This admission risk rises 10-fold over age 65 years.

Prescribing

Each GP issues 13 000 scripts per year on average; at least 50% of consultations end in prescription and 60% of the populus takes medicine each day; the average person receives 7 scripts per year (compared with 10–11 in France, Germany and Italy).

The annual cost to the NHS is about £70 000 per GP each year, or £2.3 billion (still less than 8% of the total NHS budget).

Complaints against doctors
In 1989 a total of 1361 complaints against GPs were investigated and 18% were successful. The commonest cause of complaint is 'bad manners' by GP and staff, but the commonest successful complaint is 'failure to visit'.

NHS facts and figures
NHS expenditure (1987) was £22 000 million total, i.e. £400 per head. This is 6% of the gross national product, one of the lowest costs per capita in the world. The funding is derived mainly from Government (88%) with only small contributions from National Insurance (9%) and direct payments (3%). Nearly two-thirds of this money is spent on hospitals, 10% on drugs and only 6% on general practice.

Further Reading

Recommendations for further reading can be divided into two categories: there are those books and articles which (like the claim forms of the same name) are immediately necessary and emergency 'treatments' in the urgent run-up to the examination. These are deliberately thin, concise texts that cover the bones of their subject in a straightforward and direct way, perhaps suitable in each case for a weekend's intensive study. Then there are the more expansive texts which are desirable supplementary reading for those with more time to spare. I have concentrated, in producing this reading list, for the most part on the former type of reading material, and also focused on clinical topics which constraints of space have prevented me from including elsewhere in the text.

Recommendations have been listed according to subject and is arranged in order of mention in the text. Those who have rather more time for independent reading should consult the reference list that follows.

In preparing for exams there is always more material available to read than time in which to do it. This is especially true when it comes to *journal work*, where the dramatic proliferation of published material requires doctors to acquire strategies for selective reading, weeding out the relevant and discarding the rest. Jewell (1988) has provided an excellent step-by-step catechism which should help the busy physician:

1 Does the title describe something in which I have the slightest interest?
2 Are the conclusions of limited application?
3 If true, would they alter the way in which I work?
   And only then:
4 Are the aims clearly stated?
5 Is the context clear?
6 Are the methods appropriate?
7 How complete are the data?
8 Is the result credible, rationally or intuitively?

The ruthless application of such an approach will help examinees in the endless, seemingly impossible task of cramming their quarts into pint pots!

Practice management

Ellis N. (1990) *Employing Staff* (4th edn). BMA, London.
Jones R.V.H., Bolden K.J., Pereira Gray D.J. & Hall M.S. (1990) *Running a Practice: Manual of Practice Management* (4th edn). Croom Helm, London.

Pendleton D. & Hasler J. (eds) (1983) *Doctor–Patient Communication.*
Academic Press, London.
Pendleton D., Schofield T., Tate P. & Havelock P. (1984) *The Consultation:
an Approach to Learning and Teaching.* Oxford Medical Textbooks,
Oxford.

Prevention
Lock S. (ed.) (1983) *Practising Prevention.* BMA, London.

Clinical
General
Gambrill E. (ed.) (1982) *General Practice: Tutorials in Postgraduate Medicine.*
William Heinemann Medical Books Ltd, London.

Paediatrics
Illingworth R.S. (1987) *The Normal Child: Some Problems of the Early Years
and their Treatment* (9th edn). Churchill Livingstone, Edinburgh.
GMSC & Royal College of General Practitioners (1984) *Handbook of Preventive Care for Preschool Children.* GMSC & RCGP, London.

Pharmacology
British National Formulary. British Medical Association and the Pharmaceutical Society of Great Britain, London (published annually).

ENT
Ludman H. (1988) *ABC of ENT* (2nd edn). BMA, London.

Ophthalmology
Gardiner P.A. (1979) *ABC of Ophthalmology.* BMA, London.

AIDS
Adler M.W. (ed.) (1991) *ABC of AIDS* (2nd edn). BMA, London.

Psychiatry
Bird J. & Harrison G.H. (1987) *Examination Notes in Psychiatry* (2nd edn).
John Wright, London. (Really a book for those taking the MRCPsych
examination, but concise, well laid out and, in places, very relevant.)

Dermatology
Fry L. (1984) *Dermatology: An Illustrated Guide* (3rd edn). Butterworths,
London.

Obstetrics and gynaecology
Kaye P. (1988) *Notes for the DRCOG* (2nd edn). Churchill Livingstone,
Edinburgh.

Community medicine
Donaldson R.J. & Donaldson L.J. (1987) *Essential Community Medicine.*
MTP, Lancaster.

Legal and ethical
Raffle A. (ed.) (1985) *Medical Aspects of Fitness to Drive* (4th edn). Medical
Commission on Accident Prevention.
Phillips M. & Dawson J. (1985) *Doctors' Dilemmas: Medical Ethics and
Contemporary Science.* Harvester Press, Brighton.
The General Practitioner's Yearbook. Winthrop, Winthrop House, Surbiton on
Thames, Surrey.

Epidemiology and statistics

Gore S.M. & Altman D.G. (1982) *Statistics in Practice*. BMA, London.
Jewell D. (1988) Reading scientific articles, or how to cope with the overload. *Practitioner* **232**, 720–5.
Swinscow T.D.V. (1981) *Statistics at Square One* (3rd edn). BMA, London.

Exam study books

Fry J., Bouchier-Hayes T.A., Gambill E., Moulds A. & Young K. (1988) *The MRCGP Study Book* (2nd edn). Butterworth/Update Publications, London. (Sample exam papers with worked answers.)
Moulds A., Bouchier-Hayes T.A. & Young K. (1978) *The MRCGP Examination: a Comprehensive Guide to Preparation and Passing*. MTP, Lancaster.
Sandars J.E. (ed.) (1989) *MRCGP Practice Exams* (2nd edn). Pastest, Hemel Hempstead, Herts.

Facts and figures

Fry J., Brooks D. & McColl I. (1984) *The NHS Data Book*. MTP, Lancaster.

Topical information

Consult the last 1–2 years' editorials and major review articles in *Update* magazine and the *British Journal of General Practice*.

Select Bibliography

Acres (1979) In: Edwards G. & Grant M. (eds) *Alcoholism: New Knowledge and New Responses.* pp. 324–5. Croom Helm, London.

Anderson P. (1984) What are safe alcohol levels? *Br. Med. J.* **289**, 1657–8.

Andersson I., Aspegren K., Janzon L. *et al.* (1988) Mammographic screening and mortality from breast cancer: the Malmö mammographic screening trial. *Br. Med. J.* **297**, 943–8.

Anonymous (1987) Management of hyperlipidaemia. *Drug Ther. Bull.* **25**, 89–92.

Argyle M. (1972) *The Social Psychology of Work.* Penguin, Harmondsworth, Middlesex.

Austoker J. (1990) Breast cancer screening and the primary care team. *Br. Med. J.* **300**, 1631–4.

Australian National Board (1980) The Australian Therapeutic Trial in Mild Hypertension. *Lancet* **i**, 1261–7.

Bain D.J. (1984) Deputising services: The Portsmouth experience. *Br. Med. J.* **289**, 471–3.

Bain J. (1989) Developmental screening for pre-school children: is it worthwhile? *J. R. Coll. Gen. Pract.* **39**, 133–7.

Balint M. (1957) *The Doctor, his Patient and the Illness.* Pitman Medical, London.

Banks M., Beresford S., Morrell D., Waller J. & Watkins C. (1975) Factors influencing demand for primary care in women aged 20–64 years: a preliminary report. *Int. J. Epidemiol.* **4**, 189–95.

Beardon P.H.G., Brown S.V., Mowat D.A.E. *et al.* (1987) Introducing a drug formulary to general practice — effects on prescribing costs. *J. R. Coll. Gen. Pract.* **37**, 305–7.

Beardow R., Oerton J. & Victor C. (1989) Evaluation of the cervical cytology screening programme in an inner city health district. *Br. Med. J.* **299**, 98–100.

Bernadt M.W., Mumford J., Taylor C., Smith B. & Murray R.M. (1982) Comparison of questionnaire and laboratory tests in detection of excessive drinking and alcoholism. *Lancet* **i**, 325–8.

Berne M.D. (1964) *Games People Play.* Penguin, Harmondsworth, Middlesex.

Berquist-Ullman M. & Larsen U. (1977) Acute low back pain in industry. *Acta Orthop. Scand.* Suppl. 170.

Bertakis K.D. (1977) The communication of information from physician to patient. *J. Fam. Pract.* **5**, 217–22.

Birmingham Research Group of General Practitioners (1978) Practice activity analysis. 6: visiting profiles. *J. R. Coll. Gen. Pract.* **190**, 316–17.

Bloom J.R. & Monterossa S. (1981) Hypertension labelling and sense of well-being. *Am. J. Public Health* **71**, 1228–32.

British Heart Foundation (1987) *Screening for Ischaemic Heart Disease Risk in General Practice.* British Heart Foundation, London. (Factfile.)

Brody D. (1980) An analysis of patient recall of their therapeutic regimens. *J. Chronic Dis.* **33**, 57–63.

Brown G. & Harris T. (1978) *Social Origins of Depression.* Tavistock Publications, London.

Brown G.W., Birley J. & Wing J.W. (1972) Influence of family life on course of schizophrenic disorders: a replication. *Br. J. Psychiatry* **121**, 241–58.

Brumfitt W. & Slater J.H.D. (1957) Treatment of acute sore throat with penicillin. *Lancet* **i**, 8.

Butler-Sloss E. (1988) *Report of the Inquiry into Child Abuse in Cleveland.* HMSO, London.

Byrne P.S. & Long B.E.L. (1976) *Doctors Talking to Patients.* HMSO, London.

Cartwright A. (1964) *Human Relations and Hospital Care.* Routledge & Kegan Paul, London.

Cartwright A. & Anderson R. (1967) *Patients and their Doctors: a Study of General Practice.* Routledge & Kegan Paul, London.

Cartwright A. & Anderson R. (1981) *General Practice Revisited: a Second Study of General Practice.* Tavistock Publications, London.

Cartwright A. & O'Brien M. (1976) The sociology of the NHS. In: Stacey M. (ed.) *Sociology Review Monograph No. 22.* University of Keele, Keele.

Chen E. & Cobb S. (1960) Family structure in relation to health and disease. *J. Chronic Dis.* **12**, 544–67.

Chick J., Kreitman N. & Plant M. (1981) Mean cell volume and gamma-glutamyl-transpeptidase as markers of drinking in working men. *Lancet* **i**, 1249–51.

Clark E.M. & Forbes J.H. (1979) *Evaluating Primary Care.* Croom-Helm, London.

Cockburn J., Gibberd R.W., Reid A.L. & Sanson-Fisher R.W. (1987) Determinants of non-compliance with short-term antibiotic regimens. *Br. Med. J.* **295**, 814.

Cohen J. (1986) Diagnosis and management of problem patients in general practice. *J. R. Coll. Gen. Pract.* **36**, 51.

Coleman P. (1989) The value of screening the elderly. *Family Pract. Service* **16**, 424.

Collier J. (1988) The case for and against prescribing generic drugs: generic prescribing benefits patients. *Br. Med. J.* **297**, 1596, 1598.

Colling A., Dellipiani A.W., Donaldson R.J. & MacCormack P. (1976) Teesside coronary survey: an epidemiological study of acute attacks of myocardial infarction. *Br. Med. J.* **2**, 1169.

Committee on Medical Aspects of Food Policy (COMA) (1987) *The Use of Very Low Calorie Diets in Obesity: Report on Health and Social Subjects.* No. 31. HMSO, London.

Costello R. (1975) Alcoholism treatment and evaluation, I & II. *Int. J. Addict.* **10**, 251–75, 857–67.

Court Report (1976) *Fit for the Future.* Report of the Committee on Child Health Services, Cmnd 6680. HMSO, London.

Cruickshank J.M. (1988) The case for and against prescribing generic drugs: don't take innovative research-based companies for granted. *Br. Med. J.* **297**, 1597–8.

Cumberledge Report (1986) *Neighbourhood Nursing: A Focus for Care.* Report of the Community Nursing Review. HMSO, London.

Dahl-Jorgensen K., Brinchmann-Hansen O., Hanssen K.F., Ganes T. *et al.* (1986) Effect of near normoglycaemia for 2 years on progression of early diabetic retinopathy, nephropathy and neuropathy: the Oslo study. *Br. Med. J.* **293**, 1195–9.

Davey A., Smith G., Barley M. & Blane D. (1990) The Black report on socio-economic inequalities in health 10 years on. *Br. Med. J.* **301**, 373–7.

Davis M.S. (1968) Variation in patients' compliance with doctors' advice: an experimental analysis of patterns of communication. *Am. J. Public Health* **58**, 274–88.

Department of Employment (1977) *New Earnings Survey.* HMSO, London.

Dillane J.B., Fry J. & Kalton G. (1966) Acute back syndrome — a study from general practice. *Br. Med. J.* **2**, 82–6.

Dixon R.A. & Williams B.T. (1988) Patient satisfaction with general practitioner deputising services. *Br. Med. J.* **297**, 1519–22.

Doran D.M.L. & Newell D.J. (1975) Manipulation in treatment of low back pain: a multicentre study. *Br. Med. J.* **2**, 161–4.

D'Souza M.F., Swan A.V. & Shannon D.J. (1976) A long-term controlled trial of screening for hypertension in general practice. *Lancet* **i**, 1228–31.

Dunnell K. & Cartwright A. (1972) *Medicine Takers, Prescribers and Hoarders.* Routledge & Kegan Paul, London.

Edwards G., Orford J., Egbert S., Guthrie S., Hawkes A., Hensman C., Mitcheson M., Oppenheimer E. & Taylor C. (1977) Alcoholism: a controlled trial of 'treatment' and 'advice'. *J. Stud. Alcohol* **38**, 1004–31.

Egbert L.D., Battit G.E., Welch C.E. & Bartlett M.K. (1964) Reduction of post-operative pain by encouragement and instruction of patients. *N. Engl. J. Med.* **270**, 825–7.

Ellman R. & Chamberlain J. (1984) Improving the effectiveness of cervical cancer screening. *J. R. Coll. Gen. Pract.* **267**, 537–42.

Elwood J.M., Cotton R.E., Johnson J., Jones G.M., Curnow J. & Beaver M.W. (1984) Are patients with abnormal cervical smears adequately managed? *Br. Med. J.* **289**, 891–4.

Engelhard D., Cohen D. & Strauss N. (1989) Randomised study of myringotomy, amoxycillin/clavulanate or both for acute otitis media in infants. *Lancet* **ii**, 141–3.

Epstein A.M., Hall J.A., Fretwell M. *et al.* (1990) Consultant geriatric assessment for ambulatory patients. *J.A.M.As.* **263**, 538–44.

European Working Party on High Blood Pressure in the Elderly (1985) Mortality and morbidity results from the European Working Party on High Blood Pressure in the Elderly Trial. *Lancet* **i**, 1349–54.

Forrest P. (1987) *Breast Cancer Screening.* HMSO, London.

Fowler G. (1982) Smoking: practising prevention. *Br. Med. J.* **284**, 1306–8.

Fowler G. (1988) Coronary heart disease prevention: a general practice challenge. *J. R. Coll. Gen. Pract.* **38**, 391–2.

Francis V., Korsch B.M. & Morris M.J. (1969) Gaps in doctor–patient communication: patient's response to medical advice. *N. Engl. J. Med.* **280**, 535–40.

Friedman M. & Rosenman R. (1974) *Type A Behaviour and your Heart.* Knopf, New York.

Froom J., Gilpeper L., Grob P. *et al.* (1990) Diagnosis and antibiotic treatment of acute otitis media: a report from the International Primary Care Network. *Br. Med. J.* **300**, 582–6.

Fry J. (1958) Antibiotics in acute tonsillitis and acute otitis media. *Br. Med. J.* **2**, 883.

Fry J. (1973) *Present State and Future Needs of General Practice* (3rd edn). Royal College of General Practitioners, London.

Fry J. (1979) *Common Diseases: their Nature and Incidence.* MTP Press, London.

Fulton M., Kellett R.J., MaClean D.W., Parkin D.M. & Ryan M.P. (1979) The management of hypertension — a survey of opinions among general practitioners. *J. R. Coll. Gen. Pract.* **29**, 583–7.

Gerrard T.J. & Riddell J.D. (1988) Difficult patients: black holes and secrets. *Br. Med. J.* **297**, 530–2.

Gill O.N., Adler M.W. & Day N.E. (1989) Monitoring the prevalence of HIV: foundations for a programme of unlinked anonymous testing in England and Wales. *Br. Med. J.* **299**, 1295–8.

Glover J.R., Morris J.G. & Khosla J. (1974) Back pain: a randomized clinical trial of rotational manipulation of the trunk. *Br. J. Ind. Med.* **31**, 59–64.

GMSC & Royal College of General Practitioners (1984) *Handbook of Preventive Care for Pre-school Children.* GMS Defence Fund & RCGP, London.

Goldberg D. (1981) The recognition of psychological illness by general practitioners. In: Edwards G. (ed.) *Psychiatry in General Practice*. University of Southampton, Southampton.

Gray M. & Fowler G.H. (eds) (1983) *Preventative Medicine in General Practice*. Oxford University Press, Oxford.

Grol R., Whitfield M., De Maesener J. & Mokkink H. (1990) Attitudes to risk taking in medical decision making among British, Dutch and Belgian general practitioners. *Br. J. Gen. Pract.* **40**, 134–6.

Groves J.E. (1951) Taking care of the hateful patient. *N. Engl. J. Med.* **298**, 883–5.

Gruppo Italiano per lo Studio della Streptochinasi nell' Infarto Miocardico (GISSI) (1987) Long-term effects of intravenous thrombolysis in acute myocardial infarction: final reports of the GISSI study. *Lancet* **ii**, 871–4.

Hall D.M.B. (ed.) (1989) *Health for All Children. A Programme for Child Health Surveillance*. Oxford University Press.

Hall M.H., Chng P.K. & MacGillivray I. (1980) Is routine antenatal care worth while? *Lancet* **ii**, 78–80.

Halstead C., Lepow M.L., Balassarian N., Emmerick J. & Wolinsky E. (1968) Otitis media. *Am. J. Dis. Child.* **115**, 542.

Hampton J.R., Morris G.K. & Mason C. (1975) Survey of general practitioners' attitudes to management of patients with heart attacks. *Br. Med. J.* **4**, 146–8.

Harris A.I., Cox E. & Smith C.R.W. (1971) *Handicapped and Impaired in Great Britain*. OPCS Social Survey Division, HMSO, London.

Hart J.T. (1986) Reduction of blood cholesterol in the population: can it be done? *J. R. Coll. Gen. Pract.* **36**, 538–9.

Haverkorn M.J., Valkenburg H.A. & Goslings W.R.O. (1971) A controlled study of streptococcal pharyngitis and its complications in the Netherlands. *J. Infect. Dis.* **124**, 339.

Haynes R.B., Sackett D.L., Taylor D.W., Gibson E.S. & Johnson A.L. (1978) Changes in absenteeism and psychosocial function due to hypertension screening and therapy among working men. *N. Engl. J. Med.* **299**, 741–4.

Health Education Council (1983) *That's the Limit*. HMSO, London.

Hellman G.C. (1981) Disease versus illness in general practice. *J. R. Coll. Gen. Pract.* **31**, 548–52.

Hendriksen C., Lund E. & Strømgård E. (1984) Consequences of assessment and intervention among elderly people: a three year randomised controlled trial. *Br. Med. J.* **289**, 1522–4.

Hill J.D., Hampton J.R. & Mitchell J.R.A. (1978) A randomized trial of home-versus-hospital management for patients with suspected myocardial infarction. *Lancet* **i**, 837.

Hill D., White V., Jolley D. & Mapperson K. (1988) Self examination of the breast: is it beneficial? Meta-analysis of studies investigating BSE and the extent of disease in patients with breast cancer. *Br. Med. J.* **297**, 271–5.

Hinton J. (1980) Whom do dying patients tell? *Br. Med. J.* **281**, 1328–30.

Holmes T. & Masuda M. (1974) Life change and illness susceptibility. In: Dohrenwend B.S. & Dohrenwend B.P. (eds) *Stressful Life Events: Their Nature and Effects*. John Wiley, New York.

Holmes T. & Rahe R. (1967) The social readjustment rating scale. *J. Psychosom. Res.* **11**, 213–18.

Houston H.L.A. & Davis R.H. (1985) Opportunistic surveillance of child development in primary care: Is it feasible? *J. R. Coll. Gen. Pract.* **35**, 77–9.

Howie J.G.R., Porter A.M.D. & Forbes J.F. (1989) Quality and the use of time in general practice: widening the discussion. *Br. Med. J.* **298**, 1008–10.

Hypertension Detection and Follow-up Co-operative Group (1979) Five years findings of the Hypertension Detection and Follow-up Programme. *J.A.M.A.* **242**, 2562–71.

The ISAM study group (1986) A prospective trial of intravenous streptokinase in acute myocardial infarction (ISAM). Mortality, morbidity and infarct size at 21 days. *N. Engl. J. Med.* **314**, 1465–71.

ISIS-2 (Second International Study of Infarct Survival) Collaborative Group (1988) Randomised trial of intravenous streptokinase, oral aspirin, both or neither among 17 187 cases of suspected myocardial infarction: ISIS-2. *Lancet* **ii**, 349–60.

Isles C.G., Hole D.J., Gillis C.R., Hawthorne V.M. & Lever A.F. (1989) Plasma cholesterol, coronary heart disease and cancer in the Renfrew and Paisley survey. *Br. Med. J.* **298**, 920–4.

Jelley D.M. & Nicoll A.G. (1984) Pertussis: what percentage of children can we immunise? *Br. Med. J.* **288**, 1582–4.

Kales A. (1974) Treating sleep disorders. *Am. Fam. Phys.* **8**, 158–68.

Keeble B.R., Chivers C.A. & Muir-Gray J.A. (1989) The practice annual report: post-mortem or prescription? *J. R. Coll. Gen. Pract.* **39**, 467–9.

Kenny R.A., Brennas M., O'Malley K. & O'Brien E. (1987) Blood pressure measurements in borderline hypertension. *J. Hypertension* **5** (suppl), 483–5.

Kholer L. (1984) Early detection and screening programmes for children in Sweden. In: McFarlane J.A. (ed.) *Progress in Child Health*. Churchill Livingstone, Edinburgh.

Kincey J., Bradshaw P. & Ley P. (1975) Patient's satisfaction and reported acceptance of advice in general practice. *J. R. Coll. Gen. Pract.* **25**, 558–62.

Kinlay S. & Heller R.F. (1990) Effectiveness and hazards of case finding for a high cholesterol concentration. *Br. Med. J.* **300**, 1545–7.

Knowles H.C. (1970) Control of diabetes and the progression of vascular disease. In: Ellenberg M. & Rifkin H. (eds) *Diabetes Mellitus: Theory and Practice*. McGraw-Hill, New York.

Korsch B.M. & Negrete V.F. (1972) Doctor–patient communication. *Sci. Am.* **227**, 66–74.

Kubler Ross E. (1970) *On Death and Dying*. Tavistock Publications, London.

Laing R. & Esterson A. (1964) *Sanity, Madness and the Family*. Penguin, Harmondsworth, Middlesex.

Lancet, Editorial (1990) Taking risks in general practice. *Lancet* **336**, 541.

Last J.M. (1967) Quality of general practice. *Med. J. Aust.* **i**, 780–4.

Lauritzen T., Frost-Larsen K., Larsen H.W., Deckert T. and the Steno Study Group (1983) Effects of 1 year of near normal blood glucose levels on retinopathy in insulin-dependent diabetes. *Lancet* **i**, 200–4.

Laxdal O.E., Merida J. & Trefor Jones R.H. (1970) Treatment of acute otitis media. *Can. Med. Assoc. J.* **102**, 263.

Leitch D. (1989) Who should have their cholesterol concentrations measured? What experts in the United Kingdom suggest. *Br. Med. J.* **298**, 1615–6.

Ley P., Whitworth M.A., Skilbeck C.E., Woodward R., Pinsent R., Pilce L.A., Clarkson M.G. & Clark P.B. (1976) Improving doctor–patient communication in general practice. *J. R. Coll. Gen. Pract.* **26**, 720–4.

Lowenthal L. & Bingham E. (1987) Length of consultation: how well do patients choose? *J. R. Coll. Gen. Pract.* **37**, 498–9.

Lynge E. (1981) Occupational mortality in Norway, Denmark and Finland (1971–5). In: Committee for International Co-operation of National Research in Demography (ed) *Socio-economic Differential Mortality in Industrialised Societies*. Paris, WHO.

Mant D. & Fowler G. (1990) Screening in practice: mass screening — theory and ethics. *Br. Med. J.* **300**, 916–8.

Marinker M. (1988) The referral system. *J. Coll. Gen. Pract.* **38**, 487–91.

Marsh G.N. (1985) New programme of antenatal care in general practice. *Br. Med. J.* **291**, 646–8.

Marsh G.H., Horne R.A. & Channing G.M. (1987) A study of telephone advice in managing out of hours calls. *J. R. Coll. Gen. Pract.* **37**, 301–4.

Marteau T.M. (1989) Psychological costs of screening. *Br. Med. J.* **299**, 527.

Mather H.G., Morgan D.C., Pearson N.G., Read K.L.Q., Shaw D.B., Steed G.R., Thorne M.G., Lawrence C.J. & Riley I.S. (1976) Myocardial infarction: a comparison between home and hospital care for patients. *Br. Med. J.* **i**, 925.

Maw A.R. (1983) Chronic otitis media with effusion (glue ear) and adenotonsil-lectomy: a prospective randomised control study. *Br. Med. J.* **287**, 1586–8.

Mayfield D., McLeod G. & Hall P. (1974) The CAGE questionnaire: validation of a new alcoholism screening instrument. *Am. J. Psychiatry* **131**, 1121–3.

Mazhari M. (1987) Decent paediatric care costs money. *GP Magazine*, Jan 16th, p. 17.

McGayock H.M. (1990) Developing a practice formulary. *Update* **39**, 121–4.

McGhee A. (1961) *The Patient's Attitude to Nursing Care.* E. & S. Livingstone, Edinburgh.

Mead T.W., Dyer S., Browne W., Townsend J. & Frank O. (1990) Low back pain of mechanical origin: randomised comparison of chiropracter and hospital outpatient treatment. *Br. Med. J.* **300**, 1431–7.

Milne R.I.G. & Keen S.M. (1988) Are general practitioners ready to prevent the spread of HIV? *Br. Med. J.* **296**, 533–5.

Moore A.T. & Roland M.O. (1989) How much variation in referral rates among GPs is due to chance? *Br. Med. J.* **298**, 500–2.

Morrell D.C., Gage H.G. & Robinson A. (1971) Referral to hospital by GPs. *J. R. Coll. Gen. Pract.* **21**, 77–85.

Morrell D.C., Evans M.E., Morris R.W. & Roland M.O. (1986) The five minute consultation: effect of time constraint on clinical content and patient satisfaction. *Br. Med. J.* **292**, 870–3.

Moser K.A., Fox A.J. & Jones D.R. (1984) Unemployment and mortality in the OPCS longitudinal study. *Lancet* **ii**, 1324–9.

Moulds A.J. (1985) Making the most of the Lloyd George. *Update*, 15th March.

Mourin K. (1976) Auditing and evaluation in general practice. *J. R. Coll. Gen. Pract.* **26**, 726–33.

Multiple Risk Factor Intervention Trial Research Group (1982) Multiple risk factor intervention trial: risk factor changes and mortality results. *J.A.M.A.* **248**, 1465–77.

Nachemson A. (1976) The lumbar spine: an orthopaedic challenge. *Spine* **1**, 59–71.

National Ambulatory Medical Care Survey (1980) 1977 Summary. United States, Jan–Dec 1977. Data from the National Health Survey Series 13, No. 44. Hyattsville, Md: DHEW Publication No. (PHS) 80-1795, April.

Oboler S.K. & LaForce M. (1989) The periodic physical examination in asymptomatic adults. *Ann. Intern. Med.* **110**, 214–216.

O'Dowd T.C. (1988) Five years of heartsink patients in general practice. *Br. Med. J.* **297**, 528–30.

Office of Population Censuses and Surveys (1973) *General Household Survey.* HMSO, London.

Office of Population Censuses and Surveys (1978) *Occupational Mortality,* Decennial Supplement, 1970–72, England & Wales. HMSO, London.

Parkes C.M., Benjamin B. & Fitzgerald R.G. (1969) Broken heart: a statistical survey of increased mortality among widowers. *Br. Med. J.* **1**, 740–4.

Patterson H.R. (1985) The problems of audit and research. *J. R. Coll. Gen. Pract.* **35**, 118.

Pell A.C.H., Stuart P.C., Stewart M.J. & Fraser D.M. (1990) Home or hospital care for acute myocadial infarction? A survey of GPs' attitudes in the thrombolytic era. *Br. J. Gen. Pract.* **40**, 323–5.

Peto R., Gray R., Collis R., Wheatley K. *et al.* (1988) Randomised trial of prophylactic daily aspirin in British male doctors. *Br. Med. J.* **296**, 313–16.

Pickering T.G., James G.D., Boddie C., Harshfield G.A., Blank S. & Largh J.H. (1988) How common is white-coat hypertension? *J.A.M.A.* **259**, 225–8.

Pietroni P. (1976) NVC in the GP surgery. In: Tanner B. (ed.) *Language and Communication in General Practice*. pp. 162–79. Hodder & Stoughton, Sevenoaks.

Podell R. (1975) *Physician's Guide to Compliance in Hypertension*. West Point, Merck, Pennsylvania.

Pokorny A.D., Miller B.A. & Kaplan H.B. (1972) The brief MAST: a shortened version of the Michigan Alcoholism Screening Test. *Am. J. Psychiatry* **129**, 342–5.

Polich J.M. (1980) Patterns of remission in alcoholism. In: Edwards G. & Grant M. (eds) *Alcoholism Treatment in Transition*. Croom Helm, London.

Pollak B. (1978) A two-year study of alcoholics in general practice. *Br. J. Alcohol Alcoholism* **13**, 24–35.

Rastam L., Luepker R.V. & Pirie P.L. (1988) Effect of screening and referral on follow-up and treatment of high cholesterol levels. *Am. J. Prev. Med.* **4**, 244–8.

Raw M., Jarvis M.J., Feyerabend C. & Russell M.A.H. (1980) Comparison of nicotine chewing-gum and psychological treatments for dependent smokers. *Br. Med. J.* **281**, 481.

Reader G., Pratt L. & Mudd M. (1957) What patients expect from their doctor. *Mod. Hosp.* July, 19–21.

Report of the British Heart Foundation Working Group (1989) Role of the general practitioner in managing patients with myocardial infarction: impact of thrombolytic treatment. *Br. Med. J.* **299**, 555–6.

Report of the British Hypertension Working Party (1989) Treating mild hypertension: agreement from the large trials. *Br. Med. J.* **298**, 694–8.

Roberts M.M. (1989) Breast cancer screening: time for a rethink? *Br. Med. J.* **299**, 1153–5.

Roberts M.M., Alexander F.E., Andersson T.J. *et al.* (1990) Edinburgh trial of screening for breast cancer: mortality at 7 years. *Lancet* **335**, 241–6.

Roland M.O., Bartholomew J., Courtenay M.J.F. *et al.* (1986) The five minute consultation: effect of time constraint on verbal communication. *Br. Med. J.* **292**, 874–6.

Roland M. & Dixon M. (1989) Randomised controlled trial of an educational booklet for patients presenting with backache in general practice. *J. R. Coll. Gen. Pract.* **39**, 244–6.

Rosenstock I.M. (1966) Why people use health services. *Millbank Memorial Fund Q.* **44**, 94–124.

Rotter J. (1966) Generalised expectancies for internal versus external control of reinforcement. *Psychol. Monograph* **80**, No. 609.

Royal College of General Practitioners (1972) The Future General Practitioner: Learning and Teaching. *British Medical Journal*, London.

Royal College of General Practitioners (1982) *Healthier Children — Thinking Prevention*. Report from General Practice 22. RCGP, London.

Royal College of General Practitioners (1983) The quality initiative — summary of council meeting. *J. R. Coll. Gen. Pract.* **33**, 523–4.

Royal College of General Practitioners (1985a) *Booking for Maternity Care — A Comparison of Two Systems*. Occasional paper 31. RCGP, London.

Royal College of General Practitioners (1985b) *Towards Quality in General Practice*. Council Consultation Document. RCGP, London.

Royal College of General Practitioners (1985c) *What Sort of Doctor?* Report from General Practice 23. RCGP, London.

Royal College of General Practitioners (1985d) *Quality in General Practice.* Policy Statement 2. RCGP, London.

Royal College of Psychiatrists (1979) *Alcohol and Alcoholism.* Tavistock Publications, London.

Royal Commission on the Distribution of Income and Wealth (1978) Report 6. *Lower Incomes.* Cmnd 7175. HMSO, London.

Royal Commission on the Distribution of Income and Wealth (1980) *Inequalities in Health.* HMSO, London.

Russell M.A.H., Wilson C., Taylor C. & Baker C.D. (1979) Effect of general practitioners' advice against smoking. *Br. Med. J.* **2**, 231.

Sainsbury, Lord (1967) *Report of the Committee of Enquiry into the Relationship of the Pharmaceutical Industry with the NHS.* Cmnd 3410, p. 209. HMSO, London.

Sawyer L. & Arber S. (1982) Changes in home visiting and night and weekend cover: the patient's view. *Br. Med. J.* **284**, 1531–4.

Scientific and Medical Advisory Committee of the Coronary Prevention Group (1987) *Risk Assessment: its Role in the Prevention of Coronary Heart Disease.* Coronary Prevention Group, London.

Scott T. (1985) Do we need to repeat prescribe? *J. R. Coll. Gen. Pract.* **35**, 91–2.

Secretaries of State for Social Services, Wales, Northern Ireland and Scotland (1986) *Primary Health Care: An Agenda for Discussion.* HMSO, London.

Secretaries of State for Social Services, Wales, Northern Ireland and Scotland (Nov. 1987) *Promoting Better Health: The Government's Programme for improving Primary Health Care.* HMSO, London.

Secretaries of State for Health, Wales, Northern Ireland and Scotland (1989) *Working for Patients.* HMSO, London (Cmnd 555).

Sempos C., Fulwood R., Haines C. *et al.* (1989) The prevalence of high blood cholesterol levels among adults in the United States. *J.A.M.A.* **262**, 45–52.

Shapiro S., Venet P., Strax P. & Roeser R. (1982) Ten to fourteen year effect of screening on breast cancer mortality. *J. Natl. Cancer Inst.* **69**, 349–55.

Sheldon Report (1967) *Child Welfare Centres.* Report of the Subcommittee of the Standing Medical Advisory Committee. HMSO, London.

Shepherd J., Betteridge D., Durrington P. *et al.* (1987) Strategies for reducing coronary heart disease and desirable limits for blood lipid concentrations: guidelines of the British Hyperlipidaemia Association. *Br. Med. J.* **295**, 1245–6.

Shepherd M., Cooper B., Brown A.C. & Kalton G.W. (1966) *Psychiatric Illness in General Practice.* Oxford University Press, Oxford.

Slade P.D. & Dewey M.E. (1983) The role of grammatical clues in the MCQ: an empirical study. *Med. Teacher* **2**, 146–8.

Smith D. (1976) *The Facts of Racial Disadvantage.* Political and Economic Planning, London.

Smith R. (1989) NHS Review — words from the source: an interview with Alain Enthoven. *Br. Med. J.* **298**, 1166–8.

Smith W.C.S., Konicer M.B., Davies A.M., Evans A.E. & Yarnell J. (1989) Blood cholesterol: is population screening warranted in the UK? *Lancet* **ii**, 372–3.

Social Trends No. 14 (1984) Central Statistical Office, HMSO, London.

Social Trends No. 19 (1989) Central Statistical Office, HMSO, London.

South East London Screening Study Group (1977) A controlled trial of multiphasic screening in middle-age: results of the South East London Screening Study. *Int. J. Epidemiol.* **6**, 357–63.

Stevenson J.S.K. (1982) Advantages of deputising services: a personal view. *Br. Med. J.* **284**, 947–9.

Stott P. (1989) Value for money. *Med. Monitor* 9th June p. 13.

Stott N.C.H. & Davis R.H. (1979) The exceptional potential in each primary care consultation. *J. R. Coll. Gen. Pract.* **29**, 201.

Tabar L., Fagerberg C.J., Gad A. *et al.* (1985) Reduction in mortality from breast cancer after mass screening with mammography. *Lancet* **ii**, 829–32.

Thomas K.B. (1987) General practice consultations: is there any point in being positive? *Br. Med. J.* **294**, 1200.

Thompson N.F. (1990) Inviting infrequent attenders to attend for a health check: costs and benefits. *Br. J. Gen. Pract.* **40**, 16–18.

Troup R.G. (1989) What influences doctors' prescribing. *J. R. Coll. Gen. Pract.* **39**, 259.

Tudor Hart J. (1971) The inverse care law. *Lancet* **i**, 405–12.

Tulloch A.J. (1976) *The design and evaluation of a modern medical record system.* MD Thesis, Aberdeen University.

Tulloch A.J. & Moore V. (1979) A randomised controlled trial of geriatric screening and surveillance in general practice. *J. R. Coll. Gen. Pract.* **29**, 733–42.

Tyrer P., Owen R. & Dawling S. (1983) Gradual withdrawal of diazepam after long-term use. *Lancet* **i**, 1402–6.

Tyrer P., Seivewright N., Murphy S. *et al.* (1988) The Nottingham study of neurotic disorder: comparison of drug and psychological treatments. *Lancet* **ii**, 235–40.

UK Trial of Early Detection of Breast Cancer Group (1988) First results on mortality reduction in the UK trial of early detection of breast cancer. *Lancet* **ii**, 411–16.

Vaillant G.E. (1980) The doctor's dilemma. In: Edwards G. & Grant M. (eds) *Alcoholism, Treatment in Transition,* pp. 13–31. Croom Helm, London.

Van Buchem F.L., Dunk J.H.M. & Van't Hof M.A. (1981) Therapy of acute otitis media: myringotomy, antibiotics, or neither? *Lancet* **ii**, 883–7.

Verbeck A.L.M., Hendricks J.H.C.L., Holland R., Mravunac M., Sturmans F. & Day N.E. (1984) Reduction of breast cancer mortality through mass screening with modern mammography. First results of the Nijmegan Project 1975–1981. *Lancet* **i**, 1222–4.

Veterans Administration Co-operative Study Group on Antihypertensive Agents (1970) *J.A.M.A.* **213**, 1143–52.

Waine C. (1988) *The Prevention of Coronary Heart Disease.* Royal College of General Practitioners, London.

Walker C.H.M. (1986) Child health surveillance. *Update,* 15th Nov., 906–14.

Walker J.H., Stanley I.M., Venables T.L., Gambrill E.C. & Hodgkin G.K.H. (1983) The MRCGP examination and its methods. *J. R. Coll. Gen. Pract.* **33**, 662–5.

Wallace P. & Haines A. (1985) Patients' responses to a self-administered questionnaire. *Br. Med. J.* **290**, 1949–53.

Wallis J.B. & Barber J.H. (1982) The effect of a system of geriatric screening and assessment on general practice workload. *Health Bull. (Edin.)* **40**, 125–32.

Ward A. (1974) Terminal care in malignant disease. *Soc. Sci. Med.* **8**, 233.

Weed L. (1969) *Medical Records, Medical Education and Patient Care.* Cleveland Press of Case Western Reserve University.

Whitfield M.J. & Hughes A.O. (1981) Penicillin in sore throat. *Practitioner* **225**, 234.

Wiesel S.M., Cuckler J.M., Deluca F. *et al.* (1980) Acute low back pain. An objective analysis of conservative therapy. *Spine* **5**, 324–30.

Wilkin D. & Smith A.G. (1987) Variation in GPs' referral rates to hospitals. *J. R. Coll. Gen. Pract.* **37**, 350–3.

Wilkin D., Metcalfe D.H.M., Hallam L., Cooke M. & Hodgkin P.K. (1984) Area variations in the process of care in urban general practice. *Br. Med. J.* **289**, 229–32.

Wilkins R.H. (1974) *The Hidden Alcoholic in General Practice*. Chapter 3. Elke Science, London.

Wilson A. (1989) Extending appointment length — the effect in one practice. *J. R. Coll. Gen. Pract.* **39**, 24–5.

Wilson J.M.G. (1966) In: Teeling-Smith G. (ed.) *Surveillance and Early Diagnosis in General Practice*. Proceedings of Colloquium, pp. 5–10. Office of Health Economics, London.

Wilson P., Christiansen J., Anderson K. *et al.* (1989) Impact of national guidelines for cholesterol risk factor screening. *J.A.M.A.* **262**, 41–4.

Wynder E.L., Field F. & Haley N.J. (1986) Population screening for cholesterol determination: a pilot study. *J.A.M.A.* **256**, 2839–42.

Zander L.I. (1982) Practising prevention: making a start. *Br. Med. J.* **284**, 1241–2.

Zola I. (1973) Pathways to the doctor: from person to patient. *Soc. Sci. Med.* **7**, 677–89.

Index